D0138251

FOUNDATIONS OF AUDIOLOGY
A Practical Approach

Miles E. Peterson

California State University/Los Angeles

Theodore S. Bell

California State University/Los Angeles

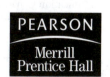
PEARSON

Merrill
Prentice Hall

Upper Saddle River, New Jersey
Columbus, Ohio

Library of Congress Control Number 2007926214

Vice President and Executive Publisher: Jeffrey w. Johnston
Executive Editor: Ann Castel Davis
Editorial Assistant: Penny Burleson
Production Editor: Sheryl Glicker Langner
Production Coordinator: Lisa S. Garboski, bookworks publishing services
Design Coordinator: Diane C. Lorenzo
Cover Designer: Kellyn E. Donnelly
Cover Image: Corbis
Production Manager: Laura Messerly
Director of Marketing: David Gesell
Marketing Manager: Autumn Purdy
Marketing Coordinator: Brian Mounts
Compositor: Aptara, Inc.

This book was set in Berkeley by Aptara, Inc. It was printed and bound by R.R. Donnelley & Sons Company. The cover was printed by R.R. Donnelley & Sons Company.

Additional Photo Credits: Figures 6.10, 6.13, 6.14 and 8.4 were supplied by the authors.

Pearson Prentice Hall™ is a trademark of Pearson Education, Inc.
Pearson® is a registered trademark of Pearson plc.
Prentice Hall® is a registered trademark of Pearson Education, Inc.
Merrill® is a registered trademark of Pearson Education, Inc.

Pearson Education Ltd.   Pearson Education Australia Pty. Limited
Pearson Education Singapore Pte. Ltd.   Pearson Education North Asia Ltd.
Pearson Education Canada, Ltd.   Pearson Educación de Mexico, S.A. de C.V.
Pearson Education—Japan   Pearson Education Malaysia Pte. Ltd.

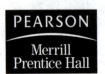

PEARSON
Merrill
Prentice Hall

10 9 8 7 6 5 4 3 2 1
ISBN 13: 978-0-13-118568-5
ISBN 10:   0-13-118568-3

To our wives,
Jann and Judy,
and to our families

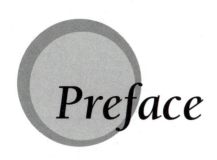

Preface

Foundations of Audiology is a concise text that presents the fundamentals of audiology with a focus on practical applications pertaining to audiometry. The text is designed for students who are not audiology majors and, as a result, is free of the more involved technical aspects of the discipline that may be inappropriate or unnecessary for this target audience. Specifically, the text was written for audiology assistants, public-school nurses, educators of the hearing impaired, speech-language pathologists, and hearing instrument specialists. Many chapters in the text include case studies that provide a better understanding of the real-world applications of audiology. In addition, numerous audiogram cases are illustrated to help facilitate comprehension of test interpretation. Each chapter ends with open-ended reflective questions that enable discussion in classroom and study groups. The text is substantiated with a volume of references and appendices with a list of suggested readings, web links for more in-depth exploration of the material, and information on professional organizations and advocacy groups.

It is hoped that this book will serve the purpose for which it is intended: to fill the need for a fundamental book for students outside the field of audiology and offer a glimpse of this profession combined with a working knowledge of the audiometric testing process.

The authors wish to express appreciation to Peter J. Ivory, Nancy E. McCoy, and Tracy L. Williams for their chapter contributions; to Edward Klein for his encouragement throughout the writing process; and to May Chin for her many years of continuous support. Also, the authors thank the reviewers of the manuscript for their insightful comments and suggestions: Rebecca Brooks, University of Alabama; Joseph E. Etienne, Western Kentucky University; Dan Halling, James Madison University; Ingred McBride, Arizona State University; Marilyn Sass-Lehrer, Gallaudet University; Renee Shellum, Minnesota State University, Mankato; Cindy Ann Simon, Florida International University; Dan Sisterhen, University of West Georgia; Joseph Smaldino, Northern Illinois University; Donna Fisher Smiley, University of Central Arkansas, and Thomas R. Zalewski, Bloomsburg University.

Brief Contents

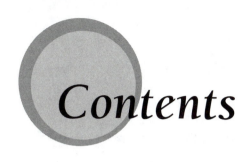

Contents

3   *Anatomy and Physiology of the Ear*   47

Theodore S. Bell and Tracy L. Williams

4   *Disorders of the Ear*   69

Peter J. Ivory

7

Physiologic Tests of the Auditory System   162

Peter J. Ivory

8

Pediatric Audiology: Screening and Evaluation   194

9   *Assessing Special Populations*   222

10   *Hearing Rehabilitation: Helping Individuals with Hearing Loss*   234

Nancy E. McCoy

Note: Every effort has been made to provide accurate and current Internet information in this book. However, the Internet and information posted on it are constantly changing, so it is inevitable that some of the Internet addresses listed in this textbook will change.

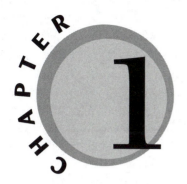

Introduction to Audiology: Serving Individuals with Hearing Loss

Key Terms

CASE STUDY

A Glimpse into the Profession

*Justin is a 4-year-old boy whose parents were concerned about his speech and language development as well as some inconsistencies in his responses to speech and other environmental sounds. He was first seen by his pediatrician, who recommended that Justin have his hearing evaluated to rule out hearing loss as the possible cause. Justin was referred to the local audiologist for a complete **audiologic evaluation**. Initially, Justin and his parents were asked a series of questions to identify particular problems and behaviors that might suggest a possible hearing loss or other disorder. The results of this **case history** revealed a normal pregnancy, no history of hearing loss in the family, and no apparent significant childhood diseases. However, the questions regarding his response to sound revealed that Justin prefers the volume of the television at a higher level than others; as well, he has a frequent need for family members to repeat themselves when communicating with him. A complete audiological evaluation was performed beginning with a visual inspection of the ear canal and eardrum, followed by a hearing test using a series of simple sounds, or **pure tones**. A measure of the ability to perceive and understand speech was also performed. Finally, the possibility of any type of middle ear disease was ruled out. Following the evaluation, the results were reviewed with Justin's parents and recommendations for intervention and a prognosis were presented.*

THE AUDIOLOGY PROFESSION

The preceding case is a sample of the type of client or patient audiologists might see and the services they would provide on a given day in their professional career. The case study will be revisited at the end of the chapter in order to provide the reader with a direct application of the material.

   This chapter is divided into two parts: the first part discusses the profession of audiology and reviews the providers of audiologic and audiometric services including requirements of employment, and the second part addresses the hearing-impaired individuals who are served by this profession. The second section includes an overview of terms used to describe hearing loss, the incidence of hearing loss in our society, some of the underlying causes and resulting effects of hearing loss, and an example of services rendered to these individuals.

AUDIOLOGISTS AND OTHER HEARING HEALTH PROFESSIONALS

The definition of **audiology** in its simplest form is the study of human hearing. But over the last 50 years, the discipline of audiology has evolved into an autonomous health care profession devoted to the evaluation of hearing and the treatment of hearing impairment. Audiology practice occurs in many arenas:

1. Clinical diagnostic and rehabilitative services in hospitals, university clinics, and other health care settings
2. Private practice providing similar services but with a particular focus on the dispensing and fitting of hearing aids and other assistive devices
3. Evaluating hearing and providing habilitation for hearing-impaired children in educational settings
4. Preventive health care through hearing conservation programs in industrial and military settings
5. Hearing screening of newborns and young children at risk for hearing loss

Audiology has also expanded to include the evaluation of the vestibular or balance system, the identification of various neurologic diseases, and monitoring the neural status of an individual undergoing a surgical procedure or during various drug treatments, such as chemotherapy for certain cancers. Regardless of the work setting, audiology is primarily concerned with the prevention of hearing loss; the identification, evaluation, and diagnosis of hearing and balance disorders; and the habilitation or rehabilitation of these disorders (American Academy of Audiology, 2004; American Academy of Audiology, 1997; American Speech-Language-Hearing Association, 2004a).

The audiology profession can be a very satisfying and rewarding career for individuals who are seeking an opportunity to help improve the quality of life for a person with a hearing impairment or balance disorder. It is a worthwhile enterprise and plays an important role in the overall general health care of society. A recent survey revealed a high level of job satisfaction for audiologists who spend a majority of their time with patients, particularly those who are in private practice (Martin, Champlin, & Streetman, 1997). Although there are many reasons for job satisfaction, the primary contribution appears to be the challenging and interesting nature of this type of work. The position of **audiologist** is rather unique in that it encompasses a whole array of employment opportunities, including clinical services, research, education, industrial hearing conservation, and the manufacturing and sale of hearing aids. In a clinical setting, audiologists provide complete diagnostic hearing evaluations, numerous special tests to differentiate various diseases related to the ear, and intervention services including the fitting of hearing aids. The audiologist in education serves as a coordinator of hearing services concerned with the screening, identification, diagnosis, and treatment of hearing loss in school-aged children; in higher education, audiologists train future professionals. In industry, hearing conservation programs are conducted by audiologists who measure the loudness levels of noise, annually test employees' hearing, and provide training on hearing loss prevention. Some audiologists specialize in training, research, customer service, sales, or marketing as a part of hearing aid manufacturing. Each of these employment choices ultimately engage the audiologist in some aspect of preventing hearing loss, evaluating hearing ability and/or balance function, or treating the impairment caused by a hearing or balance disorder.

History of Audiology

Military Rehabilitation Centers

The audiology profession can trace its beginnings back to the end of World War II when many veterans were returning home with hearing problems caused by exposure to loud sounds during military service. Prior to this time, hearing services were provided by physicians, particularly those who specialized in diseases of the ear, with the use of tuning forks and later in the 1930s with an electric **audiometer** to measure hearing sensitivity. By 1945, a substantial number of veterans were in need of rehabilitation due to the presence of noise-induced hearing loss. Physicians, speech pathologists, and psychologists worked together to create hearing rehabilitation centers at select military bases. Specifically, three main centers were established: at Deshon General Hospital (Pennsylvania), Borden General Hospital (Oklahoma), and Hoff General Hospital (California). Thus, the medical profession of otolaryngology and the rehabilitative professions of speech pathology and psychology formed the foundations on which the new discipline of audiology was built (Bergman, 2002).

Development of Training Programs

In its infancy, audiology was primarily a rehabilitation profession focusing on auditory training, lip reading, and the use of hearing aids. Testing procedures to diagnose hearing loss were limited in scope. In the 1950s, only about 500 audiologists were practicing in the United States. Typical work settings were in physicians' offices, speech and hearing centers, hospitals, or universities. Several graduate audiology programs were developed with a notable program at Northwestern University led by Raymond Carhart, PhD, who was also one of the directors at Deshon Hospital. During this time, many individuals earned PhD degrees in audiology and continued in academia, developing numerous audiology graduate programs throughout the country (Skafte, 1990). As a result of these advanced training programs, audiology practitioners continued to expand the scope of their practice, particularly in the area of diagnostic evaluation. Today, the professional scope of practice encompasses the advancement of hearing loss identification and sophisticated special auditory tests that are involved not only in diagnosis of hearing impairment but also other neurologic and balance disorders.

Hearing Aid Dispensing

Another tremendous boost to the growth of audiology occurred in the late 1970s. Prior to this time, the dispensing of hearing aids for profit was considered unethical as part of the scope of practice by the certifying body of audiology, the American Speech and Hearing Association (ASHA). The ASHA code of ethics stipulated that an audiologist's recommendation for treatment would be compromised if it involved the sale of hearing aids for profit. Hearing aid dispensing was essentially relegated to retail stores. However, the U.S. Supreme Court (*United States v. National Society of Professional Engineers*) ruled in 1977 that a professional society's code of ethics could not limit competition among its members (Skafte, 1990). Shortly thereafter, ASHA recommended a change in the ethical standard allowing audiologists to dispense hearing aids as part of comprehensive rehabilitation services, although it was not an official part of the code of ethics until 1992 (Resnick, 1993). This reversal created new opportunities for audiologists to enter private practice and renewed the profession's origins of rehabilitation with a focus on dispensing hearing aids as part of their provision of services.

The Connection to Speech-Language Pathology

Traditionally, advanced academic training in audiology led to a PhD. However, because of the current clinical and medical practice settings in which audiologists are employed, it makes sense that a professional doctoral degree similar to that obtained in optometry, podiatry, or dentistry, for example, is a more appropriate advanced degree for audiology. The awarding of a degree that has a more educational orientation (the PhD) rather than a professional degree stems from audiology's origins and its relationship to the field of **speech-language pathology**. Because of its newness as a profession, the need for audiology to gain recognition and acceptance required the academic pioneers in the field to shift from a service orientation to a research and diagnostically based discipline. The idea of establishing an independent professional school was too daunting and impractical a task and so a logical move was to become aligned with speech-language pathology (Dunn, Dunn, & Harford, 1995). Most academic programs have incorporated these two professions in the same academic departments in higher education. Therefore, the two fields historically have awarded the master's degree as the primary requirement to obtain licensure and to practice professionally. However, the unique characteristics of the two professions and the expansion in their scope of practice has caused an increase in competency requirements in each individual profession and necessitated a change in programs beyond the undergraduate level.

A Professional Doctorate

Audiology's gradual expansion over the years has caused the profession to look to a different type of advanced degree that has a more clinical focus consistent with some of the other allied health care professions. The need for an advanced professional degree that is clinical in nature was based on the fact that most audiologists work in health care settings, with fewer than 10% involved formally in audiology education (ASHA, 1999). Therefore, because audiology is primarily a clinical discipline, clinical training and education at a doctoral level appeared to be the logical direction for the profession to take in order for it to continue to advance in health care. The idea of a clinical doctorate has been of interest for more than 30 years. As the number of audiologists in private practice increased following the ruling on hearing aid dispensing, and with the founding of the Academy of Dispensing Audiologists (ADA) that same year, there was particular concern over the focus and content of audiology training programs (McCollom, 2003). At the ADA convention in 1988, 25 audiologists met to determine the feasibility of developing a professional doctorate. This degree would more closely mirror professional health care programs as a four-year professional degree following the completion of an undergraduate degree. The new degree designation was "Doctor of Audiology," abbreviated "Au.D."; it was introduced in 1989 (Goldstein, 1989).

The AuD degree began to receive considerable attention and positive recognition by most organizations in the audiology field (AAA, 1991). In the last ten years, AuD programs have been developed and as of this writing, approximately 70 audiology programs are offering the professional doctorate throughout the United States. Audiologists currently can obtain licensure and practice in most states with a master's degree, a research doctorate such as the PhD, or the new **AuD doctorate degree**. Today, audiology is recognized as an autonomous health care profession and the primary service provider of hearing evaluation and rehabilitation including hearing aid dispensing.

Audiology Subspecialties

The Audiometrist

Because of the broadening of services and/or settings in which audiologists practice professionally and the expanding demand for services, combined with the introduction of the professional doctorate, an increased need for subspecialties has emerged. The position of **audiometrist** or audiometric technician has existed for many years and still exists in some states. The primary responsibility of audiometrists is to perform hearing screening and basic hearing tests. They typically work in schools assisting audiologists with annual hearing screening programs. Because of the valuable role that speech-language pathologists and nurses occupy in the health care of children in the schools, these two professions often take on the dual responsibility of audiometrists as well. These responsibilities may include not only the actual performance of hearing screening or hearing testing, but also the administration of hearing conservation programs. Audiometrists also provide hearing conservation services in industrial work environments conducting annual testing to monitor the hearing sensitivity of workers exposed to high levels of noise. Basic hearing testing can be conducted by audiometrists in primary care or pediatric physicians' offices as a precursor to a referral to an audiologist or otolaryngologist.

Audiology Assistants

The position of **audiology assistant** has emerged recently as an extension of the audiometrist because of the broadening scope of practice in audiology and the increasing necessity for support personnel in other areas of audiology service delivery. However, the idea of an audiology assistant is not new. Over 40 years ago, the military trained corpsmen to help medical personnel by performing basic hearing testing, or **audiometry**, repairing hearing aids, and fitting earplugs for protection from noise (Northern, 2006). In the last decade, the Department of Veterans Affairs audiology clinics expanded their use of health technicians by training them to assist with numerous clerical tasks such as filing, handling of new and repaired hearing aids for shipping, equipment maintenance, and restocking inventory and hearing aid troubleshooting (Dunlop, et al., 2006). In addition to the responsibilities just indicated, other functions of an audiology assistant may include preparing specialized equipment for the purpose of conducting more in-depth audiologic or vestibular evaluations, assisting the audiologist to test infants, children, and other individuals with special needs, assessing the operation of hearing aids prior to fitting, or analyzing the functional status of hearing aids to determine the need for adjustments or repair. Specific definitions of job responsibilities that can be performed by support personnel vary by state. A consensus panel of representatives from numerous organizations including ASHA, ADA, and the American Academy of Audiology (AAA), developed a position statement and guidelines that state, in part:

> Audiology support personnel may engage in only those tasks that are planned, delegated, and supervised by the audiologist. The specific roles of audiology support personnel will be influenced by the particular needs of the audiologist and must be determined by the audiologist responsible for the support personnel's training and supervision. (ASHA, 1998)

Some audiology practices that have employed audiology assistants report an increase in efficiency and productivity without compromising patient satisfaction (Kasewurm, 2006; Beyer & Van Vliet, 2006) The recent heightened interest in utilizing audiology assistants in hearing health care settings suggests that this subspecialty will continue to expand.

Work Settings and Specialties in Audiology

The historical focus in the training of audiologists has been to provide a comprehensive regimen of course work and clinical experience so that future professionals are able to practice in a variety of settings. These settings include private practice, hospitals and skilled nursing facilities, independent and corporate-owned audiology centers, schools, universities, and industry. The distribution of audiology practice settings is displayed in Figure 1.1, with the largest number of individuals (40%) employed in a nonresidential health care facility. The "other" category is a combination of less common work facilities such as health agencies, education agencies, industry, research/scientific organizations, etc. (ASHA, 2004b). Private practice continues to be a dynamic work place for audiologists with a 20% to 30% representation of full-time professionals working in this setting (Zingeser, 2005).

For the most part, audiologists are clinical service providers regardless of their work settings, with a relatively small percent working as administrators, researchers, or in academia. Despite the primary function of this latter group, however, administrators and educators often still work as practitioners involved in direct clinical service delivery. Although practice settings are distinctly different, the specific types of hearing care

Figure 1.1 Survey results of primary employment work settings for audiologists.

Source: Reprinted with permission from *2004 Audiology Survey Report: Private Practice Salaries in Nonresidential Health Care Facilities.* Rockville, MD. Copyright 2005 by the American Speech-Language-Hearing Association. All rights reserved.

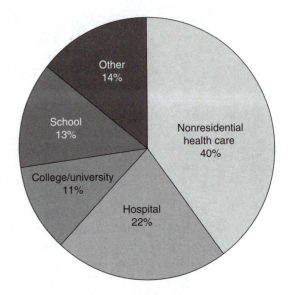

services are often quite similar. The distinction between the different specialties is typically seen in the unique job responsibilities and roles that audiologists play in the various settings. For example, the primary focus of professionals providing diagnostic hearing testing in a physician's office will be the technical expertise of administration and interpretation of these tests. Conversely, a private practitioner's major job function as owner of a retail business is practice management.

Another specialty in audiology that has shown an increase in employment is working for manufacturers of hearing instruments and other testing equipment. An audiologist in this setting is engaged in the research and development of new products, hearing instrument or equipment sales, or technical support provided to practicing audiologists who are dispensing the hearing devices of that particular manufacturer.

Despite the fact that audiology is a comparatively small health care profession, the job opportunities and choices of service provision are quite diverse. It also continues to grow as a profession; employment potential will increase dramatically in the next decade. According to the U.S. Bureau of Labor Statistics' 2002–2003 *Occupational Outlook Handbook,* "Employment of audiologists is expected to grow rapidly because the expanding population in older age groups is prone to medical conditions that result in hearing problems" (U.S. Dept. of Labor, 2003). It has also been reported that audiology is listed in the top 50 fastest growing occupations, with a projected increase in audiology jobs of 29% between 2002 and 2012 (Hecker, 2004).

Audiology Connections

Audiologists often interact with other professionals from a variety of specialties. This professional interaction may come in the form of collaboration to provide optimal intervention for an individual or a referral to a physician or other health care professional. Some of these primary connections are as follows.

Interactions with Physicians

The medical profession that specializes in treatment of ear, nose, or throat problems is formally known as **Otolaryngology—Head and Neck Surgery**. Physicians who limit their practice to treatment of diseases of the ear are thus referred to as **otologists**. Audiologists and otolaryngologists/otologists work closely together in the diagnosis and treatment of ear disorders. The audiologist relies on the physician specialist to rule out any type of disease or pathology that requires surgery or medication, and the physician relies on the audiologist to provide a complete assessment of the hearing mechanism and to assist in the diagnosis of a disease. Generally, when the hearing loss is medically treatable, the otolaryngologist becomes the primary service provider through surgery and/or medication. When the hearing loss is permanent and medical treatment is not an option, the audiologist will become the primary service provider through the selection and fitting of amplification and other therapeutic procedures. Although the roles of each professional and the scope of care can sometimes be misinterpreted, it is important to understand the specific contributions of the two disciplines and that the overlapping services are complementary and in the best interest of the patient.

Other audiology connections often include interactions with other physicians in specialties such as pediatrics, neurology, or geriatrics, and with the impact managed care has on the referral process, interactions with primary care physicians is also common. As audiologists continue to be involved in conducting specialized neurological tests, the connections to other specialties will increase.

Interactions with Speech-Language Pathologists

Audiologists also interact with **speech-language pathologists** because of the significant impact hearing loss has on communication, causing either a delay in speech and language production or speech perception. One of the first components of a speech and language evaluation for a child is to identify whether or not hearing loss is a complicating condition or possibly the underlying cause of the speech and language delay, necessitating a referral to an audiologist. Conversely, when hearing loss is identified and has shown to have a specific impact on communication, the audiologist can then make a referral to the speech-language pathologist for appropriate services. This relationship is further exemplified in the association of the two disciplines in academic departments and historically, through professional organizations previously mentioned.

Interactions with Educators

When audiology practice settings entail services to children in the public schools, collaboration occurs with **educators of the hearing impaired**, in addition to speech-language pathologists. Specially trained teachers who work with hearing-impaired children are an excellent resource in determining the particular needs of each child because of their direct daily contact with them. They in turn rely on the educational audiologist to assist the children with appropriate amplification and rehabilitative support to optimize their educational experience.

Interactions with Hearing Instrument Specialists

Prior to 1980, the dispensing and sale of hearing aids was accomplished largely by individuals who were not audiologists, but who were employed as retail sales personnel, variously called hearing aid dealers or hearing aid dispensers. Although audiologists prescribed hearing aids and evaluated hearing aid performance, they were obligated by the professional standards in place at that time to refer to hearing aid dispensers for the actual fitting of these devices. In the past 25 years, however, there has been a steady increase in the number of audiologists who dispense hearing aids as part of their professional practice. Today, the common title of a nonaudiologist dispenser is **hearing instrument specialist**. Because of the significant overlap in service and product delivery between audiologists and nonaudiologist dispensers, there has been occasional conflict with regard to changes in state licensure requirements and other regulations. But for the most part, audiologists and hearing instrument specialists espouse similar goals in providing appropriate intervention with hearing aids for the hearing impaired. The difference is the scope of practice and the depth and breadth of training required to enter the audiology profession.

PROFESSIONAL REQUIREMENTS

Academic Requirements

Audiologists

The necessary qualifications needed to practice as an audiologist are regulated by certification at the national level through ASHA, and licensure requirements in each respective state. Historically, the minimum requirement to receive a state license and national certification to practice as an audiologist has been the completion of a master's degree. With the development of the AuD professional doctorate, however, these requirements are currently in transition. The Council on Professional Standards in Speech-Language Pathology and Audiology for ASHA adopted new standards in September 1997. According to these standards, as of 2007, audiologists will need to have a bachelor's degree and complete 75 hours of credit toward a doctoral degree in order to seek certification. As of 2012, audiologists must earn a doctoral degree from an ASHA-accredited institution in order to be certified.

Audiometrists

Although the requirements to become an audiometrist are not well defined in most states, there usually are some minimal criteria that need to be met prior to employment. For example, the state of California awards an audiometrist certificate to any person who successfully completes six-semester or eight-quarter units of approved course work usually offered through state university audiology programs. In addition, public school nurses can fulfill the requirement for certification by completing one three-semester or four-quarter unit approved course.

Audiology Assistants

The education and experience requirements for an audiology assistant vary widely by state, ranging from the requirement of only a high school diploma and some additional training (15 states including Florida, Georgia, Indiana, Ohio, and Pennsylvania) to requiring a bachelor's degree (Alabama and West Virginia) or even enrollment in a master's degree program following completion of a bachelor's degree (New Mexico) (ASHA, 2005b). As of 2005, there were 32 states that officially regulate the use of support personnel, 9 of which use licensure and 23 use a form of registration. Five additional states acknowledge the use of support personnel but do not regulate their activities (ASHA, 2005a).

Clinical Requirements

A fundamental component of an audiology academic program is the inclusion of a clinical practicum experience. The required time has been set over the last few decades at 350 clinical hours in three different clinical settings, which has been sufficient to provide a well-rounded experience prior to the clinician entering the work force. However, with the addition of the AuD degree, the clinical hours have increased to several thousand hours to cover more adequately the plethora of work settings and various services that are provided by an audiologist in today's health care environment. In the past, following completion of an MA, the audiologist was required to complete the Clinical Fellowship Year (CFY). This consisted of nine months of full-time employment in a work setting supervised by a certified practicing audiologist. With the implementation of new standards, the CFY is being replaced with a 12-month full-time supervised experience that is included as part of the academic program prior to completing the AuD. Satisfactory completion of the degree and the practicum experience enables the audiologist to apply for licensure and certification immediately.

National Certification

ASHA has been the professional organization for speech-language pathology and audiology since the inception of the profession and has governed the awarding of formal certification to both professions. The specific certification is entitled the **Certificate of Clinical Competence** (CCC) with a separate designator of "A" or "SLP" distinguishing the two certifications. Traditionally, audiologists and speech-language pathologists have identified themselves professionally with the MA or PhD degree followed by the CCC-A or CCC-SLP designators signifying their academic degree and national certification. Requirements for the CCC include a master's or doctoral degree from an accredited institution, successful completion of the required clinical hours, completion of the nine-month CFY experience, and a passing score on the national examination for certification administered by the PRAXIS Series of the Educational Testing Service (ETS).

The American Board of Audiology (ABA) is an autonomous organization that was created to offer certification independent of any professional organization. It began granting voluntary certification to audiologists in 1999 (American Board of Audiology, 2005). The requirements are similar to ASHA certification, but with the addition of a minimum of 2000 hours of mentored professional practice over a two-year period. Again, the academic and clinical requirements for certification from ASHA or ABA are currently in transition with the move to a doctoral degree.

State Licensure

The requirements to obtain a license to practice audiology are quite similar from state to state, following a stringent set of requirements consistent with ASHA certification. Currently, there are 49 states that regulate the practice of audiology through licensure; the state of Colorado regulates via registration, which is not required to work as an audiologist.

The dispensing of hearing aids is categorized as an occupation separate from audiology and is regulated by its own licensure laws. Twenty states and the District of Columbia require audiologists to hold a hearing aid dispensing license while 30 states permit audiologists to dispense hearing aids under their audiology license. The requirements for this separate dispensing license vary by state, but typically include receiving a passing score on written and practical examinations prepared by the state (ASHA, 2005b).

Professional Societies

A number of professional societies have been founded to offer information, educational opportunities, and support in the sustaining of clinical practice for audiologists. A summary of the most well known organizations in which audiologists typically hold membership can be found in Appendix B.

INTRODUCTION TO THE HEARING IMPAIRED

Hearing is a primary sensory function that occurs involuntarily without requiring us to take action; in other words, it cannot be turned on and off. Hearing allows us to monitor our environment, provides a connection with others, and facilitates the process of communication. Therefore, the basic human function of communication is significantly influenced when a loss of hearing occurs. Although hearing loss is a very common problem that affects almost 31.5 million Americans (Kochkin, 2005a), it is very difficult to predict the degree to which it will cause a disabling condition for a particular individual. The reasons for the difficulty in determining the impact of a hearing loss are threefold:

1. The many ear diseases, conditions, and causes that underlie hearing loss
2. The wide variability in the specific hearing loss characteristics, such as the degree or severity of the loss that exists
3. A combination of developmental, psychosocial, and environmental factors, such as the time of onset of the loss or the time in which intervention occurs, and other multiple disabling conditions that interact with hearing loss in unpredictable ways

This section will examine the population of individuals affected by hearing impairment, the incidence of hearing loss, a general overview of approaches in management, and a summary of organizations and support groups that are available to offer assistance.

TERMINOLOGY

Variable Use of Terminology

There are various terms employed to describe hearing impairment. These terms are used to explain the disorder and interpret the results of testing to patients, parents of hearing impaired children, or other professionals such as teachers who may be involved with educating these children. Therefore, it is necessary to be consistent in our understanding of each of these terms and what they specifically describe.

First of all, it is important to recognize that the terms used will have a different connotation based on who is using that term, whether it be an educator, a clinician, medical personnel, or a parent. For example, the traditional view of hearing loss in the realm of medicine is to consider it a pathological condition implying a specific disease. Audiologists, on the other hand, emphasize the effect the hearing loss characteristics have on general communication ability. Educators may focus more specifically on the effect the impairment has on academic performance and subsequently the recommendation for educational placement. The following is a clarification of some of these terms or descriptors and their usage.

Hearing Impairment, the Hard-of-Hearing, and Deafness

World Health Organization Classification

In 1980, the World Health Organization (WHO) developed the International Classification of Impairments, Disabilities, and Handicaps (ICIDH) to define specific disabling conditions and determine the consequences of the impairments on daily living (Patterson, 2001; WHO, 1980). Based on a better understanding of disability, the classification code was revised to focus on the functional effect of impairments and other health-related issues. The current title is International Classification of Functioning, Disability, and Health (ICF), which incorporates the concepts of activity limitations involving the functional consequences of impairment on communication, participation restriction related to social and psychological consequences of the impairment, and contextual factors that are influenced by the environment (Patterson, 2001; WHO, 2005). The descriptors used to characterize hearing loss, then, should incorporate these factors of functional status when defining terminology.

Impairment, Loss, Handicap, and Disability

The terms **hearing impairment** and **hearing loss** are the general all-inclusive expressions that encompass the varying degrees and types of reduced hearing sensitivity in children and adults. These terms indicate that hearing is not within the normal range because of some problem with the physiology of the auditory system, but do not specify any of the descriptors or characteristics used to define the impairment. **Hearing disability** or **hearing handicap** are terms used to describe the functional limitations caused by a hearing loss. The contrast between a hearing loss and a hearing disability is that the first term describes the specific identification and diagnosis of reduced hearing ability, and the second characterizes the effect of the loss on everyday communication and quality of life. For example, two individuals may exhibit similar degrees of hearing impairment, but due to various underlying physiologic, psychosocial, and environmental factors, one may be able minimize and cope with the effect of the hearing loss, and the other may continue to struggle with normal day-to-day functioning even after intervention.

Deaf versus Hard-of-Hearing

The terms **deaf** and **hard-of-hearing** describe subcategories within the context of hearing impairment to delineate groups of individuals with similar hearing loss characteristics. Many years ago, at the Conference of Educational Administrators Serving the Deaf (CEASD), the following definitions were developed:

> A deaf person is one whose hearing is disabled to an extent that precludes the understanding of speech, through the ear alone with or without the use of a hearing aid.

> A hard-of-hearing person is one whose hearing is disabled to an extent that makes difficult, but does not preclude, the understanding of speech with hearing alone, with or without a hearing aid. (Frisina, 1974)

Specific to education, similar definitions are listed in the Code of Federal Regulations—34CFR 300.5:

> Deaf means a hearing-impairment which is so severe that the child is impaired in processing linguistic information through hearing, with or without amplification which adversely affects educational performance.

> Hard of hearing means a hearing-impairment, whether permanent or fluctuating, which adversely affects a child's educational performance but which is not included under the definition of "deaf" in this section" (Sanders, 1993).

In other words, these definitions are influenced by the ability of a hearing-impaired individual to maximize residual hearing in order to understand and process speech. However, other issues that may influence the use of these terms involve the cultural aspects that are specifically related to the mode of communication used. For example, the **Deaf Community** or **Deaf Culture** is identified as that group of individuals who use some visual form of manual communication, most commonly American Sign Language (ASL), to communicate. In this case, the ability to hear speech sounds in order to carry on a conversation would not be an appropriate criterion to characterize someone within this culture because of their ability to communicate using visual information. In fact, it is possible for someone who is hard of hearing to be considered a member of the Deaf Community because of a reliance on manual communication and disuse of any available residual hearing.

Conversely, many individuals who would be considered deaf because of the presence of a profound impairment may not necessarily be considered part of the Deaf Community. One reason for this apparent inconsistency is the ability of an individual with very little residual hearing to maximize that hearing to communicate orally through the use of advanced technology in **hearing aids** or surgically implanted devices called **cochlear implants**. Because of the heterogeneity of the hearing-impaired population, there tends to be a clouding of the distinction between a person who is considered deaf versus one who is considered hard-of-hearing. However, in determining the true effect of hearing impairment on a person's quality of life, the fundamental consideration is the impact that the hearing loss has on the person's ability to communicate whether it be through an oral or visual mode of communication. But for purposes of characterizing different degrees of hearing loss, the fundamental premise of how residual hearing is used to perceive and understand oral speech continues to be the primary distinction that differentiates these two categories.

The impact of deafness is typically viewed as more significant in its effect on communication as well as other psychosocial issues, but its prevalence is relatively small when compared to individuals who are hard-of-hearing. In fact, a person with deafness who is often depicted as the typical hearing impaired individual comprises less than 1% of the total number of individuals with hearing loss (National Center for Health Statistics, 1999). However, the significantly higher prevalence of the hard-of-hearing group does not negate the dramatic effect profound deafness has on someone's ability to communicate and function in society. On the contrary, individuals who are categorized in this way receive the primary intervention services in terms of academic and communicative rehabilitation. But it is also critical that the predominant hard-of-hearing group not be ignored when determining the implications of hearing impairment (Davis, 1990; Davis, Effenbein, Schum, & Bentler, 1986; Blair, Peterson, & Viehweg, 1985).

EPIDEMIOLOGY

Incidence of Hearing Loss

Hearing impairment, as previously mentioned, is estimated to affect 31.5 million Americans; this figure has more than doubled in the past 30 years (Ries, 1994; Benson & Marano, 1995; Kochkin, 2001a), and is projected to reach 50 million over the next 40 years as shown in Figure 1.2 (Kochkin, 2005a).

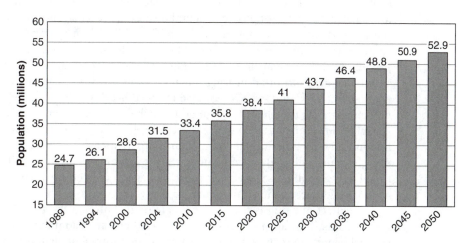

Figure 1.2   Hearing loss population (1989–2004) in millions with projections through the year 2050 based on MarkeTrak incidence of hearing loss by age group applied to U.S. Bureau of Census age population projections.

Source: From S. Kochkin 2005a, "MarkeTrak VII: Hearing Loss Population Tops 31 million People," *Hearing Review,* 12

This estimate is further magnified when the different types of temporary hearing loss are added to the incidence of hearing impairment, increasing its prevalence by several million.

Common Causes of Medically Treatable Hearing Loss

Temporary hearing loss can be the result of various ear diseases or conditions typically occurring in the outer or middle ear that can be completely overcome through medical treatment using surgery or drug therapy. The most common of these causes of temporary or fluctuating hearing loss is an infection in the middle ear called **otitis media**, which occurs frequently among infants and young children. It is estimated that 75% of all children will experience at least one episode of otitis media before the age of three, one-half of whom will have at least three infections during this same period (NIDCD, 2002a). Other examples of treatable middle ear disease are those affecting the middle ear bones such as a separation between bones called **ossicular disruption** or a calcified growth around the bones called **otosclerosis**. Surgical procedures generally can overcome or minimize hearing loss caused by these diseases. Temporary hearing loss can also occur from problems in the outer ear caused by a buildup of ear wax or cerumen, or an obstruction in the ear canal reducing sound transmission. In some cases, inner ear diseases caused by infection or allergic reaction will be temporary and recover spontaneously or with drug treatment. Although most of these causes of hearing loss can be temporary, a permanent loss can also be the result due to untimely or inadequate treatment of the disease.

Common Causes of Permanent Hearing Loss

Permanent hearing loss normally occurs in the inner ear or auditory nervous system from a plethora of causes or diseases. These causes can be associated with hereditary factors such as a genetic syndrome; a neural disorder; a vascular disorder; or infections or trauma during fetal development, at birth, in childhood, or as an adult. The two most common causes of permanent hearing loss in adults are the effects of exposure to loud sounds and the consequences of the aging process (NIDCD, 2002b, NIDCD, 1997).

About one-third of all hearing-impaired cases are at least partially attributable to hearing loss from loud sounds, or **noise-induced hearing loss** (NIH, 1990). The unit of measurement for the intensity of sound is **decibels**, or **dB**. A level of 75 decibels, which is slightly lower than typical traffic noise, is unlikely to cause permanent hearing loss. But only an increase of slightly more than 10 dB in intensity with regular daily exposure of eight hours will produce permanent hearing loss after many years (NIH, 1990). Continual increases in noise levels can cause damage to the delicate inner ear structures at a more rapid rate, as shown in Figure 1.3.

The effect of aging is the largest single contributor to the prevalence of hearing loss (Adams, Hendershot, & Marano, 1999; Benson & Marano, 1995) and consequently, elderly persons are the largest group of Americans that are hearing-impaired (NIDCD, 1996). In fact, hearing loss is the third most common chronic condition experienced by the elderly following arthritis and hypertension (Administration on Aging, 2001). The number of elderly people in the United States is increasing rapidly

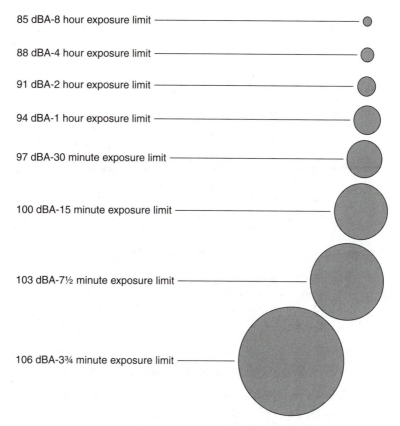

85 dBA-8 hour exposure limit

88 dBA-4 hour exposure limit

91 dBA-2 hour exposure limit

94 dBA-1 hour exposure limit

97 dBA-30 minute exposure limit

100 dBA-15 minute exposure limit

103 dBA-7½ minute exposure limit

106 dBA-3¾ minute exposure limit

Figure 1.3 Intensity comparisons with recommended permissible exposure time.
Source: Courtesy of the National Institute for Occupational Safety and Health (NIOSH)

and is expected to more than double between 2000 and 2030 (U.S Dept. of HHS, 2004). Based on the data provided by the Administration on Aging (2004), the number of persons over the age of 65 will comprise 20% of the U.S. population in just 25 years. Individuals aged 85 and older are expected to show a corresponding increase as well (see Figure 1.4).

The medical term used to describe the loss of hearing that relates to age is called **presbycusis**. Its underlying cause arises most commonly from changes in the inner ear as a result of a loss of hair cells (sensory receptors), but also can occur from changes in the middle ear or the auditory nerve pathway. Hair cell loss can be caused by the side effects of medicines, changes in blood supply to the ear from vascular disorders, compromised overall health conditions, or atrophy of the structures from aging (NDICD, 1997). The effect of age on hearing loss creates a significant dynamic in the distribution of hearing impairment (Adams, Hendershot, & Marano, 1999), as illustrated in Figure 1.5. Approximately 30% to 35% of adults over the age of 65 experience some degree of hearing loss. A detailed discussion of these and subsequent hearing disorders will be addressed in Chapter 4.

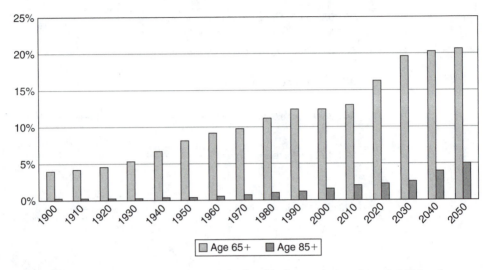

Figure 1.4 The aging of America. Growth in the elderly population through 2000 and projected increase to 2050 of individuals 65+ and 85+.
Source: U.S. Dept. of Health and Human Services Administration on Aging (2004)

The Time Factor

Time of Onset, Identification, and Intervention

Although variable causes of hearing loss have a tremendous impact on its effects, the element of time also influences the degree to which a hearing impairment creates a disabling condition. Specifically, there are three key moments in time related to a hearing loss that can potentially alter or exacerbate its impact on an individual: the time of onset of a hearing disorder, the point in time in which a hearing loss is identified and diagnosed, and the time that intervention is provided.

Figure 1.5 The percentage of individuals with hearing loss in the general population as a function of age.
Source: P. F. Adams, G. E. Hendershot, & M. A. Marano (1999), "Current Estimates from the National Health Interview Survey, 1996, National Center for Health Statistics, *Vital Health Statistics, 10*

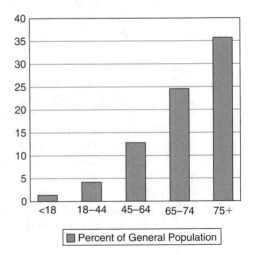

The time of a hearing impairment's onset is directly related to causal factors such as a hereditary loss present at birth, a severe childhood disease, a hearing loss from long-term noise exposure, or a presbycusic loss as part of aging. Until recently, the average age of hearing loss identification in infancy has been 30 months of age (Harrison & Roush, 1996), and for some children it is not identified until school age (Elssmann, Matkin, & Sabo, 1987). Because of the connection of hearing to normal speech and language development, time of onset of hearing loss is critical from a developmental perspective. If a hearing loss occurs prior to normal speech and language development, or **prelingually**, the disabling consequences of the loss on speech and language development potentially can be more severe than if the loss occurs after speech and language ability has been established, or **postlingually**. For more common causes of hearing loss from noise exposure or aging, the time of onset is more difficult to pinpoint because of the progressive nature of the loss and determination by an individual that hearing difficulty is sufficient to warrant pursuit of its identification.

It might be assumed that the time of identification followed by the commencement of intervention procedures would occur shortly after onset. But in many cases, there is a significant lag based on a number of factors. For example, an older adult who has developed a loss of hearing gradually over time may deny its existence and delay having a hearing evaluation or resist recommendations for intervention even after a loss has been diagnosed. Denial may also be the cause of delay in identification in an infant born with a congenital hearing impairment whose parents are unwilling to accept the presence of a problem until the lack of response to certain sounds or a delay in speech development compels them to investigate the problem. A lack of understanding regarding normal hearing and reactions to speech and other environmental sounds in an infant, or inappropriate advice received from family, friends, or professionals may also be the cause for postponing the hearing loss identification and subsequent intervention. Ideally, the three sequential events—onset, identification, and intervention—should occur successively and in a timely manner. But unfortunately, this time span often occurs over months and years, which will influence the disabling effect of a hearing impairment on communication and quality of life.

Early Identification

For infants and young children, **early identification** of hearing loss and **early intervention** are critical to maximize the development of speech and language. Early detection has been a topic of concern and interest for many years (Yoshinaga-Itano, Sedey, Coulter, & Mehl, 1998; Yoshinaga-Itano, 1995; Kenworthy,1993; Elssmann, Matkin, & Sabo, 1987), as the incidence of hearing loss has been estimated from between 1.2 and 5.7 per 1000 live births (Mauk & Behrens, 1993; Parving, 1993; Watkin, Baldwin, & McEnery, 1991), and is considered the most common birth defect (Deafness Research Foundation, 2005; Adams, Hendershot & Marano, 1999). A study by Yoshinaga-Itano and her associates (1998) has demonstrated that if a newborn with a hearing loss is diagnosed prior to six months of age and treated appropriately, higher language levels will be achieved than children with delayed diagnoses, as shown in Figure 1.6. Numerous professional organizations and state health and welfare agencies that comprise the **Joint Committee on Infant Hearing** (JCIH) advocate the implementation of universal newborn hearing screening

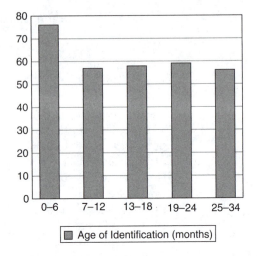

Figure 1.6 Adjusted mean total language quotients for groups based on age of identification of hearing loss.

Source: Christine Yoshinaga-Itano, Allison L. Sedey, Diane K. Coulter, & Albert L. Mehl, "Language of Early- and Later-Identified Children with Hearing Loss," *Pediatrics, 102:* 1161–1171, 1998

programs in order to minimize the negative impact of late identification of hearing loss in infants (JCIH, 2000). A detailed treatment of infant hearing screening is discussed in Chapter 8.

MANAGEMENT OF HEARING LOSS

When someone loses their ability to hear, the potential underlying causes are amazingly varied and diverse, as previously indicated. The variability of diseases of the ear requires a precise evaluation by an audiologist in order to make an accurate diagnosis and to identify the underlying source or location of the problem in the auditory pathway. But despite this diversity, the treatment for most cases of hearing loss generally falls into one of two basic categories:

1. Hearing loss that is medically treatable and commonly reversible through some form of medical (drug) or surgical intervention
2. Hearing loss that is medically nonthreatening to the health of the individual, but has characteristics that are permanent and reduce the individual's quality of life and ability to communicate effectively

The initial steps in diagnosis then involve differentiating the cause of loss in order to direct the patient toward the appropriate intervention.

If a hearing loss is medically or surgically treatable, the patient may be referred to a general practice physician or to an otolaryngologist or otologist. If the hearing loss is caused by an allergic reaction, bacterial or viral infection, or other type of disease, it often can be treated and reversed through different forms of antibiotic or steroid drug therapy. In some cases, surgery can be performed on the outer or middle portions of the ear which often results in complete recovery of hearing sensitivity.

If hearing loss is of a permanent nature, generally the patient will be referred to an audiologist to receive intervention aimed at alleviating the communication difficulties that occur. The term used to describe this type of treatment is **audiologic** (or aural) **rehabilitation** and includes the fitting of hearing aids, counseling, educating, listening training, and speechreading. In cases of congenital hearing impairment when speech and language skills have not developed, the common term is **audiologic habilitation**, and a referral for speech and language therapy and appropriate educational management also accompanies the audiologic treatment.

Hearing Loss and Communication

Because the primary means of communication for humans is through spoken language, the ability to hear speech plays a direct role in the ability to perceive and produce speech. Often, one reason that hearing loss is initially suspected in young children is their inability to develop normal speech and language. The perception of speech is based on the processing of the acoustic characteristics of a speech signal. Speech incorporates a whole array of acoustic characteristics ranging from the relatively loud low pitch of an adult male producing the vowel sound /a/, to the comparatively soft high-pitched sound that is generated by articulating the consonants /s/ or /t/. The perception of speech involves not only the loudness that is produced by vowels, but also the acoustical characteristics found in consonants that provide much of the information for discrimination and recognition of speech. The discrimination of this dynamic variation in the acoustical parameters of speech can be dramatically affected by varying types of hearing loss. Therefore, the primary goal in assisting individuals with hearing impairment is to maximize the ability to hear and understand speech, and in the case of young children, to accurately produce speech. This goal not only applies to the ability to hear and recognize the basic speech elements, but also to hear and process intonational patterns and vocal pitch that are critical to understanding a spoken message. For individuals who are hard of hearing and retain a measure of their hearing ability, the missing components of speech can be made audible through some form of amplification such as hearing aids. The most important factor in amplifying a signal is to make the elements of speech audible in order to minimize communication difficulties caused by a hearing loss. For individuals with severe to profound hearing loss or specifically those diagnosed with deafness, hearings aids can still provide benefit in many cases. However, as the severity of hearing loss worsens, the speech components critical to understanding will become less audible and the benefit derived from amplification often diminishes, further impacting the ability to communicate.

The Benefits of Amplification
The Use of Hearing Aids

The first and most important rehabilitative tool for the hearing professional to treat individuals with permanent hearing loss is the fitting of hearing aids. Hearing aids or hearing instruments are electronic devices that consist of a microphone, amplifier, speaker or receiver, and a power supply (battery) that deliver amplified sound to the impaired ear. In addition to these basic components, the advances in hearing instrument technology have generated a variety of designs and features to improve their performance and enhance sound quality. Because of these advances and the many options currently available, a primary role of the audiologist today is the selection, fitting, and programming of hearing aids. It is estimated that there are about 12.5 million hearing aids in use by over seven million individuals, 70% of whom wear two (Kochkin, 2005b). Unfortunately, of the millions of individuals who are candidates for hearing aids, less than 25% actually take advantage of the benefit derived from wearing them (Kochkin, 2005b; Popelka, Cruickshanks, Wiley, Tweed, Klein, & Klein, 1998; Stephens, Callaghan, Hogan, Meredith, Rayment, & Davis, 1990).

Hearing Aid Benefit

Hearing aids are well known to provide significant benefit with numerous studies verifying their capacity to overcome or minimize the deleterious effects of hearing impairment (Humes, Garner, Wilson, & Barlow, 2001; Humes, Christensen, Thomas, Bess, Hedley-Williams, Bentler, 1999; Newman & Sandridge, 1998; Humes, Christensen, Bess, Hedley-Williams, 1997; Kochkin, 1996; Mulrow, Tuley, & Aguilar, 1992; Mulrow, Aguilar, Endicott, Tuley, Velez, Charlip, Rhodes, Hill, & DeNino, 1990). In addition to these studies that report improved speech perception, the benefit of hearing aid use is also perceived by hearing aid users as reported in satisfaction ratings.

A recent consumer survey by Kochkin (2005a) revealed a customer satisfaction rating of 77.5% (see Figure 1.7), which places hearing aids in the top one-third of products and services in the United States. The significant improvement observed in the level of satisfaction in recent years may be due to several variables, some of which are the advancements in hearing aid technology such as digital signal processing and the use of multiple microphones (Kochkin, 2002; Kochkin, 2001; Kochkin, 1996).

Figure 1.7   U.S. overall customer satisfaction trends for hearing instruments that are 1–4 years old.

Source: From S. Kochkin 2005a, "MarkeTrak VII: Hearing Loss Population Tops 31 Million People," *Hearing Review, 12*

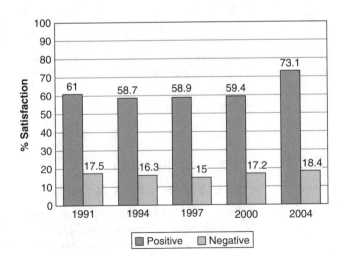

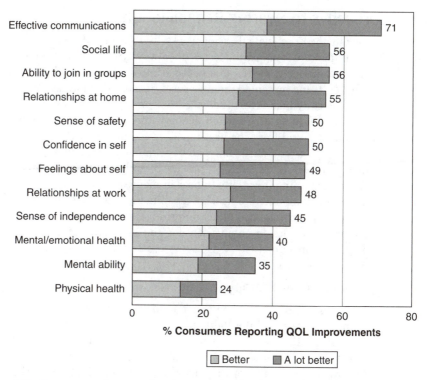

Figure 1.8 Percentage of current hearing instrument users reporting improved quality of life (QOL) due to hearing instrument use.

Source: From S. Kochkin 2005b, "MarkeTrac VII: Customer Satisfaction with Hearing Instruments in the Digital Era," *Hearing Journal, 58*

In addition to improved speech perception and high levels of customer satisfaction, hearing aid use has also been shown to enhance the overall quality of life and well-being of adults with hearing loss (Bridges & Bentler, 1998; Crandell, 1998; Mulrow, Tuley, & Aguilar, 1992). A 1999 study by the National Council on Aging evaluated the effects of untreated hearing loss and the benefit of hearing aids on the quality of life for adults and their families. In summarizing this exhaustive research, Kochkin and Rogin (2000) stated:

> Hearing instruments are clearly associated with impressive improvements in the social, emotional, psychological and physical well-being of people with hearing loss in all hearing loss categories from mild to severe. As such, these findings provide strong evidence for the "value" of hearing instruments in improving the quality of life of people with hearing loss.

Figure 1.8 displays the results of the most recent consumer survey indicating percentage of individuals who have experienced an improvement in their quality of life with hearing instrument use (Kochkin, 2005b).

Other Approaches to Hearing Rehabilitation

Despite the beneficial effects of successful hearing aid use, a complete resolution to the disabling impact of hearing loss is not always achieved. It is important to note that when amplification is provided to a hearing-impaired listener, the increased intensity of the sound is being presented, in most cases, to a damaged inner ear. It is difficult to provide a consistently high level of satisfaction from hearing aid use for all users due to the fact that normal inner ear function is not restored merely by amplifying sound. Rather, the amplified sound from the hearing aid is essentially forcing the remaining normal sensory receptors and nerve fibers to be stimulated in an attempt to overcome those areas that have been damaged. This process often lends itself to a less than satisfactory conclusion regarding the ability to hear in many difficult listening environments. Thus, an important component of hearing rehabilitation involves appropriate counseling regarding realistic expectations of hearing aid use and therapeutic intervention to provide additional strategies to compensate for the communicative difficulties not resolved by amplification alone.

Rehabilitation Therapy

Audiologic rehabilitation therapy in individual or group settings includes **speechreading** training to maximize the ability to use visual cues, observe body language, and develop lipreading skills. A variety of communication strategies can also be taught in therapy and can then be employed in everyday situations. For example, an increased awareness of the environment can allow a person with hearing loss to control or manipulate the listening situation in simple ways like reducing background noise at home or work, changing seating arrangements while watching television, or selecting a location in a restaurant with optimal lighting and minimal noise. These, and other techniques, serve to help fill the gap between an ideal communicative interchange and inadequate benefit provided by amplification.

Speech and Language Development

When children are born with or acquire a hearing loss at an early age, the absence or lack of normal speech language development is often the primary motivator for parents or other professionals to seek an evaluation of hearing. An intact hearing mechanism is essential for normal feedback of auditory speech cues, which in turn are required to develop normal speech and language production. Once a hearing loss is identified in a child, adequate support for speech and language development must be included as part of the overall rehabilitative process. Speech-language pathologists and deaf/hard-of-hearing educators then become primary service providers in supplying the appropriate intervention for speech, language, and academic development.

Assistive Listening Devices

A particular communication environment that has shown the lowest rate of satisfaction among hearing aid users is listening in noisy surroundings (Kochkin, 2000). A method of overcoming and managing hearing loss when communicating in a difficult listening environment is with the use of electronic devices other than hearing aids called **assistive listening devices.** An example of this type of system is a wireless frequency-modulated or **FM system** that can be coupled to hearing aids or used independently. A remote microphone is worn by a speaker, such as a teacher, lecturer, or minister, and the speech signal is transmitted directly to a receiver worn by the hearing-impaired listener. The difference between the signal and the background noise is improved because of this transmission and the listener is able to better utilize the amplified signal with less interference. **Infrared systems** are also a popular type of device using the same concept of sound enhancement as the FM system to help improve the signal, but employing infrared light waves similar to a television remote control to transmit the signal. These systems are commonly used when the source of the desired signal is stationary such as in movie theaters or with the television. Amplifiers and telecommunication devices can also be attached to the telephone to improve that particular communicative situation. Amplification devices are continuously being developed to improve the ability to hear and communicate in specific listening situations when the amplification from hearing aids is not sufficient.

Cochlear Implants

Another approach to improving audibility is with the use of a device called a cochlear implant. Individuals who are deaf and unable to benefit from hearing aid amplification are now able to perceive sound through this device. The implant is comprised of an external microphone, amplifier, and speech processor connected to an array of electrodes that are surgically implanted in the inner ear. Cochlear implants have continued to be refined and currently allow for audibility and processing of sound with unprecedented fidelity and quality—speech in particular—for children and adults with severe to profound hearing loss. A detailed discussion of hearing rehabilitation strategies through the use of hearing aids, assistive devices, cochlear implants, and audiologic rehabilitation/habilitation therapy can be found in Chapter 10.

Advocacy for the Hearing Impaired
Individuals with Disabilities Education Act (IDEA)

In the 1970s, educators and professionals providing services to children with disabilities determined that the state educational systems were not meeting these children's educational needs. In 1975, Congress enacted public law 94-142, which was known as the Education for All Handicapped Children Act. It is currently referred to as the **Individuals with Disabilities Education Act (IDEA)** (Tucker, 1997). The main purpose of IDEA is to ensure that all children with disabilities receive a free, appropriate, public education that emphasizes special education and related services designed to meet their unique needs in the least restrictive environment. According to IDEA, the placement of children in an academic environment that is most appropriate is based on their particular needs. In some cases, this has been interpreted as meaning that each child with a disability should be mainstreamed into a regular classroom under the assumption that this placement is the least restrictive and provides a sense of normalcy to the education of all

Table 1.1 Change in classroom types for hearing impaired children toward more mainstreamed educational placements over an 11-year period, including comparisons with all other disabilities.

	Change in Educational Placements			
	Regular Class	Resource Room	Separate Class	Separate Facility
Hearing Impaired:				
1985–86	20%	22.4%	32.6%	24.9%
1996–97	37.5%	18.3%	26.6%	17.5%
All Disabilities:				
1996–97	46.2%	26.8%	22.4%	4.5%

Source: U.S. Dept. of Education, 22nd Annual Report to Congress, Appendix A, Table AB8, 2000

children. However, upon implementation of the IDEA, it was discovered that many disabled children, and particular to our discussion, children with hearing loss, could not properly function in a regular classroom and the assumption that a regular classroom presented the least restrictive environment was challenged. A 1997 amendment to the IDEA clarified classroom placement by stating that, "a child with a disability is to be removed from the regular educational environment only when the nature or severity of the disability is such that education in regular classes with the use of supplementary aids and services cannot be achieved satisfactorily" (IDEA, 1997). The 2000 Office of Education Report to Congress clearly confirmed the shift of hearing-impaired children toward the regular classroom between 1986 and 1997 as shown in Table 1.1 (U.S. Dept. of Ed., 2000). The goal of the IDEA is to favor the integration of hearing-impaired children in the regular classroom but with the priority being the provision of an "appropriate" education even if it requires an alternative approach to **mainstreaming**.

No Child Left Behind

More recently, Public Law 107-110 has increased the services to children. Commonly called the No Child Left Behind Act of 2001 (NCLB), its purpose is to improve the academic achievement of the disadvantaged and "ensure that all children have a fair, equal, and significant opportunity to obtain a high-quality education and reach, at a minimum, proficiency on challenging state academic achievement standards and state academic assessments." (U.S. Dept. of Ed., 2000).

Americans with Disabilities Act (ADA)

Another legislative act that has had a significant impact on services to the hearing impaired as well as all disabled individuals is the **Americans with Disabilities Act (ADA)**, signed into law in 1990. The primary intent of this law was to eliminate discrimination against anyone who is disabled. It was established with four components that address the equal opportunity for these individuals in the areas of employment, public services, public access, and telecommunications. Specific to the hearing impaired, the ADA ensures that a hearing loss cannot be used to rule out an individual to be considered for employment as long the job tasks can be performed. It requires employers to make accommodations for the hearing loss such as providing amplifiers for the telephone or other assistive devices (EEOC, 1991). It also guarantees that a public agency such as a local or state government or transportation service be required to provide accommodations for disabled individuals to receive services just as any other member of the public. In addition, the ADA requires that any goods or services be provided without discrimination by supplying auxiliary aids or devices to assist with or overcome the disabling condition. Examples of this requirement are the provision of assistive listening devices in movie theaters to offer an amplified signal to the hearing-impaired consumer and the requirement of all new telephones to be hearing aid compatible (DOJ, 1991). The telecommunications component of the ADA involves, in part, the creation of telephone relay services that allow a severely hearing impaired individual to communicate with others through a specially trained operator who serves as an intermediary to transfer the information between parties (FCC, 1991). This service is in addition to the already existing requirement that all new telephones be hearing aid compatible as specified in the Hearing Aid Compatibility Act (FCC, 1988). Recently, this requirement was revised to include cell phones as well (FCC, 2003). The implementation of the ADA has created an increased awareness of the particular needs of people with disabilities and provided greater opportunities for employment and access to public services in the community.

Support Groups

Another source of advocacy has been the development of consumer groups. In 1979, a national organization called Self Help for Hard of Hearing People, Inc. (SHHH) was formed. Its name was recently changed to Hearing Loss Association of America. It has local chapters located throughout the country with the goal of offering support, social interaction, and advocacy to the hearing-impaired population. With the advent of cochlear implant use, another group called Cochlear Implant Club International (CICI) was formed. Its purpose is to provide a forum for interaction among cochlear implant users, their families, and professionals who work with them. In addition, numerous other organizations have been created for the purpose of support, advocacy, and education. A summary of the largest and most well known organizations is listed in Appendix B.

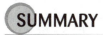 **SUMMARY**

A Glimpse into the Profession Revisited

The beginning of this chapter presented a case study. The audiologist conducted a complete evaluation with the aid of an audiology assistant due to the age of the patient. From the results of the hearing evaluation, Justin was diagnosed with a permanent hearing loss that is moderate in its degree of severity. This result identifies Justin as a child who is hard-of-hearing of unknown cause. The fortunate aspect of Justin's case is that his hearing loss is only of a moderate nature, leaving him with substantial residual hearing ability. He has already been able to compensate to some degree and has developed speech and language despite the hearing loss. However, this type of loss does create some delay in his language ability and some errors in his articulation of certain speech sounds. Following an examination by the otolaryngologist to rule out the possibility of medical treatment, the first intervention process for Justin would be to provide amplification through the use of hearing aids to compensate for the hearing loss. The future prognosis for Justin, with proper intervention, is normal auditory listening capability and the likelihood of regular classroom placement with the use of an FM system coupled to his hearing aids. He will also need support from a speech-language pathologist and possibly an educator of the hearing impaired to assist with speech and language development and academic tutoring. Justin should be successful with hearing aid use throughout his life and able to function normally in society using oral speech effectively to communicate.

CHAPTER REVIEW

❏ Audiology is a health care profession devoted to the evaluation of hearing, the prevention of hearing loss, the diagnosis of hearing impairment, and the treatment of hearing-related problems.

❏ Audiology emerged in the last century as a new profession at the intersection of the medical field of otolaryngology and the rehabilitative fields of speech-language pathology and psychology. It has grown to be a well-recognized autonomous profession with its own professional organizations, providing a wide range of services.

❏ Audiologist assistants and audiometrists are subspecialties of audiology and offer increased effectiveness and productivity in a hearing health care practice. This type of position increases the opportunities for employment in an audiology work setting.

❏ Audiology offers many specialties in a variety of practice settings including, but not limited to, independent clinics, hospitals, private practice, education, and industry.

❏ Audiologists interact directly with physicians and other health care providers, speech-language pathologists, and psychologists, as well as educators both in elementary and secondary education.

❏ Presently, audiologists typically practice with a master's degree but the profession is in transition to an entry-level degree of a clinical doctorate designated as the AuD.

❏ Hearing impairment affects over 31 million Americans, with a variety of causes that can have a significant impact on a person's communicative function.

❏ Hearing impairment is the general term used to describe this type of difficulty, but it can be separated into categories identified as hard-of-hearing and deafness based on a number of variables, but in particular the use of residual hearing and the ability to hear and develop speech.

❏ There are numerous underlying causes of a hearing impairment, the two most common of which are exposure to loud sounds and presbycusis, which is part of the aging process. In fact, the elderly constitute over one-half of all individuals who are hearing-impaired, forecasting an ever-increasing number of hearing impaired coincident with the aging of America.

❏ The loss of hearing has a significant disabling effect on the ability to communicate, which generally worsens concurrent with the severity of the impairment.

❑ Communication ability and the impact of hearing loss are also affected by the age of onset the hearing loss occurs, the time that it is first identified, and the time when some type of intervention is provided.

❑ The management of hearing loss is dependent on whether the loss is temporary and can be treated medically or surgically or whether it is permanent.

❑ The first and most important rehabilitative tool in treating permanent hearing loss is maximizing the remaining hearing ability with the use of hearing aids, cochlear implants, or assistive listening devices.

❑ Audiologic rehabilitation and speech and language therapy can assist hearing-impaired adults or children adjust to their hearing loss, maximize their listening skills, and develop their speech and language ability.

❑ In support of individuals who have been disabled by hearing loss, some key legislation has been enacted to provide appropriate education and services in the community and the general public. Specifically, the Individuals with Disabilities Education Act (IDEA) was specifically designed to place hearing-impaired children in a least restrictive environment in order to optimize their educational experience. The Americans with Disabilities Act (ADA) was also passed to offer access to public services as well as telecommunication to individuals who are disabled.

❑ Numerous support and advocacy groups have also been formed to assist the hearing impaired understand and deal with their disability in attempting to improve their quality of life.

ACTIVITIES FOR DISCUSSION

1. Case Study: Assuming that Justin receives appropriate intervention, how quickly do you think he will be able to overcome his speech/language delay and are there any other services he might need?

2. What does the future look like for the profession of audiology with regard to growth, jobs, and salaries particularly in view of the increase in the elderly population, the implementation of universal newborn hearing screening programs, and the advances in testing procedures and intervention technology?

3. What effect will the professional doctorate have on employment opportunities, not only for audiologists, but also for audiometrists and audiology assistants?

4. Why is the time factor so important when determining the extent of hearing disability?

REFERENCES

Adams, P. F., & Marano, M. A. (1995). Current estimates from the National Health Interview Survey, 1994. National Center for Health Statistics. *Vital Health Statistics, 10*, 193.

Adams, P. F., Hendershot, G. E., & Marano, M. A. (1999). Current Estimates from the National Health Interview Survey, 1996. National Center for Health Statistics. *Vital Health Statistics, 10*, 200.

American Academy of Audiology (2004). Audiology: Scope of Practice. Audiology Documents, [online]. http://www.audiology.org

American Academy of Audiology (1997). Audiology: Scope of practice. *Audiology Today, 9*(2), 12–13.

American Academic of Audiology (1991). Position statement: The American Academy of Audiology and the professional doctorate (AuD). *Audiology Today, 3*(4), 10–12.

American Board of Audiology (2005). Application Handbook [online]. http://www.americanboard-ofaudiology.org

American Speech-Language-Hearing Association (2005a). State Regulation of Support Personnel: An Overview [online]. http://www.asha.org.

American Speech-Language-Hearing Association (2005b). State licensure trends, www.asha.org

American Speech-Language-Hearing Association. (2004a). Scope of practice in audiology. ASHA Supplement 24.

American Speech-Language-Hearing Association (2004b). 2004 Audiology Survey Report: Survey methodology, respondent demographics, and glossary. Rockville, MD: Author.

American Speech-Language-Hearing Association (1999). Demographic survey of ASHA member and non-member certificate holders in audiology only, for the period January 1 through December 31, 1998.

American Speech-Language-Hearing Association (1998). Position statement and guidelines on support personnel in audiology. *ASHA, 40* (Spring, Suppl. 18), 19–21.

American Speech-Language-Hearing Association (ASHA). (1996). Scope of practice in audiology. *ASHA*, Suppl. 16, 12–15.

Benson, V., & Marano, M.A. (1995). Current estimates from the National Health Interview Survey, 1993. *National Center for Health Statistics.* Vital Health Stat 10(190).

Bergman, M. (2002). American Wartime Military Audiology. *Audiology Today*, Monograph 1.

Beyer, C., & Van Vliet, D. (2006). The use of supportive personnel in the corporate network. *Audiology Today, 18*(1), 31–32.

Blackwell, D. L., Collins, J. G., & Coles, R. (2002). Summary of Health Statistics for U.S. Adults: National Health Interview Survey, 1997. *National Center for Health Statistics.* Vital Health Stat 10(205).

Blair, J. C., Peterson, M. E., & Viehweg, S. H. (1985). The effects of mild hearing loss on academic performance among school-aged children. *The Volta Review, 87,* 87–94.

Bridges, J., & Bentler, R. (1998). Relating hearing aid use to well-being among older adults. *Hearing Journal, 51*(7), 39–44.

Crandell, C. (1998). Hearing aids: Their effects on functional health status. *Hearing Journal, 51*(2), 2–6.

Davis, J. (1990). *Our Forgotten Children: Hard of Hearing Pupils in the Schools (2nd ed.).* Washington, DC: Self Help for the Hard of Hearing.

Davis, J., Effenbein, J., Schum, R., & Bentler, R. (1986). Effects of mild and moderate hearing impairments on language, educational, and psychosocial behavior of children. *Journal of Speech and Hearing Research, 51*(1), 53–63.

Deafness Research Foundation (2005). Early detection and intervention [online]. http://www.drf.org/WCHH/Hearing_Loss/early_detection.htm

Department of Justice (DOJ) (1991). Nondiscrimination on the basis of disability in state and local government services and by public accommodations and in commercial facilities: Final rule, 28 Code of Federal Regulations Part 35 and 36. Federal Register, 56 (144).

Dunlop, R. J, Beck, L. B., Dennis, K. C., Gonzenbach, S. A., Abrams, H. B., Berardino, J. T., Styer, S. A., & Hall, A. (2006). Support personnel in VA audiology, *Audiology Today, 18*(1), 24–25.

Dunn, H. H., Dunn, D. R., & Harford, E. R. (1995). *Audiology Business and Practice Management.* San Diego: Singular.

Elssmann, S. A., Matkin, N. D., & Sabo, M. P. (1987). Early identification of congenital sensorineural hearing impairment. *The Hearing Journal, 40,* 13–17.

Equal Employment Opportunity Commission (EEOC) (1991). Equal employment opportunity for individuals with disabilities: Final rule, 29 Code of Federal Regulations Part 1630. Federal Register, 56 (144).

Federal Communications Commission (FCC) (2003). Telecommunications services for hearing and speech disabled: Final rule, 47 Code of Federal Regulations, Part 68.317. Federal Register.

Federal Communications Commission (FCC) (1991). Telecommunications services for hearing and speech disabled: Final rule, 47 Code of Federal Regulations, Parts 0 and 64. Federal Register, 56(148).

Federal Communications Commission (FCC) (1988). Telecommunications services for hearing and speech disabled: Final rule, 47 Code of Federal Regulations, Part 68.112. Federal Register.

Frisina, R. (1974). Report of the committee to redefine deaf and hard of hearing. Washington, DC: Conference of Executives of American Schools for the Deaf (CEASD).

Goldstein, D. P. (1989). AuD degree: The doctoring degree in audiology. *Asha, 31.* 33–35.

Harrison, M., & Roush, J. (1996). Age of suspicion, identification and intervention for infants and young children with hearing loss: A national study. *Ear and Hearing, 17,* 55–62.

Hecker, D. E. (2004). Occupational employment projections to 2012. *Monthly Labor Review Online, 127*(2), 80–105.

Humes, L. E., Christensen, L. A., Bess, F. H., & Hedley-Williams, A. (1997). A comparison of the benefit provided by well-fit linear hearing aids and instruments with automatic reduction of low-frequency gain. *Journal of Speech, Language, and Hearing Research, 40*(3), 666–685.

Humes, L. E., Christensen, L., Thomas, T., Bess, F. H., Hedley-Williams, & Bentler, R. (1999). A comparison of the aided performance and benefit provided by a linear and a two-channel wide dynamic range compression hearing aid. *Journal of Speech, Language, and Hearing Research, 42*(1), 65–79.

Humes, L. E., Garner, C. B., Wilson, D. L. & Barlow, N. N. (2001). Hearing-aid outcome measures following one month of hearing aid use by the elderly. *Journal of Speech, Language, and Hearing Research, 44*(3), 469–486.

Individuals with Disabilities Education Act (IDEA) (1997). Amendments to the IDEA: Final Rule, 34 Code of Regulations, 300.550. Federal Register.

Joint Committee on Infant Hearing (2000). Year 2000 Position Statement: Principles and Guidelines for Early Hearing Detection and Intervention Programs, *Audiology Today.* Special Issue.

Kasewurm, G. A. (2006). The positive impact of using audiologist's assistants, *Audiology Today, 18*(1), 26–27.

Kenworthy, O. T. (1993). Early identification: Principles and practices. In J. G. Alpiner and P. A. MacCarthy, *Rehabilitative Audiology: Children and Adults,* Baltimore: Lippincott, Williams & Wilkins.

Kochkin, S. (2005a). MarkeTrak VII: Hearing loss population tops 31 million people, *Hearing Review, 12* (7), 16–29.

Kochkin, S. (2005b). MarkeTrak VII: Customer satisfaction with hearing instruments in the digital age, *Hearing Journal, 58* (9), 30–43.

Kochkin, S. (2002). MarkeTrak VI: 10-year customer satisfaction trends in the U.S. hearing instrument market. *Hearing Review, 9* (10).

Kochkin, S. (2001). MarkeTrak VI: The VA and direct mail sales spark growth in hearing aid market. *Hearing Review, 8*(12), 16–24, 63–65.

Kochkin, S. (2000). MarketTrak V: Customer satisfaction revisited. *Hearing Journal, 53* (1).

Kochkin, S. (1996). Customer satisfaction and subjective benefit with high-performance hearing instruments. *Hearing Review, 3*(12), 16–26.

Kochkin, S., & Rogin, C. M. (2000). Quantifying the obvious: The impact of hearing instruments on quality of life, *Hearing Review, 7* (12).

Martin, F. N., Champlain, C. A., & Streetman, P. S. (1997). Audiologists' professional satisfaction. *Journal of the American Academy of Audiology, 8,* 11–17.

Mauk, G. W., & Behrens, T. R. (1993). Historical, political, and technological context associated with early identification of hearing loss. *Seminars in Hearing, 14,* 1–17.

McCollom, H. F. (2003). A brief history of the AuD. *Advance for Audiologists, 5*(4), 14–15.

Mulrow, C. D., Aguilar, C., Endicott, J. E., Tuley, M. R., Velez, R., Charlip, W. S., Rhodes, M. C., Hill, J. A., & DeNino, L. A. (1990). Quality-of-life changes and hearing impairment. A randomized trial. *Annals of Internal Medicine, 1,* 113(3), 188–94.

Mulrow, C. D., Tuley, M. R., & Aguilar, C. (1992). Sustained benefits of hearing aids. *Journal of Speech and Hearing Research, 35*(6), 1402–1405.

National Center for Health Statistics. (1999). [www.cdc.gov/nchs/fastats/disable/htm]

National Institute on Deafness and Other Communication Disorders (NIDCD) (2002a). Otitis Media. NIH Pub. No. 97-4216 [online]. http://www.nidcd.nih.gov/health/hearing/otitism.asp.

National Institute on Deafness and Other Communication Disorders (NIDCD) (2002b). Noise-Induced Hearing loss. NIH Pub. No. 97-4233 [online]. http://www.nidcd.nih.gov/health/hearing/noise.asp

National Institute on Deafness and Other Communication Disorders (NIDCD) (1997). Presbycusis. NIH Pub. No. 97-4235 [online]. http://www.nidcd.nih.gov/health/hearing/presbycusis.asp

National Institute on Deafness and Other Communication Disorders (NIDCD) (1996). National Strategic Research Plan: Hearing and Hearing Impairment. Bethesda, MD: HHS, NIH.

National Institutes of Health. Noise and Hearing Loss. NIH Consens Statement Online 1990 Jan 22–24 [cited 2005, Aug. 23]; 8(1), 1–24

Newman, C. W., & Sandridge, S. A. (1998). Benefit from, satisfaction with, and cost-effectiveness of three different hearing aid technologies. *American Journal of Audiology, 7*(2), 115–128.

Northern, J. L. (2006). Look around: The audiology assistants are here!, *Audiology Today, 18*(1), 5.

Parving, A. (1993). Congenital hearing disability: epidemiology and identification: A comparison between two health authority districts. *Int J Pediatr Otolaryngol, 27,* 29–46 [Medline].

Patterson, N. M. (2001). A Tutorial: Use of the WHO ICIDH-2 for Determining Aural Rehabilitation Goals. *Research Project, University of South Florida* [online]. http://etd.fcla.edu/SF/SFE0000012/etd.pdf

Popelka, M. M., Cruikshanks, K. J., Wiley, T. L., Tweed, T. S., Klein, B. E., & Klein, R. (1998). Low prevalence of hearing aid use among older adults with hearing loss: The Epidemiology of Hearing Loss Study. *J Am Geriatr Soc, 46*(9), 1075–1078.

Resnick, D. M. (1993). *Professional Ethics for Audiologists and Speech-Language Pathologists.* San Diego: Singular.

Ries, P. W. (1994). Prevalence and characteristics of persons with hearing trouble: United States, 199–91. *National Center for Health Statistics.* Vital Health Stat 10(188).

Sanders, D. A. (1993). *Management of Hearing Handicap: Infants to Elderly.* Englewood Cliffs, NJ: Prentice Hall.

Skafte, M. D. (1990). Fifty years of hearing health care. *Hearing Instruments,* Commemorative Issue, *41*(9).

Stephens, S., Callaghan, D., Hogan, S., Meredith, R., Rayment, A., & Davis, A. (1990). Hearing disability in people aged 50–65: Effectiveness and acceptability of rehabilitative intervention. *Brit Med J, 300*(6723), 508–511.

Tucker, B. P. (1997). *IDEA Advocacy for Children Who Are Deaf or Hard of Hearing.* Singular: San Diego.

U.S. Department of Education (2001). Public Law 107-110, No Child Left Behind Act of 2001, an amendment to the Elementary and Secondary Education Act of 1965 (20USC-6301).

U.S. Department of Education (2000). 22nd Annual Report to Congress, Appendix A, Table ABS.

U.S. Department of Health and Human Services Administration on Aging (2004). A Profile of Older Americans. A Research Report [online]. http://www.aoa.gov/prof/Statistics/profile/2004/profiles2004.asp

U.S. Department of Health and Human Services Administration on Aging (2001). A Profile of Older Americans. A Research Report [online]. http://www.aoa.gov/prof/Statistics/profile/2001/profiles2004.asp

U.S. Department of Labor (2003). Bureau of Labor Statistics, *Occupational Outlook Handbook*: Audiologists [online]. http://www.bls.gov

Watkin, P., Baldwin, M. & McEnery, G. (1991). Neonatal at risk screening and the identification of deafness. *Archives of Diseases in Childhood, 66,* 1130–1135.

World Health Organization (2005). *ICF: International Classification of Functioning, Disability, and Health.* Full Version [online]. http://www.who.int/icidh.

World Health Organization (1998). *Towards a Common Language for Functioning and Disablement: ICIDH-2* [online]. http://www.who.int/icidh.

World Health Organization (1980). *International Classification of Impairments, Disabilities, and Handicap.* Geneva. Author.

Yoshinaga-Itano, C. (1995). Efficacy of early identification and intervention. *Seminars in Hearing, 16,* 115–120.

Yoshinaga-Itano, C., Sedey, A., Coulter, D. K., & Mehl, A. L. (1998). Language of early- and later-identified children with hearing loss. *Pediatrics, 102,* 1161–1171.

Zingeser, L. (2005, March 22). Trends in private practice among ASHA constituents, 1986 to 2003. *The ASHA Leader,* pp. 10–11, 14.

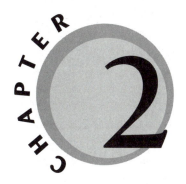

Acoustics and Psychophysics

Theodore S. Bell and Tracy L. Williams

Key Terms

ACOUSTICS

Acoustics is the branch of the physical sciences that pertains to sound and vibration. The ability to detect acoustical disturbances in our surroundings is an important, even critical, capability that many species rely on for survival. For humans, however, acoustical energy underlies our most unique and significant ability—speech. In textbook diagrams, sound is frequently depicted with a series of concentric circles radiating from a vibrating source. This pattern arises because sound originates from movement generated in an elastic medium traveling in the form of an omnidirectional wave of mechanical energy with alternating high- and low-pressure regions. The principles used to describe the propagation and behavior of sound are the same principles that govern many other phenomena in which wave motion, vibration, or oscillation are involved such as hydrodynamics, magnetism, and electricity. Acoustics must be considered when we study speech and hearing. The approach employed in this text is driven primarily by applications to audiologic practice, room acoustics, speech, measurement and calibration, hearing conservation, noise control, hearing aids, and related fields such as speech-language pathology and psychology.

CHARACTERISTICS OF SOUND

The propagation of sound in air is the result of the movement of air particles. In the atmosphere, molecules bounce off one another, causing them uniform dispersion in space. This property of gases, to disperse uniformly, is the basis for the restoring force needed for sound to propagate in air. The molecules provide the mass. As the molecules in the air are moved from their equilibrium position, they are pushed or pulled back into equilibrium by a restoring force. When air molecules are packed closely together, the density per unit of area is greater than normal—a condition called **compression** or **condensation**. When the molecules are less dense than the equilibrium state, the condition is called **rarefaction**.

Wave Motion

Sound waves radiate in all directions, like an expanding sphere. As the sphere gets larger and larger, its surface, for all practical purposes, can be treated like plane. This is the mathematical model used most often for the sake of simplicity. **Reflection** and **diffraction** are two important aspects of wave motion as sound travels in space encountering objects in its path. When an **incident wave**, or first arriving wave, encounters an obstruction, it is reflected back onto itself. If a wave encounters an object that only partially obstructs its path, it will continue past the object, changing its shape as it wraps around the obstruction—a phenomenon known as diffraction. If a hole exists in an object, the wave will continue on its path through the opening. This characteristic of sound waves poses a particular problem in the soundproofing of spaces. The ear is so sensitive that even the tiniest of holes will transmit audible energy into or out of an enclosure.

A reflected wave may interfere with later incident waves and, depending on the particular geometry, either cancel or sum with the incident waves. If a sound wave hits a reflective barrier head-on at 180°, then it will reflect back onto itself, interfering with subsequent wave fronts. If the reflected wave and the next incident wave happen to align such that the peaks add together, amplitude increases, called **constructive interference**. If the reflections and incident waves combine such that the positive peak aligns with the negative peak, then the waves will cancel each other out, called **destructive interference**. Acoustical interference of two waves of the same frequency traveling in opposite directions results in a **standing wave** pattern where in some locations sound intensity is reinforced, and a short distance away, intensity may be dramatically reduced.

Refraction is the bending of a sound wave. This phenomenon occurs when the speed of the sound is altered, usually by a temperature difference or a change in the impedance of a medium. This effect is demonstrated visually with a rod that seems to abruptly bend at the point at which it enters a pool of water. With acoustical waves, diffraction is most often due to changes in atmospheric pressure or temperature, but can also occur when a medium changes with respect to its velocity.

Absorption is another related concept. When a sound wave encounters a barrier, a small portion of the energy is absorbed by the surface of the obstruction, while most of the energy is reflected. The acoustical measure of sound absorption is called the absorption coefficient—simply the ratio of absorbed energy to total energy of the incident wave. Different materials have different absorption characteristics. Typically, hard surfaces reflect better than soft ones. Architects carefully select building materials to control the amount of absorption in their designs. When there are no reflections, a space is called **anechoic,** meaning that there are no detectable echoes. Enclosed spaces are not naturally anechoic because there are always some reflections present. These reflections are perceived as **reverberation.** In fact, sound that does not include some reverberation is perceived as unnatural. Two types of wave motion are expressed in **transverse waves** and **longitudinal waves.** A transverse wave rises and falls periodically in space like a rope held at one end and sharply snapped. The wave generated travels from the secured end down the length of the rope. The membranes of the inner ear vibrate in the same fashion. Sound in air, by contrast, takes the form of a longitudinal wave. Air molecules move, back and forth in the same plane, along an axis aligned with the direction of sound emanation. Both transverse and longitudinal wave displacement are described by the same equations and relationships.

Vibrating Systems

The trading back-and-forth of energy between the inertia generated by a moving mass and a restoring force is a critical concept in understanding acoustics. This concept is illustrated by the pendulum, a simple oscillating system, in which the pendulum bob (weight at the end of the pendulum arm) provides mass and gravity provides the restoring force. The pull of gravity causes the bob to accelerate toward the midline of the pendulum whenever it is displaced from perpendicular. Gravity also causes the mass to decelerate after it passes the midline; technically, this is called negative acceleration. As the mass falls, it gains inertia, meaning that as it accelerates and increases in force (recall, $F = ma$). At the midline of the pendulum, the point at which the force of gravity is equalized, it is inertia that keeps the mass moving, only to be dissipated by the effects of gravity.

In a simple spring-mass system, a single mass is attached to a spring. The mass provides momentum and the spring provides the restoring force. The pull or push of the spring is proportional to the distance the mass is deflected, a relationship known as **Hooke's law.** As a mathematical relationship, $F = -kx$, where F is force, and x is distance.

Impedance is described as the net effect of all forces that oppose vibration: **resistance, mass reactance,** and **compliant reactance.** Resistance is friction. In the case of sound in air, resistance is the effect of air molecules bumping into one another and losing energy to heat. Loss of energy to heat causes the sound wave to diminish gradually over time—a phenomenon called **damping.** Damping is described in terms of reduction in amplitude over time.

Mass reactance is a form of stored energy related to the inertia inherent in any moving mass. In the case of sound in air, mass is supplied by air molecules, and the inertial energy caused by the molecules accelerating is the stored energy termed reactance. Compliant reactance is another form of stored energy in an oscillating system. For sound in air, the restoring force is due to the air molecules' tendency to disperse uniformly. Mass reactance and compliant reactance complement one another, trading back and forth as the oscillation progresses through its cycle. **Admittance** is the inverse of impedance, describing how well sound allow entry into a medium.

SINUSOIDS

Frequency

The simplest type of sound wave is called a **sine wave, sinusoid,** or pure tone. Pure tones are like those produced by a tuning fork. Sinusoids (plotted as pressure variation against time) are used to describe sounds in the air and vibration in general. A sinusoid is described in terms of its wavelength, frequency, amplitude, and phase. **Wavelength** (λ) is the distance from peak to peak of one wave to the next. This representation of maximum pressure, to minimum, and back to maximum is also called a **cycle**. The unit of one cycle per second is known as a **Hertz** (Hz) in honor of the German physicist, Heinrich R. Hertz. **Frequency** is defined as the number of times per second that a cycle occurs (cycles per second, or cps). The subjective attribute of **pitch** is correlated with frequency, such that the higher the frequency the higher the pitch. A sound that produces a pitch is known as a tone. A pressure wave that repeats itself 1000 times in one second would be called a 1000-Hz tone. If that tone were to continue for 10 seconds, then 10,000 cycles would pass in that time frame.

Phase

The individual points of a sinusoid are identified in terms of circular motion, described in degrees or **radians**. There are 360° in a circle corresponding to 2π radians. Pi (π) is the transcendental number that describes the ratio of the circumference of a circle to its radius, constant for any circle. The circumference of a circle is $2\pi r$ where r is the radius. One-fourth of the way around a circle is 90° or $\pi/2$ radians, and one-half of the way around a circle is 180° or π radians, and so forth. Figure 2.1 shows a circle on an x-y graph with the horizontal axis corresponding to the diameter of the circle. Rotating the radius counterclockwise, the maximum y-value is at 90°, then at 180° it is zero again. Continuing around, 270° is minimum value of the y-axis and at 360° it is back to zero. The angle between the x-axis and the rotating radius is called the **phase angle**. In terms of radians, the angular distance traveled is 2π. The angular velocity is expressed as radians per second. For a more detailed explanation, refer to Kinsler and Frey (1962).

If two pure tones coincide in the same place in their respective cycles, they are said to be in phase. If the cycles do not coincide, the tones are out of phase. Two tones are 90° out of phase when one tone is at its peak at 90° and the other is at 180° crossing zero. Two tones that are 180° out of phase have one tone at maximum while the other is at minimum amplitude. If these two tones share the same amplitude, they cancel each other out (active noise suppression).

The amount of time required for the completion of one cycle is called a period. For sounds, this is usually measured in milliseconds. Notice that the period (seconds/cycle) is the reciprocal of frequency (cycles/second). Given that sound in 0°C air at sea level travels 331 meters/second, a 100-Hz wave travels 3.31 meters in one cycle (331 meters/second) / (100 cycles/second) = 331/100 meters/cycle.

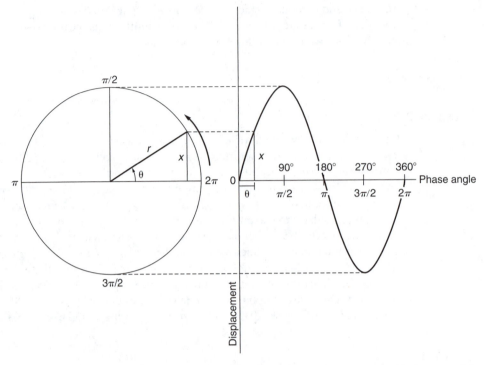

Figure 2.1   Sinusoid generated from the rotation of a vector (*r*). Instantaneous displacement (*x*) plotted as a function of the phase angle subtended by *r* and the *horizontal axis.*

Amplitude

The range of displacement of a wave from its point of equilibrium is called its **amplitude**, which can represent a distance or a pressure. The point at which the displacement is greatest is called maximum displacement, or peak amplitude. There is a positive and a negative peak on every wave. Average amplitude is measured using what is known as a **root-mean-square** (**RMS**) average, simply the square root of the average squared displacement. The RMS value is always positive, corresponding to 0.707 times the peak amplitude of a simple sine wave. The average would be zero if the numbers were not squared before averaging, because the negative region of the wave would cancel the positive when summed.

As initially stated, the science of sound is concerned with pressure, defined as force per unit area. This measurement is called the **Pascal** and is equivalent to one **newton** of force applied to one square meter of area. A newton is formally defined as the force required to accelerate one kilogram of mass from zero meters/second to one meter per second in one second. In the **centimeter-gram-second** (**cgs**) system of measurements, the unit of force measured is called the **dyne**. Because pressures associated with audible sound are so small in magnitude, they are referred to in millionths of a Pascal, or **microPascal** (μ**Pa**). Pressure may also be described in dynes per square centimeter.

INTENSITY OF SOUND

The Decibel

The **decibel (dB)** often uses 20 µPa as its reference pressure, representing the approximate threshold of sound detection for the human ear (see Killion, 1978). The decibel scale is simply a relative measure of intensities or pressures. It is based on a ratio in which the numerator is an observed quantity and the denominator is a reference quantity. Different references are employed in various acoustical applications, although with sound intensities, a value of 10^{-12} watts/m^2 is typically used to represent the approximate threshold of human hearing sensitivity. The range of intensities that the human ear can detect is very large, approximately 10^{12} to 1 (a trillion to one) from the threshold of delectability to the threshold of pain (for a discussion of loudness discomfort level, see Morgan, Wilson, and Dirks (1974). For convenience, the scale of the range of sensitivity is converted using logarithms, or powers of ten. Log to the base ten and powers of ten are inverse functions. Thus, log (10^{12}) is 12 and $\log(10^0) = \log(1) = 0$. By performing the log transformation, the trillion-unit scale is reduced to a 12-unit scale ranging from 0 to 12. For even greater convenience, the resulting scale is multiplied by 10, thereby transforming the range of practical sound intensities into a 0 to 120 scale.

The prefix *deci* means one-tenth, thus the decibel scale corresponds to the **bel** scale by a factor of ten. In other words, one decibel is equivalent to one-tenth of a bel. Conversely, one bel equals 10 decibels. The bel and decibel scales are described by the following equations:

$$\text{bel} = \log (I_{obs}/I_{ref}) \qquad \text{decibel} = 10\log (I_{obs}/I_{ref})$$

where I_{obs} is the observed intensity level and I_{ref} is the reference intensity level. Intensity is measured in watts/cm^2. When the quantities are expressed as sound pressures, a slightly different form of the decibel equation is used:

$$\text{decibel} = 20\log (P_{obs}/P_{ref})$$

P represents the observed and reference pressures. When the specific value of 20 µPa is employed as the reference pressure, the specification dB$_{SPL}$ (dB sound pressure level) is used. Note that the scaling factor of 10 has been replaced with a factor of 20 in the equation when pressures are described. It is actually the same equation, but because pressures are the squares of intensities, the exponent becomes a multiplier in the logarithmic transformation. Sound pressure level is thus given by the following equation in the MKS (meter-kilogram-second) system:

$$\text{dB}_{SPL} = 20\log (P_{obs}/20 \; \mu\text{Pa})$$

In terms of the centimeter-gram-second (cgs) system of units, the relationship is expressed as:

$$\text{dB}_{SPL} = 20\log (P_{obs}/0.0002 \text{ dynes/cm}^2)$$

Both of the dB equations are equivalent to each other; only the scale of the units has changed.

Decibel Scales

There are many different decibel scales in common usage. In audiologic settings, the reference pressure is frequency specific and represents the threshold for sound detection by normally functioning human ears at particular frequencies. This decibel variant is called **dB hearing level (dBHL)**. Audiometric standards are given by the American National Standards Institute publication ANSI S3.6-2004, revision of ANSI S3.6-1996. The difference between observed and reference pressures in dBHL indicates the amount of observed hearing loss or the amount of pressure above the normal threshold for a particular frequency. A related term, **dB sensation level (dBSL)**, uses a subject's actual hearing sensitivity threshold as its reference level. This concept is discussed further in a subsequent chapter. Another decibel scale commonly used in industrial and community noise settings is called the dBA scale (and related dBC, dBD scales). Engineering and electrical applications commonly use 10^{-18} watts/cm^2 as the reference intensity, resulting in the **dB intensity level (dBIL)** scale. For further discussion see Knudsen (1932), Beranek (1988), Tonndorf (1980), or Peterson and Gross, (1967).

Sound loses energy as it travels. The relationship between distance that sound travels and energy it loses is known as the **inverse square law.** As the name implies, intensity diminishes in proportion to the square of distance traveled. In decibels, the intensity of a wave can be described as $-dB = 20 \log (d1/d2)$, where d1 and d2 refer to distances from the source. For example, the drop in decibels from one meter to two meters away from a stationary source would be 20 log (1/2), or $20 \times (-0.3) = 6$ dB. Consequently, when distance is doubled intensity diminishes by 6 dB.

COMPLEX SOUNDS

Fundamental and Harmonic Components

Sound waves are not always simple sine waves. In nature, pure tones rarely occur in isolation. Instead, there are almost always interactions with other waves resulting in periodic repeating waveforms with complex shapes. Complex sounds can be characterized through the analysis of their simple wave components. This method of analysis, called **Fourier analysis** after French scientist J. B. J. Fourier, deconstructs the periodic waveform into a set of sine waves that facilitate understanding speech perception. The auditory system performs a mechanical Fourier analysis on complex sounds that is known as **Ohm's acoustical law.**

Complex waves are integer multiples of the lowest frequency component of the wave known as its **fundamental** frequency. Higher wave components are called **harmonics** or **overtones**. See Figure 2.2. Various proportions of harmonics relative to each other and the fundamental give each sound its characteristic tonal quality, a psychological property called **timbre**. These differences in harmonic content allow easy differentiation between one voice and another or between the sound of a saxophone and that of a trumpet.

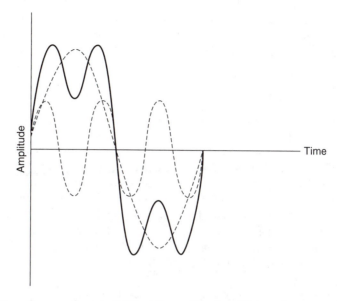

Figure 2.2   Complex waveform (solid line) formed by the addition of two pure tones (dashed lines), both initiated at a phase of 0°.

When the harmonics are not integer multiples of the fundamental frequency, the sound is inharmonic. If two tones of different frequencies that are not harmonically related are heard together, an amplitude distortion resulting in an additional frequency that is the difference between the original two frequencies is detected. This fluctuation in amplitude is called **beats** (Wever, 1929). The phenomenon is not subtle and is commonly referred to by musicians as being "out of tune." When tuning instruments or matching voices to instruments, adjustments to pitch eliminate the beat frequency (see Backus, 1969). When there are many inharmonic components present in a sound, the sounds are heard as noise. When a sound contains all frequencies of sound simultaneously, it is termed **white noise**, analogous to white light, which contains all frequencies of light. White noise sounds like static or a hissing sound. Some of the consonants in our language are noises—the *s* or *sh* sounds, for example. Noises are commonly used in hearing evaluations because they contain all frequencies of sound (Speaks, 1999).

Reverberation

As sound travels through space and reflects off objects, subsequent reflections travel farther than the incident wave or earlier reflections, progressively losing intensity over distance and time. The brain fuses reflections and incident waves together into a single percept, meaning that are not perceived the immediate echoes even though they are physically present. This fusion of the individual waves into a single perception is called the **precedence effect** in psychology. Architects measure reverberation in terms of the number of seconds it takes for a sound to reduce its intensity by 60 decibels. This measure is called T_{60}. Musical spaces usually have T_{60} measures in the range of 2 to 4 seconds. Good speech intelligibility requires considerably shorter T_{60} times, usually less than one second. Individuals with hearing impairment or receptive language problems require even less reverberation for good speech intelligibility.

Frequency Selectivity

The ability of the auditory system to resolve sinusoidal components of a complex tone is referred to as frequency resolution, or frequency selectivity, and is demonstrated by masking processes. **Masking** is defined as an increase in threshold for a sound in the presence of another sound. Masking occurs when the pattern of neural excitation obscures excitation caused by the signal. Masking can have both a sensory component (refractory period of neurons) and a memory component (parallel processing). The brain stem uses phase difference information between the two ears to separate the signal from the ground noise. The effect of a mismatch in phase is a release from masking and a resulting improvement in threshold sensitivity. This binaural effect is called masking level difference (MLD). Masking level differences are greatest for low frequencies.

The selective passing of specific frequencies is called **resonance** or **filtering**. Resonance characteristics depend primarily on the length of the chamber or tube through which the sound travels. The acoustical properties of the ear canal are of particular importance to audiologists. The ear canal is open at one end, but closed at the other by the eardrum. The closed end forces a **node** (minimum pressure point) while the open one forces an **antinode** (maximum pressure point). The corresponding wavelength is one-quarter of a cycle between the node and antinode. Thus the resonance frequency produced by the tube is four times the length of the tube; for humans, this frequency corresponds to approximately 3000 Hz. Other arrangements of openings and closures produce different resonance characteristics. Sometimes, a broad range of frequencies is allowed to resonate, while at other times, the filter can be quite narrow. Filters or resonators are described in terms of their **center frequency characteristic** and the steepness, or sharpness of the filter, a quantity that is sometimes termed the "Q" of a filter. Preferred frequencies for acoustical measurements are given in ANSI S1.6-1984, Revised 1987.

PSYCHOPHYSICAL CONCEPTS

Psychoacoustics

Acoustics relies on understanding the relationship between the mechanical properties of sound and the manner in which they are represented in the auditory system. The relationship between auditory stimuli and sensation is termed **psychoacoustics**. Psychoacoustics is a subset of the larger field of **psychophysics** pioneered by Gustav Fechner in 1850. To facilitate explaining the relationship between physical stimuli and subjective experience, Fechner devised ways to measure: (1) minimum perceptual intensities, called **detection**, (2) how different stimuli have to be to no longer appear the same, called **discrimination**, and (3) sensation intensity, termed **scaling**. Fechner also identified **absolute threshold** as the minimum level (magnitude) at which a stimulus can be detected, or the stimulus intensity at which detection occurs 50% of the time. For auditory stimuli, this critical intensity level at 1000 Hz is approximately 6.5 dB_{SPL} for monaural hearing (Yost and Killion, 1997).

Measurement of Absolute Threshold

The measurement of absolute threshold is accomplished in several ways. The **method of constant stimuli** presents a fixed set of tones differing in intensity, one at a time. The perceiver responds "yes" when detecting the tone, and "no" when the tone is not audible. The **method of limits** presents an audible tone in a descending series, decreasing the tone until the listener reports that it cannot be heard, and then increases audibility in an ascending series, each series providing an estimate of absolute threshold that falls somewhere between the last two stimuli. **Adaptive testing** allows for a more accurate tracking of threshold over time, as it does not end the series at the last two stimuli presented, but rather continues several series reversals around reported threshold in a **staircase method** of measurement.

The inherent problem with each of these methods of measuring absolute threshold arises in conditions of uncertainty, or whether a weak stimulus was present in a series. Listeners who may not want to appear hard of hearing or may wish to appear especially sensitive will respond "yes" on almost every trial. To control for such response strategies, a **catch trial**, in which no stimulus is presented, is inserted into the series. The catch trial alone, however, is not enough to account for motivational or expectation effects that may bias the listener's decision-making process in conditions of uncertainty.

Signal Detection Theory

Signal detection theory (SDT) makes it possible to separate changes in performance related to sensation from those associated with the decision criterion by representing these variations across time as a probability distribution (Green & Swets, 1966). In SDT, there is no absolute threshold because it assumes that the internal noise in our sensory system and the external noise in the environment is ongoing and fluctuating, so that for each trial, the listener must separate the signal from the background of noise. As a result, the listener reports that the signal is either present or absent, leading to four possible outcomes: a hit ("yes" on a signal present trial), a false alarm ("yes" on a signal absent trial), a correct negative ("no" on a signal absent trial), or a miss ("no" on a signal present trial). The outcomes are mapped into distributions of equal variances representing the noise and the signal plus noise conditions. The area of overlap is the error, either miss or false alarm. The **criterion** (β), or response bias, is a cognitive component and can be adjusted based on consequences or payoff. A person's criterion may be neutral (equal probability of miss or false alarm), liberal (high rate of false alarms and hits), or conservative (low rate of hits, high rate of misses, few false alarms). **Sensitivity** (d'), based on keenness of detection, is indicated by the separation between the means of the two distributions described in terms of standard deviations, such that the greater the distance between means, the greater the sensitivity and the less probability for errors.

Just Noticeable Difference

When discriminating between stimuli, a standard is established to which all other stimuli will be compared. There is a point of **subjective equality** wherein stimuli are perceived to be exactly the same. When differences are reported 50% of the time, halfway between the point of subjective equality and perfect discrimination, a **difference threshold** is noted. The difference threshold is the result of dividing the interval of uncertainty (between 0.25 and 0.75) by 2. Difference threshold varies over time and conditions. The smallest difference in frequency that is distrainable is called the **just noticeable difference** (JND) or **difference limen** (DL). JNDs characterize the input/output behavior of the auditory system such that if discrimination is good then the difference threshold will be small. There are difference limen for both frequency (DLF) and intensity (DLI). JNDs are larger for larger standards. The relationship between the difference threshold and the magnitude of a standard is expressed in **Weber's law:**

$$\Delta I = kI$$

where ΔI is the difference threshold, I is the magnitude (intensity) of the stimulus, and k is a constant (0.048 for sound) indicating the proportion by which a standard must be changed to be detected 50% of the time.

Stevens (1951, 1956) generated an equation that describes the relationship of physical intensity to estimations of magnitude. Magnitude scales are typically logarithmic, that is, based on power functions. Also known as the power law, **Stevens' law** is:

$$S = aI^{m}$$

where S is a measure of sensation intensity, a is a constant, and m is the characteristic exponent for that sensory experience. For sound S would be indicative of loudness (L) and m would equal 0.60. Steven's law suggests that the magnitude of the perceived sensations provided by specific stimulus intensities depends on the size of the exponents.

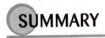 SUMMARY

CHAPTER REVIEW

❏ Sound is vibration or changes in mechanical pressure in an elastic medium. Vibration causes compression and rarefaction of molecules, creating waves of mechanical energy that lose energy over distance. This relationship between distance and energy loss is known as the inverse square law. The reduction of energy due to friction is called dampening.

- The first wave to arrive from the sound source is known as the incident wave. Two waves of the same frequency traveling in opposite directions create a standing wave pattern.

- Impedance is net effect of forces that oppose vibration (resistance, mass reactance, and compliant reactance). Admittance is the inverse of impedance. Wave energy encounters: absorption, reflection, diffusion, refraction, suppression, and resonance or filtering described in terms of the center frequency characteristic.

- Reflections are perceived as reverberations; their absence is termed anechoic. The fusion of reflections and the incident wave into a single percept is known as the precedence effect.

- Wave motion can be either longitudinal or tranverse. The simplest sound wave is known as a sinusoid, sine wave, or pure tone. The sound wave is described in terms of its wavelength (λ), cycle, and frequency.

- Frequency is expressed in Hertz (Hz), equivalent to one cycle per second, and has its psychological correlate of pitch. Measured in radians, the sine wave is described in terms of its amplitude, phase angle, and period.

- Sound pressure level, a measure of intensity or loudness, is expressed in decibels (dB), and the pressure of audible sound, in microPascals (μPa).

- Wave interaction results in complex waveforms. Complex waves are integer multiples of the lowest frequency component of the waves known as the fundamental.

- Higher wave components are known as harmonics or overtones. The relationship of harmonics to each other and their fundamental result is the tonal quality termed timbre. Harmonics that are not integer multiples of their fundamental are called inharmonic and have amplitude fluctuations called beats. Multiple inharmonic components result in white noise.

ACTIVITIES FOR DISCUSSION

1. What is the difference between dB, SPL, and dBIL?

2. What is the difference between dBHL and dBSL?

3. Approximately what length in meters is one cycle of each of the following?

   100 Hz sinusoid

   1,000 Hz sinusoid

   10,000 Hz sinusoid

4. Estimate the reverberation characteristics of the room that you are in. Which surfaces are reflective and which are absorptive? How could this room be improved?

5. What are the perceptual correlates to: frequency, intensity, and harmonic content?

6. What are the measures of pressure in the cgs and MKS systems?

7. Make a diagram of two waves: in phase 0°, out of phase, 90°, 180°, 270°.

8. Describe a simple signal detection experiment and the ways in which a person can be correct or in error. What do d' and β measure?

9. If you were speaking to someone at a distance of 1 meter, then moved to a distance of 2 meters, what would be the drop in decibels? What would be the drop at:

   4 meters

   8 meters

REFERENCES

ANSI S3.6-2004 (2004). Specifications for audiometers American National Standards Institute. New York: ANSI.

ANSI S1.6-1997 (1997). American National Standards Institute (1997). Preferred frequencies, frequency levels, and band numbers for acoustical instruments. New York: ANSI.

Backus, J. (1969). *The Acoustical Foundations of Music*. New York: W. W. Norton & Co.

Beranek, L. L. (1988). *Acoustical Measurements* (2nd ed.). New York: American Institute of Physics.

Green, D. M., & Swets, J. A. (1966). *Signal Detection theory and Psychophysics*. New York: John Wiley & Sons.

Killion, M. C. (1978). Revised estimate of minimum audible pressure: Where is the "Missing 6dB." *Journal of the Acoustical Society of America, 63,* 1501–1505.

Kinsler, L. E., & Frey, A. R. (1962). *Fundamentals of Acoustics*. New York: John Wiley & Sons.

Knudsen, V. O. (1932). *Architectural Acoustics*. New York: John Wiley & Sons.

Ladefoged, P. (1962). *Elements of Acoustic Phonetics*. Chicago: University of Chicago Press.

Morgan, D. E., Wilson, R. H. & Dirks, D. D. (1974). Loudness discomfort level: selected methods and stimuli. *Journal of the Acoustical Society of America, 56,* 577–581.

Peterson, A. P. G., & Gross, E., Jr. (1967). *Handbook of Noise Measurement*. West Concord, MA: General Radio Co.

Speaks, C. E. (1999). *Introduction to Sound: Acoustics for Hearing and Speech Sciences* (3rd ed.). San Diego: Singular Publishing Group.

Stevens, S. S. (1956). The direct estimation of sensory magnitude—loudness. *American Journal of Psychology, 69,* 1–25.

Stevens, S. S. (1951). Mathematics, measurement, and psychophysics. In S. S. Stevens (Ed.), *Handbook of Experimental Psychology* (pp. 1–49). New York: John Wiley & Sons.

Tonndorf, J. (1980). Physics of sound. In M. M. Paparella & D. A. Shumrick (Eds.), *Otolaryngology: Vol. 1. Basic Sciences and Related Disciplines* (2nd ed.), pp. 177–198). Philadelphia: W. B. Saunders Co.

Wever, E. G. (1929). Beats and related phenomena resulting from the simultaneous sounding of two tones. *Psychological Review, 36,* 402–423.

Yost, W. A., & Killion, M. C. (1997). Quiet absolute thresholds. In M. Crocker (Ed.), *Handbook of Acoustics*. New York: Wiley.

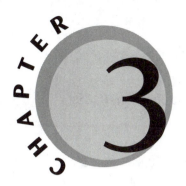

Anatomy and Physiology of the Ear

Theodore S. Bell and Tracy L. Williams

Key Terms

OVERVIEW OF THE EAR

Our ears are amazing organs. They are keenly sensitive to minute changes in the atmospheric pressure around us, with each part of the ear accentuating and transforming these vibrations as we sense and perceive them. Our ears are especially sensitive to those vibrations that comprise our vocabulary of spoken words. As sound waves travel from a vibrating sound source to the ear, the external ear funnels the waves into the middle ear where the sound is amplified. The energy of the waves moves from the air into the fluid-filled inner ear, which contains specialized sensory cells that convert the mechanical energy of the pressure waves into electrical impulses. Following this conversion of mechanical energy into electrical energy, better known as transduction, the information is encoded into patterns of activity in the auditory nerve to be subsequently analyzed in higher brain centers.

The ear is naturally described by three divisions derived from its anatomical components: the outer ear, the middle ear, and the inner ear. See Figure 3.1. The outer ear, or external ear, more formally called the **auricle**, is composed of the visible part of the

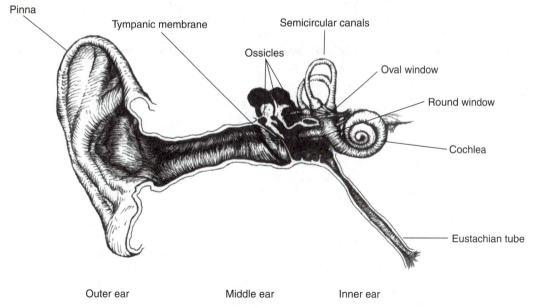

Pinna

Tympanic membrane

Semicircular canals

Ossicles

Oval window

Round window

Cochlea

Eustachian tube

Outer ear   Middle ear   Inner ear

Figure 3.1   **Overview of the ear.** Illustrated by Tracy L. Williams.

ear, the **pinna**, and the ear canal, the **external auditory meatus**. The boundary between the outer ear and the middle ear is the **tympanic membrane (TM)**, or eardrum. The middle ear is an air-filled cavity where three tiny bones connect the TM to the inner ear. The inner ear is called the **cochlea**, which contains the transducer cells that convert mechanical energy into neural messages. The ear is embedded in the **temporal bone** on each side of the skull, which contains tiny air-filled pockets and has important support structures and boundary walls for the ear. The bony canals that the inner ear occupies in the temporal bone are called the **labyrinth**. The labyrinth contains the semicircular canals and **vestibule** of the vestibular system (sense of balance), as well as the cochlea.

TERMINOLOGY

Medical vocabulary is easy to comprehend because its terms usually describe shape, location, or function. Although modern language translations are now commonly employed, many older Latin terms still persist in common usage. For example, **medial** is a Latin term that indicates a location in the middle or towards the midline of body, while **lateral** designates a position that is away from the midline. In the anatomy of the ear, the medial wall of the middle ear is formed by the cochlea, whereas the lateral wall of the middle ear is the tympanic membrane, or eardrum. **Superior** and **inferior** indicate positions above and below, respectively. *Superficial* implies that something is near the surface, whereas *deep* refers to structures farther away from the surface. **Anterior** means forward, or toward the front, and **posterior** means towards the rear; sometimes **ventral** (toward the belly) and **dorsal** (toward the back) are used to describe the same orientation. A structure is **peripheral** when it is at the surface or away from the center, whereas **central** is toward the center. The related terms *external* and *internal* describe an outer or inner surface, respectively. **Distal** and **proximal** are terms that correspond to something being farther away or nearer to some particular reference.

There are three orthogonal planes of reference in anatomy, meaning that they are each at right angles to one another. The **frontal plane**, sometimes called the **coronal plane**, is a slice that divides the body into front and back sections. The **sagittal plane** divides the body into left and right sides. Finally, the **transverse plane**, also called the **horizontal plane**, runs perpendicular to the coronal and sagittal planes cutting the body into horizontal cross sections.

THE EXTERNAL EAR

Anatomy of the Pinna and Ear Canal

The anatomy of the external ear can be traced with the finger. The **sebaceous** (fatty) flap of tissue called the lobule, or ear lobe, is very pliable, having no internal bone or cartilage support. There are both attached and free-hanging types of ear lobes. The ridge above the outer edge of the pinna is called the **helix**, due to its helical contour. Toward the top of the curvature is a small mound called **Darwin's tubercle**. This part of the helix also has an indented fold underneath it in the shape of a keel of an upside-down boat, hence is called scaphoid fossa. *Scaphoid* refers to the shape and *fossa* refers to the indentation itself.

The helix tracks downward into the fleshy bowl of the **concha**. This is referred to as the **crus**, or leg, of the helix. Just superior and anterior to the lobule are two smaller, more rigid mounds of tissue. These are called the **tragus** and **antitragus**. The tragus is larger and is located very near to the auditory canal opening. In fact, one can occlude the opening by gently pressing on the tragus until it seals the canal opening completely. The antitragus is smaller and closer in proximity to the lobule. The prefix *anti* may be translated as *adjacent*.

Beyond the crus is another fold of tissue that courses upward, splitting into two distinct branches. This structure, termed the **antihelix**, runs adjacent to the helix. The two branches of the antihelix are called the **crura of the antihelix** and the triangular-shaped indentation formed by the branches is called the **triangular fossa**. The two bowl-shaped chambers around the opening of the canal are called the concha. The larger inferior chamber is called the **cavum** and the smaller superior section is called the **skiff**. Deeper in the ear canal are sweat glands and cerumenal glands, where **cerumen**, or earwax, is produced.

Functions of the External Ear

In everyday terms, the ear is one of two fleshy protrusions on the side of the head that collect sound. Some erroneously consider the external ear to be of little importance in human hearing. The auricle does in fact serve a significant role in our perception of sound. The external ear is unique to each human in terms of its precise turns and folds—much like a fingerprint. The overall shape of the auricle is based on an underlying piece of springy cartilage that has an elasticity and consistency of plastic. This cartilage is covered in tissue and fat. The visible part of the ear that protrudes from the head is called the pinna. The pinna and ear canal serve as a resonator, an aid to sound localization, and even as a cushion for the delicate spongy temporal bone, in which the inner ear and the vestibular system, our sense of balance and motion, are embedded. Recent studies have shown that the superficial topography of these folds produce cues that the brain interprets for depth perception and sound localization (e.g., Kuhn, 1979; Shaw, 1974; Wright, Hebrank & Wilson, 1974).

THE MIDDLE EAR

The Tympanic Membrane

The middle ear is a kidney-shaped space separating the external auditory meatus from the cochlea. The lateral limit is the tympanic membrane and the medial wall contains the oval and round windows of the cochlea. The cavity itself is normally filled with air, and the pressure equilibrium with the ambient outside pressure is maintained via the **Eustachian tube**, which courses from the floor of the middle ear to the back of the throat, an area called the **nasopharynx**.

The tympanic membrane is actually a compound collection of tissues with a blood supply and innervation. The largest part of the tympanum itself, called the **pars tensa**, consists of three layers. The pars tensa is relatively stiff, and actually vibrates in response to sound. There is a more dense part of the TM at the superior margin called the **pars flaccida**, because it is more flaccid by comparison. The lateral (outermost) layer is a covering of skin, continuous with the surrounding ear canal. The middle layer is composed of fibrous tissue, actually two layers of spiral and radial fibers. The medial layer (inner-most) is a mucous membrane (for further discussion see Yost, 1994). The most obvious function of the tympanum is to transduce the sound pressures into mechanical vibra-tions by transforming the deflections of the membrane into the middle ear. In order to do this the tympanum must be flexible, able to move with tiny fluctuations in air pres-sure, and also must be coupled directly to the tiny middle ear bones, the **ossicles**.

The Ossicular Chain

The ossicles are three bones that comprise the ossicular chain in the middle ear and are attached to the tympanic membrane. See Figure 3.2. This attachment is at the footplate of the hammer, or malleus, the most lateral of the three ossicles. The attachment is made with an oval-shaped ligament that securely binds them together but does not offer any substantive support.

The **malleus**, or "hammer," is connected to the tympanum by the long process, or ex-tension, of the malleus called the **manubrium**. The point of attachment is visible through the translucent grey-colored membrane, and is called the **umbo**. The head of the malleus is connected to the **incus**, or "anvil," and together they take up about half of the space in

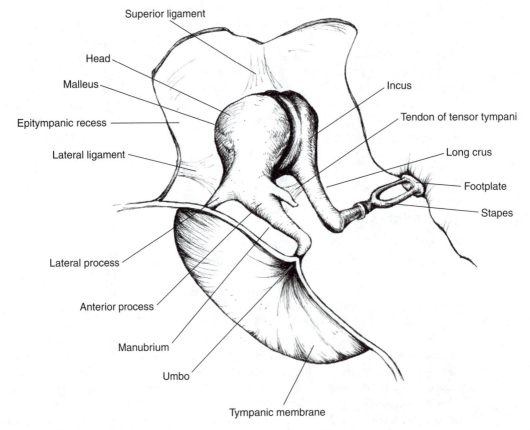

Figure 3.2 Ossicular chain. Illustrated by Tracy L. Williams.

the middle ear. The malleus in humans is approximately 8 mm in total length, and the incus about 7 mm in length along its major axis. The incus is attached to the stapes, or footplate, by a small annular ligament. The **stapes** is the smallest bone in the body, weighing only 2 to 4 mg. Its name derives from its shape, like a stirrup. The shape actually allows it to transmit energy into the ear most efficiently due to its low mass. The footplate of the stapes is attached to the cochlea at the oval window with an elastic annular ligament around the perimeter of the footplate. The area of the footplate is on average slighter greater than 3 mm^2. Thus, there is a continuous linkage from the tympanum to the oval window (for further discussion see Glasscock & Shambaugh, 1990).

The Middle Ear Muscles

The ossicles are further held in place by the **stapedius muscle** and the **tensor tympani.** The tensor tympani connects to the upper part of the manubrium and courses parallel to the eustachian tube. The stapedius muscle, the smallest in the body, attaches to the head of the stapes. Both muscles act in concert to modify the alignment of the ossicles when stimulated by the acoustic reflex in order to provide protection from loud sounds being transmitted into the ear. For soft sounds, the ossicles produce amplification. In response to sustained loud sounds, muscle tension acts on the typannic membrane and repositions the ossicles to pull back the stapes lessening the force on the oval window. The range between the threshold of hearing and the threshold of pain is known as the dynamic range of the auditory system.

Functions of the Middle Ear

Impedance is defined as the sum of all the energy that opposes the transmission of sound. If the impedances of two media are unequal, the sound will not easily transmit from one to the other. The important point here is that more energy is required to produce a wave in the fluid chambers of the ear than in the atmosphere where the sound originates. The middle ear overcomes the impedance mismatch between air and fluid in two ways. First, there is a difference in the area of the tympanic membrane relative to the area of the stapes footplate; this difference allows about 25 dB of improved sound transmission by focusing the vibratory area onto the smaller footplate. Second, there is a leverage created by the geometric configuration of the ossicles contributing about another 12 or 13 dB of amplification. Further, the ossicles do not vibrate equally well at all frequencies and intensities; this characteristic is thought to provide some additional protection for the cochlea. Some authors suggest that another function of the ossicles is to reduce the amount of bone conduction, or direct vibration of the skull, due to chewing or swallowing.

THE INNER EAR

The Cochlea

The cochlea is where the actual transduction of mechanical to electrical energy takes place in the ear. The cochlea derives its name from its shell-like shape. See Figure 3.3. The oval window, where the stapes footplate is connected to the cochlea, is the point at which the mechanical energy from the middle ear transmits its vibration into the fluids of the cochlea. As the fluid is disturbed, it causes a deflection of the membranes in the cochlea, which in turn causes the membranes to move and thereby stimulates tiny hair cells that ultimately transmit electrical signals to the brain. The cochlea is basically a sealed coiled tube larger at the base than at the apex, or tip. The cochlea's inner wall is called the **modiolus**, from which the spiral lamina, a small bony shelf, protrudes. The **basilar membrane** (BM) spans beyond this shelf via the spiral ligament to form a division of the cochlea into two chambers, or scalae. The two scalae, filled with **perilymph**, are connected at the apical end in a small opening called the **helicotrema**. The channel above the basilar membrane is called the **scala vestibuli**, and the lower chamber is called the **scala tympani**. The **oval window** transmits vibration into the scala vestibule, while the **round window** is the terminus of the scala tympani, which forms a boundary with the middle ear cavity. These perilymph-filled chambers are connected and do not compress, so that when the oval window pushes inward, the round window reacts by pushing outward, and vice versa. The basilar membrane is the base of support for the hair cell transducers contained in a triangular fluid-filled sac called the **cochlear duct**, or **scala media**, that runs the entire length of the cochlea. The cochlear duct is separated from the scala tympani by the basilar membrane and from the scala vestibuli by a thin membrane called **Reissner's membrane** that is only one or two cells in thickness. The side of the cochlear duct contains the blood supply to the organ, called the **stria vascularis**. The stria vascularis is responsible for maintaining the metabolic processes and balance within the cochlea; without it, the transduction process cannot be accomplished.

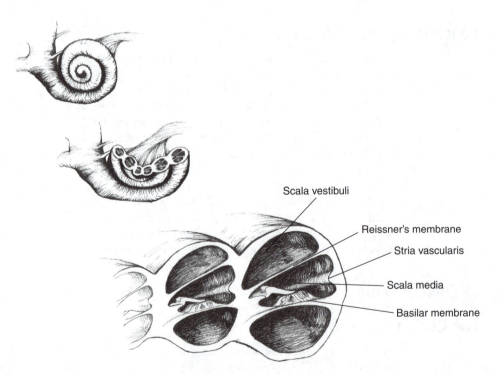

Scala vestibuli

Reissner's membrane

Stria vascularis

Scala media

Basilar membrane

Figure 3.3 **Cochlea cross-section.** Illustrated by Tracy L. Williams.

The cochlear duct contains a fluid, called **endolymph**, which differs from perilymph in the relative proportions of sodium and potassium ions.

The Organ of Corti

Central to the structure of the inner ear is the **organ of Corti**. The integrity of this structure is sustained by the pillars of Corti, sometimes called the rods of Corti, which are rigid structures that resemble two pillars leaning towards each other, forming a triangular-shaped tunnel through the interior space, called the **tunnel of Corti**; it is filled with a fluid called cortilymph, which very much resembles cerebrospinal fluid in its chemical composition. See Figure 3.4

The **inner hair cells** (IHCs) align in a single row along the inner (medial) side of the pillars of Corti. There are about 3500 IHCs in humans, arranged in small bundles of 40 to 60 **stereocilia** in a U-shaped cluster. The supporting cells surround the base in a cuplike fashion. These cells, called **Deiters cells**, have an upward coursing appendage that gives vertical support to the hair cell (e.g., see Lawrence, 1980). Other cells, called the **cells of Hensen**, press laterally on the sides of the cells to further secure them in place.

On the other side of the pillars of Corti are three to five rows of **outer hair cells** (OHCs). The 12,000 or so OHCs, each containing about 150 stereocilia in a more angular V or W shape. The tallest stereocilia come in contact with the thin gelatinous membrane called the

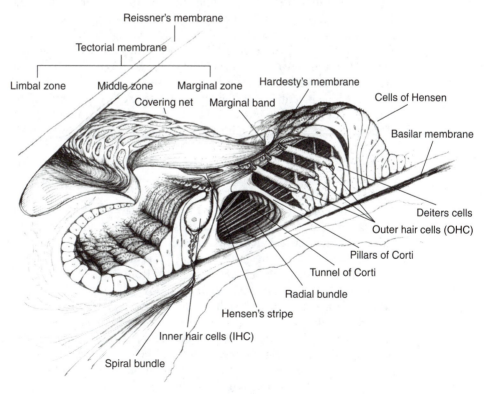

Figure 3.4   Organ of Corti Illustrated by Tracy L. Williams.

tectorial membrane. Individual stereocilia are linked together by small **cross links** and **tip links** helping to keep them rigid and moving together. See Lim (1980) for a discussion of cochlear anatomy as it is related to cochlear micromechanics.

Mechanical Characteristics of the Cochlea

The basilar membrane is wider and thicker at the apical end of the cochlea, and is under less tension as well. These characteristics cause it to vibrate in concert with the input sound pressure. As the fluid is displaced by the motion of the stapes footplate at the oval window, it generates a pressure wave in the fluid that travels along the basilar membrane. The mechanical characteristics of the basilar membrane cause it to deflect as the traveling wave travels from base to apex. The point of maximal deflection of the basilar membrane is dependent on the frequency of the input; high frequencies produce maximal deflection at the basal end (near the footplate) and the lower frequencies produce a maximum at the apical end (near the helicotrema).

Electrical Activity in the Cochlea

The electrical potentials observed in the inner ear are the result of mechanical disturbances. The origin of these potentials is likely the hair cells. When vibration sets the oval window in motion, the pressure differential on the BM causes it to change its orientation with respect to the tectorial membrane, stimulating the hair cell bundles. As a result, tip links tighten and hair cells torque, opening channels that allow an influx of potassium ions (K+). See Figure 3.5. The depolarization of the cell releases neural transmitters that stimulate the spiral ganglion and generate an action potential that travels up the auditory nerve (e.g., see Geisler, 1991, 1993).

The resting potential of the endolymph of the scala media, termed the **endocochlear potential (EP)**, is approximately 80 millivolts (mV). The intracellular resting potential of the hair cells is −70 mV. The 150-mV range between the two constitutes the largest voltage differential in the body, providing a "battery" that ensures electrical transduction is most effective. The stria vascularis is responsible for maintaining this potential, thus any damage to the stria will reduce this differential and subsequently interfere with the transduction process.

The **cochlear microphonic (CM)** is an alternating current that is only observable when a stimulus is present. A characteristic of the CM it that it mimics the acoustical input with an electrical analog that has the same intensity and frequency characteristics (Dallos, 1975). The magnitude of the CM is proportional to the displacement of the basilar membrane, and is believed to originate from the hair cells. The CM is easily measured outside the cochlea at the round window. The **action potential** (AP) arises outside of the cochlea as the result of the **VIIIth nerve** firing. It is the sum of many individual neurons firing nearly simultaneously within a bundle of nerves. The AP is negative early on, and then gradually becomes positive in charge, then again negative as the apical neurons get summed. It reflects the gross electrical activity of the cochlea, primarily from the first turn. Deviations from normative results, even for such gross activity, are of diagnostic significance given the ease of recording. The **summating potential** (SP), like the resting potential, is also a dc potential, but it only occurs when

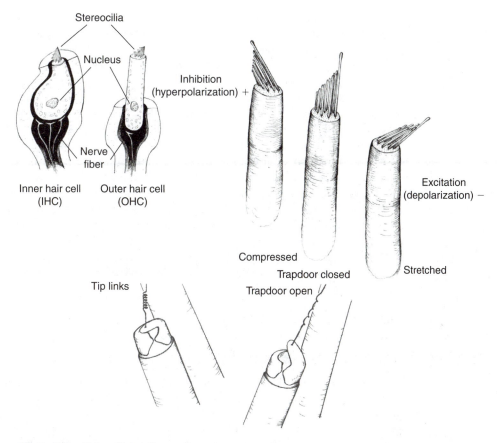

Figure 3.5   **Hair cell detail.** Illustrated by Tracy L. Williams.

there is acoustic stimulation. The SP may be positive or negative, shifting the overall baseline of the response. Its origin is not well understood (Dallos, 1981).

Outer Hair Cell Activity

The bending, twisting, and torquing of the stereocilia by the basilar and tectorial membranes gives rise to the basic stimulation of the hair cells that causes them to depolarize and transmit their information on the central nervous system (Ades & Engstrom, 1974). Whereas the OHCs are physically touching the tectorial membrane, the IHCs are more likely stimulated by fluid motion. When the tips of the stereocilia are displaced, the permeability of the cell membrane changes to allow ions to flow into and out of the cell changing its polarity and eventually causing it to depolarize.

In recent years, research has been conducted on an interesting phenomenon concerning the OHCs called hair cell **motility** (e.g., see Dallos, 1992). The OHCs expand and contract with the polarity of the cochlea. IHCs do not demonstrate this property. The change in size occurs in two time frames, one very rapidly, in tenths of milliseconds, the other more slowly, over several seconds. These movements have identified OHCs as "dancing hair cells," indicative of their motility. Not only do the OHCs change in length, but because they are attached to the tectorial membrane, they also change the overall mechanical stiffness of the basilar and tectorial membranes.

Most of the nerves from the cochlea emanate from the inner hair cells, providing the primary mechanism for sensitivity and frequency resolution. The outer hair cells provide feedback though motility to improve sensitivity and create amplification for small vibrations. The motility of OHCs is responsible for phenomena related to **cochlear emissions** (Kemp, 1978). **Otoacoustic emissions** (OAEs) are an active process of amplification in the ear. Also known as cochlear echoes or Kemp echoes, OAEs are narrowband acoustic signals generated in the inner ear of normal-hearing individuals. The mechanisms responsible for OAEs are the same as those that govern ability to detect low-level sounds. OAEs vary and can occur in the absence of stimulation (spontaneous emissions) or in response to stimulation (evoked emissions). Most forms of hearing impairment are characterized at onset by the weakening or loss of this feedback mechanism. A noninvasive procedure that involves the placement of a tiny microphone at the entrance of the ear canal is used to measure these emissions and provides useful data for evaluating inner ear function.

THE AUDITORY NERVOUS SYSTEM

The Peripheral Auditory Nervous System

The cochlea is enervated with both **afferent** and **efferent nerve fibers.** Afferent fibers are sensory nerves emanating from the hair cells within the cochlea; they are arranged tonotopically; that is, each frequency is restricted to a specific region of the basilar membrane. Efferent fibers emanate from higher regions of the nervous system and carry information to the cells from above. There are two types of afferent fibers, called type I and type II. Neither variety of nerve has a protective myelin sheath within the organ of Corti. Fibers from the apex (low frequencies) of the cochlea are in the middle of the nerve bundle, whereas higher-frequency fibers, emanating from the basal portions of the cochlea, are on the outside of the bundle. After the auditory nerve exits the cochlea and merges with the vestibular fibers to form the VIIIth nerve, it travels on to the cochlear nucleus.

The type I fibers are **radial fibers,** comprising about 85% of the total innervation of afferents, whereas the lesser type II fibers are called outer **spiral fibers.** The type I fibers are connected to the IHCs one- or two-to-one; that is, each IHC transmits its information along a dedicated nerve, but each IHC may be innervated by up to 20 type I fibers. The type II fibers innervate mostly the first row of OHCs in a one-to-many fashion; that is, each nerve attaches to many OHCs. The afferents leave the cochlea via the **habenula perforata,** an opening in the spiral lamina.

The Central Auditory Nervous System

The VIIIth cranial nerve serves the hearing and balance senses. Upon exiting the habenula perforata, the nerve becomes myelinated and produces neural spikes that travel along the nerve to the cochlear nucleus. From the cochlear nucleus nerve tracts rise both ipsilaterally (same side) and contralaterally (opposite side), forming a complex network of pathways ascending to the areas of the cortex associated with sound. All the fibers that exit the cochlea synapse at the cochlear nucleus. The cochlear nucleus is not well understood in its function, although it is arranged tonotopically; that is, particular frequencies are associated with specific areas of the nucleus. It is also interconnected with all the other higher nuclei in the ascending auditory nervous system. The nucleus may be involved in tuning the stimulation to assist in auditory image formation.

Exiting the cochlear nucleus, nerve impulses travel to the **olivary complex.** Olivary refers to its shape, which is like an olive. This junction is particularly significant because it is the first point in the nervous system where the two ears communicate with one another. The olivary complex allows for the localization of sound in space and correlation of the signals from the two ears (binaural hearing) to assist in figure-ground separation (i.e., separating signal and noise). The **inferior colliculus** receives input from each of the lower nuclei, the cochlear nuclei and the olivary complex. Some cells respond to only one ear, while others respond binaurally. Recent research implicates the olivary complex as a source of central auditory processing deficits (for further reading see: Spoendlin, 1978; Durrant, 1983; Phillips, 1988; Perrott, Briggs, & Perrott, 1970).

From the superior olive, the neural transmission passes upward through the inferior colliculus to the **lateral lemniscus** ("ribbon"), and onward to the **medial geniculate** ("knee-shaped" nuclei) where it is gated into the appropriate areas of the cortex, **Heschel's area** and **Wernicke's area.** There are also connections to the cerebellum (locomotion) and to the reticular formation (arousal). See Figure 3.6.

The efferent nervous system associated with hearing descends from the cortex and many points below, finally emanating from the olivary complex to bypass the cochlear nucleus and connect directly with the hair cells. The efferent system is largely inhibitory in its function. These fibers innnervate both the IHCs and the OHCs.

SOUND PROCESSING IN THE EAR

Adaptation, Fatigue, and Recruitment

Intense exposure to sounds for an extended duration produces changes in the auditory system's responsiveness. When first stimulated, an auditory nerve neuron responds vigorously. However, if steady stimulation continues, the neuron's firing rate drops until its energy output is balanced by its input. A shift in threshold resulting from a reduction in sensitivity of a group of receptors is termed a temporary threshold shift (TTS). The decline in receptor response is known as neural adaptation. The psychological component of adaptation is a decline in the perceived magnitude of the stimulus at onset followed by a perceived magnitude that remains roughly constant. Fatigue occurs when sensitivity is reduced and absolute threshold increases after exposure. Fatigue can be transient for low exposure but permanent and pathological for very intense sounds (see Moore, 1997). Abnormally rapid growth of perceived loudness in response to sensation level increases is known as loudness recruitment, and although it usually occurs in the impaired ear, a similar phenomenon can occur in normal hearing. Loudness recruitment is generally connected to cochlear outer hair cell damage and is usually absent in conductive or retrocochlear deafness.

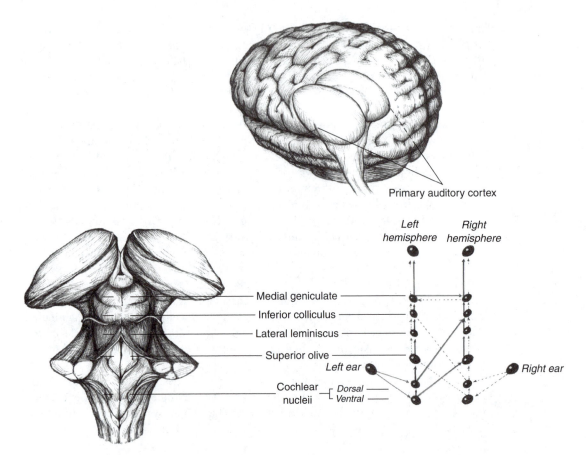

Primary auditory cortex

Left hemisphere   Right hemisphere

Medial geniculate
Inferior colliculus
Lateral leminiscus
Superior olive
Left ear
Cochlear nucleii   Dorsal
Ventral
Right ear

Figure 3.6   Illustration of the auditory pathway from the cochlear nuclei to the primary auditory cortex. Illustrated by Tracy L. Williams.

The Coding of Loudness

Increases in sound intensity stimulates larger areas of the basilar membrane. The ear codes loudness through the firing rates (spikes/sec) of neurons. The rate of loudness differs for tones of varying frequencies, 2000 Hz receiving maximal response. Some fibers are sensitive near threshold (the lowest sound level where a change in response can be measured), while others range from 20–30 dB up to 80–90 dB maximum. Neurons with high thresholds (wide dynamic ranges) have low spontaneous firing rates and less sensitive synapses; consequently, a large increase in sound level is required to increase BM displacement to the point where the neuron saturates (fatigue). The dynamic range for neurons with high spontaneous firing rates is quite small, 15–30 dB. For further discussion see Jesteadt, Wier, and Green (1977).

Firing frequency is usually a logarithmic function of stimulus intensity. Although it is roughly true that tones of equal SPL are perceived as equally loud, loudness grows more rapidly at low frequencies than middle frequencies. This phenomenon is demonstrated by the shapes of equal loudness contours generated by Fletcher and Munson (1933). Equal loudness contours do not directly indicate how loud a sound appears to the listener, but rather how intense a 1000-Hz tone must be to sound equally loud. A 1000-Hz tone is presented simultaneously with another tone and adjusted until it reaches a level at which it is perceived as equally loud. This level is measured in **phons**, units that represent equal loudness contours.

Stevens (1956) generated an equation that describes the relationship of physical intensity to estimations of magnitude. Also known as the power law, Stevens' law suggests that the magnitude of the perceived sensation provided by a specific stimulus intensity depends on the size of the exponent. Stevens offered the **sone** as the unit of loudness measurement. The sone is defined as the loudness of a 1000-Hz tone at 40 dB SPL. For further reading on basic correlates of the auditory stimulus, see Licklider (1951).

The Coding of Pitch

A curious illusion results when the fundamental is removed from a complex sound. When a fundamental is greater than 50 Hz, the pitch of a sound without the fundamental is perceived as the same as the sound presented with its fundamental intact. The missing fundamental illusion is central to two classic theories of basilar membrane motion. The earliest theory, the place principle advanced by Helmhotz, proposed that the fibers of the basilar membrane were arranged like the strings of a harp; specific regions vibrating in sympathy with low-frequency tones and others with high frequencies. Békésy (1960) modified place theory with his discovery that the narrower tighter base of the basilar membrane near the oval window, experiences maximum displacement with high-frequency tones, while regions of the BM at the wider apex respond maximally to low tones. In the case of the missing fundamental illusion, Békésy assumed that the BM responded as if the missing fundamental were present. If this assumption held true, then the BM would be masked by presence of stimulation in the same region. Masking, in fact, does not occur when noise centered on the same frequency as a missing fundamental is inserted into a complex sound. What happens is that the perceived pitch of that sound turns out to be the same as the missing fundamental.

An alternative to the place theory, the frequency principle, suggests that pitch corresponds to the overall pattern of neural impulses evoked by the stimulus. Neurons fire at peak compression of the sound wave (phase locking), such that 500 Hz produces 500 bursts of spike potentials per second in the auditory nerve. According to the frequency principle, adding or masking the fundamental frequency for tones below 4000 Hz does not alter the pattern of neural firing, because whether neurons are firing at the fundamental or not makes little difference to the pattern of bursts produced by the harmonics.

The volley principle, proposed by Wever and Bray (1937), explains: (1) how the auditory nerve can carry spike potentials of up to 4000 Hz when the absolute refractory period of the neuron limits its frequency resolution and, (2) how pressure (loudness) and frequency (pitch) can be coded separately at the auditory nerve. The volley principle states that neurons fire in groups, each neuron firing at a specific phase of the sinusoid, resulting in a burst of activity at each pressure peak of the sound input. An increase in sound pressure does not change volley frequency, rather it increases the number of neurons firing at each pressure peak. Frequency is coded by the frequency of volleys and pressure by the number of responses per volley.

Aspects of each of the theories cited above are used to explain pitch perception. The human ear demonstrates peak performance at frequencies between 5000 Hz and 4000 Hz where both frequency and place principles apply. Frequencies outside of this range depend on one mechanism and subsequently have poorer resolution. For frequencies below 500 Hz, pitch perception is explained by the frequency principle. Frequencies from 4000 Hz to 20,000 Hz are mediated by the place principle (Békésy, 1960; Green, 1976).

The Critical Band

Fletcher (1940) proposed that the basilar membrane behaves like a narrowly tuned bank of filters covering the range of audible sound, each filter having a different center frequency and bandwidth. These BM filters are not fixed, instead they are continuous and can be mapped in various positions by the brain. A pitch maximally stimulates a restricted region of the BM "tuned" to that frequency; however, it also stimulates adjacent areas corresponding to a band of frequencies, or the effective total bandwidth, called the **critical band** (CB). The collective output of the filters is not the product of a single stimulation, but rather a series of stimulations that span the frequency range of hearing (see Zwicker, Flottorp, & Stevens, 1957; Bilger, 1976).

The CB varies as a function of frequency. Patterson and Moore (1986) constructed a series of experiments demonstrating that the CB is a band of frequencies to which adding tones does not facilitate detection. From the overall spectrum of a noise, Patterson deleted a specific frequency and inserted a tone in the middle of the resulting gap, measuring for thresholds of the tone. The narrow gap masked the tone, necessitating that tone intensity increase to be detected. Widening the gap improved threshold until a critical point where frequencies on either side of the tone have no effect on its percept and the signal threshold asymptotes.

Temporal Resolution

The ability to detect changes over time, either gaps between stimuli or amplitude modulation, is termed temporal acuity or temporal resolution. Temporal resolution depends on the analysis of patterns in envelope of sound, that is, in the overall changes in magnitude spectrum rather than the finer structural changes of the sound (Green, 1971). Both the time pattern within each frequency channel and a comparison across channels are analyzed. For further discussion refer to Takahashi and Bacon (1992).

Hearing loss and age are almost always confounded in the study of temporal acuity. Age-related performance deficits in temporal processing are largely independent of hearing loss, reflecting central auditory dysfunction rather than peripheral loss. Older listeners not only take longer to process sound information, they are more susceptible to interference; thus the evidence of age effects are more robust with complex stimuli. The ability to detect brief gaps between stimuli, or **gap detection**, improves with age at both higher and lower frequencies; although this improvement may reflect a developmental factor rather than changes to peripheral auditory fine tuning. For broadband noises, normal threshold for detecting a gap is 2–3 milliseconds except at very low levels. Elderly listeners are less sensitive to modulation. Complex sequential patterns demonstrate cognitive and central processing factors associated with uncertainty and familiarity. Duration discrimination examines temporal ability by measuring difference limen for changes in stimulation. Elderly listeners show poorer duration discrimination than the young (see Fitzgibbons Gordon-Salant, 1994, 1995).

Localization and Binaural Hearing

Binaural is the term that refers to the condition of having two ears. Because in humans the ears are located on opposite sides of the head, sound waves can arrive at the ears at different times due to the difference in path length from ear to ear. When the stimulus is identical at the two ears, it is called **diotic**; when it is different at the two ears it is **dichotic**. **Monaural** describes the condition where sound is detected in only one ear.

When one ear receives sound that is not directly in front, behind, above, or below the head, the other ear is in the sound shadow, receiving waves that are bent around the head or body. The direction of sound sources is defined relative to three planes that intersect at right angles roughly in the center of the head. The horizontal plane and frontal planes pass through the upper margins of the ear canals and the lower margins of the eye sockets, and the median plane defines central points equidistant from both ears. The direction of arriving sounds is described by azimuth and elevation. Sounds on the horizontal plane are at 0° elevation. A sound directly in front of a person is at 0° azimuth and 0° elevation. Sounds opposite the left ear are at 90° azimuth and 0° elevation and those at 180° azimuth are behind the head.

When a sound source is aligned with the median plane, there is no amplitude and/or phase difference in the arrival of the sound at the two ears. For all other conditions, an **interaural time difference** (ITD), or when defined in decibels, an **interaural level difference** (ILD) can provide cues to sound localization. Low-frequency sounds have wavelengths longer than the width of the head; as a result, they bend (diffraction) easily around the head. In contrast, the tiny waves of high-frequency sounds produce shadows. Consequently, ITDs are most useful at low frequencies, while ILDs are useful in localizing sound at high frequencies. This two-process theory of sound localization is known as the **duplex theory**. At middle frequencies, neither cue proves particularly useful. The smallest spatial separation between sequential sounds that can be detected is known as the **minimum audible angle**.

As mentioned, the spectral changes in the sound wave produced by the pinnae help to amplify and localize sound; however, the head and other body parts can also help with localization through unique patterns of dampening or delaying of the sound. The combined effects of individual differences in anatomical topography provide cues for the localization of complex sounds that are summarized in a mathematical description called the **head-related transfer function (HRTF)**.

THE VESTIBULAR SYSTEM

Our vestibular organs sense balance and equilibrium. Some fluids and nerves of the vestibular system are shared with those of the auditory system. In addition, the vestibular sensory transducers that sense movement and orientation are surprisingly similar to those of the hearing sense. Although these similarities exist between the two systems, the vestibular organ interacts little with our auditory sense, but it is intimately related to vision and visceral sensations.

The vestibular system is composed of three semicircular canals, roughly at right angles to each other, stemming from a fluid-filled sac called the vestibule. Each of the canals has a bulge near one of its attachments with the **utricle**, part of the vestibule. The bulge is called the **ampulla**; it contains the receptor organs called the **cristae ampulares**. The semicircular canals are called the superior, posterior, and horizontal canals and rotational movement in a particular direction causes a fluid flow to stimulate the receptor organ as it flows through the ampulla. The **sensory epithelium** of the vestibular system is similar to that of the auditory system. Tiny hair cells are deflected by the fluid motion and generate a nerve impulse to the brain as the result. Linear motion is sensed by another section of the organ known as the **saccule**. The saccule contains the **macula**, where hair cell transducers are present, stimulated by movement of fluid through the organ due to inertia (Honrubia, Strelioff, & Sitko, 1976). The macula is covered with a gelatinous substance containing tiny crystals called **otoliths**. The otoliths provide mass that facilitates the movement of the macular cells in response to linear motion. The fluids of the vestibular system, endolymph and perilymph, are continuous with those of the auditory system, and the oval window, where the stapes footplate comes in contact with the cochlea, is located in the vestibule. The vestibular nerve from each sensory transducer joins the cochlear nerve soon after leaving the organ to form the VIIIth nerve.

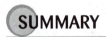

SUMMARY

CHAPTER REVIEW

- ❑ Unique sound-localizing properties of the pinna channel sound waves into the external auditory meatus, which amplifies specific frequencies through resonance. In humans, frequencies common to speech benefit the most from this amplification.

- ❑ At the tympanum, vibrations are transmitted to a succession of three tiny bones that further amplify the sound in the middle ear: the malleus, incus, and stapes.

- ❑ Air in the middle ear is equalized with the surrounding atmosphere via the Eustachian tube. The stapes applies pressure at the membrane-covered opening of the fluid-filled cochlea called the oval window. Amplification of sound waves in the middle ear results in pressure of the stapes at the oval window to be about 15 times greater than that at the tympanum.

- ❑ The oval window lies on the boundary of the middle and inner ear and at the base of one of three tubes in the cochlea called the vestibular canal. The apex, or far end of the vestibular canal, is connected at the helicotrema to the tympanic canal. The tympanic canal has a membrane separating it from air called the round window. The round window flexes in response to movement in the perilymph. The third canal of the cochlea, the scala media, is contained by two membranes—Reissner's and the basilar membrane (BM), and filled with endolymph, a fluid more viscous than perilymph.

❏ The basilar membrane is tapered to facilitate the transfer of energy from middle to inner ear. The organ of Corti, which contains the hair cells that transduce mechanical energy into neural signals, lies along the length of the BM.

❏ The tips of the outer hair cells (OHCs) are embedded in the tectorial membrane, which extends into the cochlear duct from the Reissner's membrane. While inner hair cells (IHCs) are stimulated by fluid motion, the torquing of OHCs results in depolarization.

❏ Fibers emanating from the hair cells form the spiral ganglion. Axons of the spiral ganglion form the auditory nerve. The auditory nerve exits the cochlea and merges with vestibular fibers to form the VIIIth nerve, which travels on to the cochlear nucleus.

❏ Nerve impulses travel to the olivary complex and from the superior olive to the inferior colliculus, the lateral lemniscus, and then onward to the medial geniculate where it is gated to the Heschel's and Wernicke's areas of the cerebral cortex.

❏ Neuron firing rates account for loudness perception while pitch, a function of frequency, and is explained by aspects of the place, frequency, and volley theories.

❏ The critical band describes the behavior of the basilar membrane as a series of auditory filters with a regions responding maximally to corresponding frequencies.

❏ Sound localization is achieved through the resolution of interaural time and intensity differences in binaural hearing in the olivary complex but is aided by the topography of the pinna, head, and body.

❏ The vestibular organs, contained in the same bony labyrinth as the cochlea, maintain the sense of balance and equilibrium.

ACTIVITIES FOR DISCUSSION

1. Track the path of a sound stimulus through the structures of the outer, middle, and inner ear.

2. How do structures of the ear overcome the impedance mismatch between air and fluid media?

3. Describe activity on the basilar membrane. What is the critical band?

4. When considering low- and high-pitched tones, which are better at maskers? Why?

5. Explain the specifics of where and how transduction takes place.

6. How are the outer and inner hair cells different in function? What is motility?

7. Diagram the ascending pathway.

8. What is the missing fundamental illusion and how does it contribute to theories of pitch perception.

9. Which mechanisms of the ear are involved in sound localization?

10. Which cues, ITDs or ILDs, provide the most useful information for localizing low-frequency sounds? Why?

REFERENCES

Ades, H. W., Engstrom, H. (1974) Anatomy of the inner ear. In W. D. Keidel W. D. Neff (Eds.), *Handbook of Sensory Physiology, Auditory System: Anatomy, Physiology (Ear),* (vol. V/1, pp. 125–158). Berlin: Springer-Verlag.

Békésy, G. V. (1960). *Experiments in Hearing.* In E. G. Wever (Ed. Trans.), New York: McGraw-Hill.

Bilger, R. C. (1976) A revised critical-band hypothesis. In S. K. Hirsh S. R. Silverman (Eds.), *Hearing and Davis: Essays Honoring Hallowell Davis* (pp. 191–198). St. Louis: Washington University Press.

Dallos, P. (1992). The active cochlea. *The Journal of Neuroscience, 12*(12), 4575–4585.

Dallos, P. (1981). Cochlear physiology. *Annual Review of Psychology, 32,* 153–190.

Dallos, P. (1975). Electrical correlates of mechanical events in the cochlea. *Audiology, 14,* 408–418.

Durrant, J. D. (1983). Fundamentals of sound generation for auditory evoked responses. In E. J. Moore (Ed.), *Bases of Auditory Brain Stem Evoked Responses* (pp. 15–49). New York: Grune & Stratton.

Fitzgibbons, P. J., & Gordon-Salant, S. (1995). Age effects on duration discrimination with simple and complex stimuli. *Journal of the Acoustical Society of America,* Dec. 98(6), 3140–3145.

Fitzgibbons, P. J., & Gordon-Salant, S. (1994). Age effects on measures of auditory duration discrimination. *Journal of Speech and Hearing Research,* June, 37(3), 662–70.

Fletcher, H. (1940). Auditory patterns. *Review of Modern Physics, 12,* 47–65.

Fletcher, H., & Munson, W. A. (1933). Loudness, its definition, measurement, and calculation. *Journal of the Acoustical Society of America, 5,* 82–108.

Geisler, C. D. (1993). A model of stereociliary tip-link stretches. *Hearing Research, 65,* 79–82.

Geisler, C. D. (1991). A cochlear model using feedback from motile outer hair cells. *Hearing Research, 54,* 105–117.

Glasscock, M. E., & Shambaugh, G. E. (1990). *Surgery of the Ear* (4th ed.). Philadelphia: W. B. Saunders Co.

Green, D. M. (1976). *An Introduction to Hearing.* Hillsdale, NJ: Lawrence Erlbaum Associates.

Green, D. M. (1971). Temporal and auditory acuity. *Psychological Review, 73,* 540–551.

Honrubia, V., Strelioff, D., & Sitko, S. T. (1976). Physiological basis of cohclear transduction and sensitivity. *The Annals of Otology, Rhinology & Laryngology, 85,* 697–710.

Jesteadt, W., Wier, C. C., Green, D. M. (1977). Intensity discrimination as a function of frequency and sensation level. *Journal of the Acoustical Society of America, 61,* 169–177.

Kemp, D. T. (1978). Stimulated acoustic emissions from within the human auditory system. *Journal of the Acoustical Society of America, 64,* 1386–1391.

Kuhn, G. F. (1979). The pressure transformation from a diffuse sound field to the external ear and to the body and head surface. *Journal of the Acoustical Society of America, 65,* 991–1000.

Lawrence, M. (1980). Inner ear physiology. In M. M. Paparella & D. A. Shumrick (Eds.), *Otolaryngology: Basic Sciences and Related Disciplines* (2nd ed., vol. 1, pp. 216–240). Philadelphia: W. B. Saunders Co.

Licklider, J. C. R. (1951). Basic correlates of the auditory stimulus. In S. S. Stevens (Ed.), *Handbook of Experimental Psychology* (pp. 935–1039). New York: John Wiley Sons.

Lim, D. J. (1980). Cochlear anatomy related to cochlear micromechanics. [Review]. *Journal of the Acoustical Society of America, 67,* 1686–1695.

Moore, B. C. J. (1997). *An Introduction to the Psychology of Hearing* (5th ed.). London: Academic Press.

Patterson, R. D., & Moore, B. C. J. (1986). Auditory filters and excitation patterns as representations of frequency resolution. In B. C. J. Moore (Ed.), *Frequency Selectivity in Hearing* (pp. 123–176). London: Academic Press.

Perrott, D. R., Briggs, R., & Perrott, S. (1970). Binaural fusion: Its limits as defined by signal duration and signal onset. *Journal of the Acoustical Society of America, 47,* 565–568.

Phillips, D. P. (1988). Introduction to anatomy and physiology of the central nervous system. In A. F. Jahn & J. Santos Sacchi (Eds.), *Physiology of the Ear* (pp. 407–429). New York: Raven Press.

Shaw, E. A. G. (1974). The external ear. In W. D. Keidel & W. D. Neff (Eds.), *Handbook of Sensory Physiology. Auditory System: Anatomy, Physiology (Ear),* (vol. V/1, pp. 455–490). Berlin: Springer-Verlag.

Spoendlin, H. (1978). The afferent innervation of the cochlea. In R. F. Naunton & C. Fernandez (Eds.), *Evoked Electrical Activity in the Auditory Nervous System* (pp. 21–41). New York: Academic Press.

Stevens, S. S. (1956). The direct estimation of sensory magnitude—loudness. *American Journal of Psychology, 69,* 1–25.

Takahashi, G. A., Bacon S. P. (1992). Modulation detection, modulation masking, and speech understanding in noise in the elderly. *Journal of Speech and Hearing Research,* Dec, 35(6), 1410–1421.

Wever, E. G. & Bray, C. W. (1937). The perception of low tones and the resonance-volley theory. *Journal of Psychology, 3,*101–114.

Wright, D., Hebrank, J. H., & Wilson, B. (1974). Pinna reflections as cues for localization. *Journal of the Acoustical Society of America, 56,* 957–962.

Yost, W. A. (1994). *Fundamentals of Hearing: An Introduction* (3rd ed.). San Diego: Academic Press.

Zwicker, E., Flottorp, G., & Stevens, S. S. (1957). Critical bandwidth in loudness summation. *Journal of the Acoustical Society of America, 29,* 548–557.

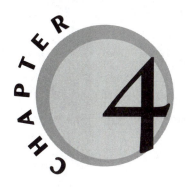

Disorders of the Ear

Peter J. Ivory

Key Terms

CASE STUDY

A Glimpse into the Profession

Caitlin is a cute three-year-old whose parents are complaining that she doesn't seem to pay attention when they call her and that she prefers television, music, and DVDs louder than they do. Her parents have no concerns regarding her speech and language development and, in fact, noted that Caitlin likes to have books read to her, although she insists that the reader talks loud. Her parents stated that Caitlin had several ear infections with fever and associated pain when she was one year old but none recently. She appears in good health. Although there is no family history of hearing loss, Caitlin's parents are concerned about this as a possibility.

OVERVIEW OF CONDITIONS OF THE EAR

In a medical model, a test result has only two interpretations: (1) *Normal:* what is expected for the majority of persons who are without disease or structural difference; or (2) *Abnormal:* what a result is called if it departs from normal. In medical terms, another word for abnormality is **pathology.** In audiology, a measurable departure from normal results on audiometric testing is referred to as **hearing loss.**

It is likely the case that most persons with hearing loss do not have their hearing loss due to "disease" as this word is typically understood. Truly, there are cases in which hearing loss is an indication that the person has a significant health problem and therefore, needs medical treatment; however, there are many more cases in which hearing loss is simply a confirmation of a nonmedically significant condition that does not require medical attention—for example, in the hearing loss of an older adult.

A critical concept in further consideration of dysfunction of the auditory mechanism is the possibility that multiple and different pathologies or differences may coexist simultaneously in different locations in the auditory system, an occurrence referred to as **coexisting lesions.** Having a pathology or difference in one part of the system does not preclude the possibility of having a pathology or difference in another part of the system. With this in mind, and in order to simplify this discussion, all pathology or difference will be discussed in this chapter in isolation, understanding that actual patients may present with one or more auditory system pathologies or differences at any given time.

Description and quantification of hearing loss are usually based on audiometric test results, which are discussed in detail in Chapter 6 of this text. When pathology located in the outer and/or middle ears causes hearing loss, that hearing loss is called a

conductive hearing loss. When pathology located in the inner ear and/or the auditory nerve causes hearing loss, that hearing loss is called a **sensorineural hearing loss.** When coexisting pathologies occur causing both a conductive hearing loss and a sensorineural hearing loss, that hearing loss is called a **mixed hearing loss.** In addition to the audiometric tests described in Chapter 6, audiologists also employ tests of the physical function of parts of the auditory system—for example, acoustic immittance testing (primarily tests of middle ear function, such as tympanometry), otoacoustic emissions (primarily, a test of inner ear function) and the auditory brainstem response (a test of auditory nerve response). These tests are discussed further in Chapter 7.

Audiometric test results may trigger any number of consequent actions in both the medical context (for example, recommendation for/against surgery) and in the legal context (for example, determination of financial compensation for industrial or military hearing loss). Therefore, audiometric test results must be reliable and valid estimates of the person's organic hearing status. However, audiometric test findings could possibly hide the fact that the tests were performed incorrectly or even that the person being tested did not understand what to do or even intended to demonstrate hearing loss when their hearing status was actually normal. Conventional audiologic testing is structured to recognize and therefore minimize these outlying possibilities. In this way, audiologic test procedures remain a valuable tool in hearing assessment and in determining appropriate intervention for persons with hearing loss.

Normal Hearing Status

While it may seem unusual to mention "normal hearing status" in a chapter on disorders and conditions of the ear, it should be always remembered that in most clinical situations, many hearing tests will yield results that are classified as "within normal limits." The capable audiologist understands what "normal" is, understands how the results of one test correlate with another test, and, just as importantly, understands how people with normal hearing behave. The audiologist performing the testing and the equipment used to complete audiologic tests must also be "normal." Incompetent test administration or the use of equipment that does not meet calibration standards will also yield data that could be misinterpreted as hearing loss, when in fact the person had hearing within normal limits.

Medical Model (Pathology) versus Cultural Model (Difference)

When audiologists work in medical environments, they are part of a medical model that describes results/patients as either normal or abnormal. In the medical model, the action plan is clear: if abnormal, find the cause (**etiology**) of the abnormality; treat the cause with an appropriate remedy; minimize spread of cause and abnormality; and monitor the patient to a level of acceptable function. For hearing losses that are caused by infectious disease processes that have the potential to progress and erode adjacent tissues and even be fatal, the medical model seems to be an appropriate way to view hearing loss, especially for a person who, predisease, had normal hearing.

However, there are many individuals who may have significant hearing loss but no pressing medical need. These individuals likely identify with the cultural model of

Deafness (Lane, 1992). In the cultural model of Deafness, hearing status is viewed simply as a physical difference in a person, but not one which defines that person. Although culturally Deaf people may receive very little useful information through sound, they do not view themselves as abnormal or infirm in the medical sense and typically do not seek treatment for their Deafness but simply view themselves as different in terms of language preferences and needs.

CONDITIONS AFFECTING THE OUTER EAR

The function of the outer ear is simple: to passively collect sound waves at the auricle and funnel them into the external ear canal. The auricle, owing to its exposed position on the surface of the skull, is subject to a variety of injuries and conditions that are medically significant but rarely cause significant hearing loss. The auricle is frequently affected by both sharp trauma (lacerations; animal/human bites) and blunt trauma; posttraumatic vascular complications; frostbite; and burn injuries (due to fire; hot liquid; electrical; chemical; or excessive sun exposure). A long-term complication of excessive sun exposure is malignancy; not surprisingly then, the auricle is a common location for malignancies of the skin, especially in older, fair-skinned people (Storper, Canalis, & Lambert, 2000). Clinically significant hearing loss due to a problem in the outer ear is caused by blockage or absence of the air pathway of the external ear canal. Additionally, the external ear canal is often the site of infection, which may not cause hearing loss but which may be unpleasant due to the possibility of associated pain and discharge.

Outer Ear Malformations: Microtia and Atresia

Congenital (that is, present at birth) structural differences in the outer ear are usually caused by genetic/inherited factors. In the otology literature, external and middle ear malformations are classified into three groups depending on the degree of severity of malformation and number of affected structures: Group I—minor malformations; Group II—moderate malformations; and Group III—severe malformations (Mattox, Nager, & Levin, 1991). Group II—moderate malformations—accounts for the majority of external ear malformations, including a continuum of malformation of the auricle, **microtia**—literally, "small ear." Microtia itself is subdivided based on severity into three types: microtia type I (auricle partly recognizable); microtia type II (auricle in grossly undeveloped state); and microtia type III (the structures that are present have no correspondence to a normal auricle). The severest form of auricle malformation is part of Group III and is anotia, the complete absence of the auricle. In many cases of microtia, plastic surgery can be performed to achieve a cosmetic improvement (Ruder, 2000).

Many ears with microtia also have another malformation, **atresia**—literally, "no hole," which is the absence of an external ear canal. Unilateral atresia is stated to be six times more common than bilateral atresia (Maceri & Lambert, 2000). For reasons unknown at this time, atresia is more common in males and affects the right ear more frequently than the left ear (Mattox et al., 1991). Assuming that the inner ear is normal, an ear with atresia will have a maximum conductive hearing loss (hearing loss in the range of 60–65 dB). Therefore, a newborn with a bilateral atresia will be at significant risk for delay in speech and language development without intervention, specifically amplification. A child with a unilateral atresia should develop speech and language without significant delay, although like others with only one functionally hearing ear, this child will have difficulty in auditory localization and will have difficulty in understanding speech in situations with significant background noise.

Microtia and atresia are often part of a larger set of structural differences that most likely include malformation of the middle ear structures and possibly include structural differences in other bones of the skull. Additionally, there may be malformations also of physically distant structures—for example, fingers, toes, and the kidneys. Less likely, but possible, are associated malformations of the inner ear.

Obstructions in the External Ear Canal

A normally developed external ear canal is vulnerable to obstruction throughout the entire life span. Because the outer portion of the ear canal contains glands that produce a fatty, protective secretion called cerumen and because the ear canal is lined with skin that is constantly shedding, these substances can accumulate into a completely occluding plug in the ear canal, typically causing a significant conductive hearing loss. Additionally, some people develop a benign bony growth, such as an **osteoma** or an **exostosis** in the ear canal, which usually partially occludes the ear canal. These benign bony growths are prominent on otoscopic inspection of the ear canal and only become clinically significant if they enlarge sufficiently to occlude the ear canal.

Foreign objects of all types can get lodged in the ear canal causing an occlusion. When there is a **foreign body** in the ear canal, there is always risk that the foreign body could cause damage to the tympanic membrane at the deep end of the ear canal either on its own or during unskilled attempts at removal. Foreign bodies containing caustic chemicals (for example, hearing aid batteries) could lead to additional trauma. Objects that are impacted deep in the ear canal or organic materials that expand due to absorption of moisture (for example, kernels of corn or seeds) can cause significant pain in the ear (**otalgia**). A crawling or flying live insect in an ear canal typically causes significant anxiety and pain and usually needs to be subdued prior to removal.

Significant accumulations of ear canal debris or foreign bodies placed in the ear canal may cause an itching sensation and pain. Treatment is removal of the source of the occlusion with monitoring, which may include medicated eardrops to promote healing.

Infections in the External Ear Canal

Because the external ear canal is an exteriorized cavity, it is exposed to all the typical organisms that are on the surface of the body and in the environment. Occasionally, an opportunistic organism might flourish in the ear canal leading to inflammatory changes as the body fights the intrusion of the organism. The general term for an inflammation of the external ear canal is **otitis externa**. Inflammatory consequences during otitis externa may include swelling, pain, and drainage from the ear. If swelling and drainage lead to occlusion of the ear canal, there may be hearing loss also. Otitis externa usually is caused by one of several types of common bacteria. However, an otitis externa could also be caused by a fungus, in which case it is called **otomycosis**. Treatment for otitis externa typically includes the administration of appropriate medications to fight the source of the infection and to minimize the spread of infection and the use of topical steroids to reduce swelling of the inflamed ear canal tissues. Persons who are immunosuppressed or are diabetic are at higher risk for contracting an otitis externa. For the older person with diabetes, there is an associated and potentially lethal type of external ear canal infection, conventionally referred to as malignant otitis externa, that requires quick and aggressive medical care to prevent the infection from spreading throughout the adjacent base of the skull.

CONDITIONS AFFECTING THE TYMPANIC MEMBRANE

The tympanic membrane is an important structure in the auditory system because it is the first transducer structure, converting sound waves into mechanical movement. Even though it is located at the medial (deep) end of the external ear canal, the tympanic membrane is exposed to the air of the world and so, when sound waves propagating through the air strike it, it moves in response to those sound waves. The functional placement of the tympanic membrane, recessed on average in the adult human 2 to 3 cm and fronted by a typically S-shaped curvature of an external ear canal, provides some degree of passive protection from injury. Changes to the mechanical integrity of the tympanic membrane will likely cause some conductive hearing loss.

The tympanic membrane will function optimally when there is equal air pressure on both sides of it. Yawning, sneezing, and swallowing will cause the eustachian tube to open and consequently equalize the pressure in the middle ear spaces. The eustachian tube can also be forcefully opened by closing the nose and mouth and blowing air (Valsalva maneuver). Any condition that reduces the presence of air in these two spaces will compromise the ability of the tympanic membrane to move and cause a conductive hearing loss. Because the tympanic membrane is attached to the ossicular chain of the middle ear, conditions that affect the ossicles and middle ear will influence the function of the tympanic membrane. These conditions will be discussed in the next section.

Perforations of the Tympanic Membrane

The most common and most serious change to the mechanical integrity of the tympanic membrane is when there is a **perforation** or hole in the tympanic membrane. Perforations of the tympanic membrane are medically significant for two reasons: first, the perforation likely causes some degree of hearing loss; second, and perhaps more important, the perforation opens up the middle ear space to direct intrusion from elements of the external environment, including water and skin from the ear canal. Water intrusion through a perforation and into the middle ear spaces is a potential problem because water typically contains multiple life forms and other contaminating material, any of which could be a probable agent for an inflammation or infection in the middle ear spaces. Therefore, all persons with known perforation are advised to keep water out of the ear with the perforation. Ear physicians refer to this as "strict water precautions." The issue of external ear canal skin invading the middle ear space through a perforation is a medically serious concern (this is discussed later).

A spontaneous perforation may occur during an episode of a middle ear infection due to the accumulation of fluid on the medial side (the middle ear side of the tympanic membrane) and thus, the perforation serves to release that fluid into the external ear canal. Typically, these types of perforations heal on their own without a permanent effect on hearing, although these sites may be later marked by a tympanosclerotic plaque (see below). However, if causative middle ear disease continues, the perforation may not close and the person ultimately would be left with a permanent perforation and its consequences, including hearing loss.

Perforations are also caused by trauma due to many different types of acute incidents and roughly fall into four categories: direct trauma; concussive injury from an explosion or a blow to head that caused a sudden compression of air in the ear canal; barotrauma; and temporal bone fractures (Canalis, Abemayor, & Shulman, 2000).

Direct trauma is typically caused by the careless use of instruments utilized for the purpose of cleaning the ear canal (ear swabs, bobby pins, paper clips) or foreign bodies pushed into the tympanic membrane accidentally. Another type of a direct trauma occurs in the industrial work of the welder who is in a field of flying, hot beads of metal (slag). When a piece of hot metal encounters the tympanic membrane, perforation and burn and subsequent additional infection may occur.

There are several types of concussive incidents that have caused perforations. A hand-cup or slap to the side of the head in an assault has been described as a common cause of concussive trauma (Hough & McGee, 1991). Another type of concussion occurs with explosions, such as bombs and firing of artillery in combat situations. Additionally, trauma secondary to waterskiing has been cited as commonly causing perforation.

Barotrauma refers to damage caused by changes in the pressure surrounding the tympanic membrane; typically, this would occur during descent during scuba diving. Finally, the tympanic membrane may suffer perforation as part of a fracture of the bone it is housed in (that is, the temporal bone).

Audiometric findings in tympanic membrane perforation typically include some degree of a conductive component to the hearing loss, which could range from slight (10 dB) to moderate (50 to 60 dB). In general, it is difficult to correlate degree of conductive loss to the physical changes at the tympanic membrane (namely, size and location of perforation).

Tympanosclerosis

Tympanosclerosis is the name given to irregular, white plaques that are commonly seen on tympanic membranes. Tympanosclerosis refers to the benign, nonprogressive, degenerative changes in the connective tissue layer of the tympanic membrane following repeated inflammatory disease of the middle ear and also following placement of **tympanostomy tubes** (Brown & Meyerhoff, 1991). The primary change to the connective tissue (collagen) of the tympanic membrane is an abnormal deposition of calcium, contributing to an unambiguous white appearance of the plaques.

Tympanosclerosis typically affects only the tympanic membrane; when this is the case, usually there is no effect on hearing, although tympanometry may reveal an increase in static acoustic admittance (see Chapter 7). In cases in which the tympanosclerosis affects the ossicles of the middle ear, their ability to move may be restricted and may show some conductive hearing loss and reduced static acoustic admittance.

CONDITIONS AFFECTING THE MIDDLE EAR

The middle ear serves as a mechanical interface between the air of the world and the fluid of the inner ear. Without the middle ear, humans would have a significant (60 dB) conductive hearing loss affecting the ability to hear sounds through air conduction. It has been argued that the development of the middle ear represents a significant advancement in phylogeny because animals with a functioning middle ear system are better adapted to life in the air (as opposed to life in the seas).

There are two requirements for optimal function of the middle ear. First, there needs to be air on both sides of the tympanic membrane, that is, in the external ear canal and also in the middle ear spaces on the medial side of the tympanic membrane. Secondly, the three middle ear bones (the ossicles) need to be able to move. Because the middle ear is bound on one side by a normally intact tympanic membrane and because the rest of its surfaces are bone, there needs to be an air supply to the middle ear for ventilation and maintenance of optimal air pressure equalization. This air supply comes from a tube (the eustachian tube) that runs from the back of the throat up to the front wall of the middle ear. The eustachian tube has two ends: one is relatively large, is generally always open, and is in the front (anterior) wall of the middle ear cavity; the other opening, in contrast, is relatively small, is usually closed, and is in the soft tissue of the back of the throat (specifically, the area called the nasopharynx).

In general, middle ear dysfunction is caused by: problems in air pressure equalization and subsequent poor ventilation of the middle ear spaces; problems that affect the mobility of the tympanic membrane and the ossicles; and also, significant structural differences that reduce or eliminate mechanical function.

Eustachian Tube Dysfunction

As already stated, the primary role of the normally functioning eustachian tube is to ventilate the middle ear spaces. This ventilation optimizes the mechanical motion of the tympanic membrane and ossicles. There are a variety of conditions that can prevent the eustachian tube from opening. These can be categorized as either: inflammatory tissue change in the nasopharynx; conditions of physical difference in the anatomy of the nasopharynx; or growth of a mass in the nasopharynx (Bluestone, 1991). When the tissue in the back of the throat swells, as it does in a variety of conditions (sinusitis; adenoiditis; tonsillitis; or in cases of allergy), the eustachian tube is prevented from opening. When the eustachian tube cannot ventilate the middle ear space, the mucosal lining of the middle ear cavity absorbs all available air and eventually creates a vacuum, that is, a negative pressure relative to the air on the lateral side of the tympanic membrane. This negative pressure in the middle ear space creates a pressure differential that is greater toward the middle ear side. This negative pressure differential pulls the tympanic membrane medially and disrupts its optimal mechanical function but usually there is no significant effect on hearing. If there is hearing loss, it will be a slight conductive hearing loss. This sequence of events is generally called **eustachian tube dysfunction (ETD)**. When ETD causes a significant negative pressure in the middle ear spaces, cells in the tissues lining those spaces can break down and exude fluid (see below).

Otitis Media

Otitis media is a general term for an inflammation or infection of the middle ear spaces, possibly including the mastoid cavities that are posterior to the middle ear. There are many different etiological entities that could be referred to as otitis media. In the medical literature, there are several categorization schemes that are beyond the scope of this chapter. However, there are three main defining characteristics of otitis media as follows: (1) fluid will be present in the normally air-filled middle ear space; (2) this fluid may or may not be infected with some infectious agent, typically bacteria; and (3) there may be consequential degenerative changes to the tissues of the middle ear.

In the medical literature, one type of fluid found in otitis media is called effusion. Effusion has two components: exudate and transudate. Inflammatory processes break down cell membranes of blood cells and cells in the mucosal lining of the middle ear such that their intracellular fluids leak out or exude (this is called active exudate). Negative pressure secondary to ETD affecting similar cells pulls fluids normally contained within those cells out, resulting in transudate fluid (Handler & Magardino, 2000). Exudate and transudate fluids are not by themselves infectious; these are normally intracellular fluids that were forced out of their original cells. Effusion is simply the accumulation of these intracellular fluids in a space not typically designed to contain fluid, such as the normally air-filled middle ear spaces.

When an infection is present, the body responds by sending white blood cells (leukocytes) to the site of the infection. The interaction of the white blood cells with the infection yields a fluid-like substance referred to as pus (leukocytes plus dead cell debris). This process, the formation of pus, is referred to as **suppuration**. The resulting fluid that contains pus is referred to as **purulent** fluid. A final concept important to the understanding of otitis media and its effects on hearing is the consistency (viscosity) of the fluid, which can range from thin and watery (also known as "serous") to thick and glue-like. With these concepts in mind, several of the classic types of otitis media can be further described and better understood.

Otitis media with effusion (OME) is a common version of otitis media and one of the most common conditions affecting the auditory systems of children. In the United States, more than two million episodes of OME occur annually, with a total cost of care estimated to be over $4 billion (American Academy of Family Physicians, 2004). In OME, there is an accumulation of fluid (effusion) in the middle ear space, but without the presence or signs of infection. Because the effusion in OME is often thin in consistency, this type of otitis media is also referred to as serous otitis media (SOM). Also because this type of OME does not imply infection, it is also sometimes referred to as "nonsupperative otitis media." An untreated and unresolved OME may continue without active infection but in this time course, the effusion may considerably thicken, resulting in a state described as "glue ear." In OME, there may be minimal conductive hearing loss in SOM with a greater degree of conductive hearing loss as the fluid approximates a thicker consistency. An OME in a glue ear state may have a 30- to 35-dB conductive hearing loss. Because there is no active infection in OME, it may be present for a long period of time. OME is typically a disorder affecting young children and persons with differences in nasopharyngeal structure and function (as examples: those with Down's syndrome or cleft palate).

Acute otitis media (AOM) (also known as acute suppurative otitis media) refers to an episode of the presence of an infected fluid in the middle ear. In the United States, AOM is the most common infectious condition in children requiring the administration of antibiotic medications (American Academy of Family Physicians & American Academy of Pediatrics, 2004). An episode of AOM will typically have the hallmarks of infection (fever, pain, accumulation of white blood cells or leukocytes to fight the infection, and secondary body effects) and typically results from bacterial infection (Bluestone, 1991). The inflammation from AOM in turn leads to ETD, which in turn, causes a consequent OME (Handler & Magardino, 2000). The most common predisposing factor in AOM is prior upper respiratory infection (Canalis and Lambert, 2000a). As with OME, AOM primarily affects children. Audiometric findings are also variable depending on the status of the infection. When hearing is involved, there will be a mild conductive hearing loss. As with OME, audiometric results will depend on the presence and thickness of effusion in the middle ear spaces.

Chronic Ear Disease and Cholesteatoma

Chronic ear disease, also known as **chronic otitis media (COM)**, refers to unresolved infection of the middle ear spaces, including the mastoid spaces as well as of the mucosal lining of these spaces, with a nonintact tympanic membrane and discharge. COM typically implies an infectious, permanent, progressive, and erosive/destructive process. Because of the physical proximity of the middle ear spaces to other important structures (for example, the inner ear, the facial nerve, the brain), an unchecked erosive infection has the capacity to cause consequential damage to these structures (Hashiaki, 2000). Often, a patient with COM will have an acute incident precipitated by the consequential damage—for example, erosion through the wall of the inner ear causing an episode of extreme and debilitating dizziness requiring hospitalization. For these reasons, medical management of COM is critical and often requires multiple surgeries for removal of infected tissues. In COM, there is usually mild to moderate conductive hearing loss and, additionally, there may be evidence of associated sensorineural hearing loss due to spread of infection to the inner ear as well.

A common consequence of middle ear disease and tympanic membrane perforation is a growth in the middle ear spaces, which is the accumulation of dead, exfoliated skin cells from the external ear canal and the lateral surface of the tympanic membrane. This growth is called a cholesteatoma. Otologic authorities have pointed out for decades that this term, cholesteatoma, is an inaccurate and misleading description of this growth (strictly speaking, the preferred term is keratoma) (Schuknecht, 1993) but the term cholesteatoma remains in common use.

Typically, exfoliated skin cells accumulate in a pocket of decaying, erosive organic materials that may be continually enlarging as more dead skin cells are deposited. This pocket can form at any perforation site (although more likely for a perforation on the edge of the tympanic membrane, that is, a marginal perforation) or in the upper area of the tympanic membrane when it is pulled into the middle ear space because of negative pressure (due to ETD), causing what is called a *retraction pocket*. These growths have a smooth, white, pearl-like appearance and may eventually envelope the entire chain of ossicles.

Cholesteatoma is medically significant, not only because it can erode the chain of ossicles, but it could also enlarge superiorly and erode into the brain cavity. Cholesteatoma may possibly cause only a mild, conductive hearing loss. In part, this finding is explained by the fact that the cholesteatoma forms a bridge between the tympanic membrane and the inner ear, thus permitting mechanical transmission of energy. Typically, surgical removal of the cholesteatoma is performed with the likely outcome that the patient may require use of a hearing aid after its removal.

Otosclerosis

Otosclerosis is a progressive disorder of bone regrowth found solely in the bony walls of the inner ear (the bony labyrinth); it has as its primary clinical sign a progressive conductive hearing loss due to involvement and ultimate fixation of the stapes bone as it rests in the oval window membrane of the bony labyrinth. The typical onset of this disorder is in the third decade of life. The exact cause of otosclerosis is unknown although its histologic stages have been documented and described (Schuknecht, 1993; Goodhill, Harris, & Canalis, 2000). In otosclerosis, vascular and enzymatic activity initially degrade old, "good" bone, which is then replaced by new bone that is structurally different in its cellular content. This bone regrowth pattern does not affect all areas of the bony labyrinth equally or simultaneously, but rather, has sites of active involvement. The name for a site of involvement is a "focus."

When the focus of the otosclerotic neo-bone growth is at the footplate of the stapes bone, then it becomes clinically evident. Otosclerosis is a bilateral disorder; however, due to the eccentricities of the bone regrowth process, it usually does not demonstrate identical hearing loss in each ear. On audiometric testing, otosclerosis shows a progressive conductive hearing loss that can range from mild to a maximum conductive loss (60 dB). The severity of hearing loss is directly related to the degree of fixation of the stapes (Schuknecht, 1993). In the classical audiometric description of otosclerosis, there is relatively less conductive hearing loss at 2000 Hz, a finding called the **Carhart notch** in recognition of the audiologist who initially described it (Carhart, 1950). Persons with otosclerosis may be candidates for surgery that attempts to decrease the fixation of the stapes or to replace it with a prosthesis. In addition, a person with conductive hearing loss due to otosclerosis would function well with hearing aid amplification.

Consequences of Trauma: Ossicular Discontinuity

The three middle ear bones (malleus, incus, and stapes), which form the ossicular chain, laterally attach via the malleus in the tympanic membrane and terminate with the attachment of the stapes into the oval window membrane of the inner ear. In addition to these two attachments, there are two bone joints (one joining the malleus and incus; and the second joining the incus and stapes). This chain can be disrupted by trauma of different types, resulting in a discontinuity or disconnection. Because of the attachment in the tympanic membrane, any trauma to the tympanic membrane is a potential trauma also to the ossicles. In addition, a closed-head injury, especially one that results in a fracture of the temporal bone (the bone that houses the auditory system), may cause a disconnection of the ossicular chain. Typically, the site of the disconnection is the joint between the incus and the stapes. When there is a complete ossicular disconnection, there will be a maximum (60 dB) conductive hearing loss. Following the resolution of any acute aspects of the trauma, surgery to reconnect the ossicular chain can be considered.

Congenital Genetic Conditions

There are many well-documented, genetic syndromes that involve abnormalities of the outer and middle ears, with probable associated conductive hearing loss. A **syndrome** is a group of medical or physical characteristics that occur together with the same cause (Arnos et al., 1996), constituting a recognizable pattern in persons not related to one another. The suspicion of a syndrome is important because then, the presence of other features can be considered. In this way, the documentation of one feature of a syndrome often leads to the identification of other features. This type of information is valuable in considering the natural course and progression of the syndrome and, as appropriate, in genetic counseling.

As discussed earlier, anomalies of the outer ear with genetic etiology include microtia and atresia. Anomalies of the middle ear with genetic etiology include: absence of the middle ear itself; absence of ossicles; and ossicular malformations, such as abnormal fusion of ossicles and other bony abnormalities. Usually, these types of bony abnormalities will cause some degree of conductive hearing loss. There are many syndromes that involve the outer and middle ears (Toriello et al., 2004). Three example syndromes will be discussed because they demonstrate striking, multiple anomalies at both near and far body locations.

Branchio-oto-renal (BOR) Syndrome is an inherited condition that has been mapped to the EYA1 gene on human chromosome 8q13.3 (Kemperman et al., 2002). The clinical features of this syndrome are variable in their manifestation and include: conductive hearing loss due to ossicular abnormality or fixation; fistulas, cysts, and clefts along the distribution of the second branchial arch (roughly, on the neck); malformed auricles (microtia); and kidney involvement ranging from minor anomalies to possibly a complete absence of a kidney (renal agenesis). Abnormal bone structure of the auditory mechanism can also affect the bony labyrinth and therefore also cause problems in inner ear function.

Treacher Collins Syndrome is an inherited syndrome that has been mapped to the TCOF1 gene on the long arm of human chromosome 5. The clinical features include bilateral conductive hearing loss due to bilateral atresia and bilateral ossicular malformation or fixation; auricular malformations (microtia); abnormalities in the eyelids (coloboma); downward slanting eyelids; underdevelopment of the jaw; and cleft palate.

Apert Syndrome is one example of a group of syndromes involving craniosynostosis (abnormal skull bone fusion) with associated conductive hearing loss (Toriello et al., 2004). Syndromes with craniosynostosis have skull bone abnormalities (this, in part, explains the involvement of the middle ear structures) that include bulges in areas of the skull and widely spaced eyes. Apert Syndrome has the additional feature of having fused fingers and toes, a condition known as **syndactyly**.

CONDITIONS AFFECTING THE INNER EAR

Most communicatively significant hearing loss is attributable to a problem in the inner ear(s). The inner ear contains the sensory organs for both balance and hearing and therefore it is not unusual for a person to have both balance problems and hearing problems. The portion of the inner ear that contains the sensory organ for hearing is the cochlea. Hearing loss with its origin in the cochlea is specifically referred to as sensory hearing loss, although the broader term, sensorineural hearing loss (SNHL) is in greater general use. As a category, SNHL includes hearing loss due to dysfunction in the inner ear (the "sensori" part) as well as due to dysfunction along the hearing nerve pathway (the "neural" part).

Unlike the previously described conductive losses that have a maximum loss around 65 dB (HL), SNHL can range from very slight (25 dB) to profound (120 dB +) in terms of severity of loss. Again, unlike conductive hearing loss in which speech understanding remains unaffected and excellent, SNHL often has residual deficits in speech understanding. Unlike conductive hearing losses, which often have excellent medical or surgical interventions for the restoration of hearing, SNHL rarely is amenable to medical or surgical treatment that restores hearing, leaving electronic amplification as the treatment of choice. Accordingly, most candidates for hearing aid amplification have SNHL (Cheple, 1991).

SNHL may be congenital (that is, present at birth), early onset, delayed in onset, or may occur at any time during the person's lifetime. SNHL may affect one ear only (unilateral hearing loss) or both ears (bilateral hearing loss). SNHL may be due to genetic inheritance or due to the effects of acute trauma, infectious disease, or even as a consequence of certain medications. SNHL often occurs for reasons that cannot be explained, but which may be genetic in origin or due to an interaction of genetically determined susceptibility and environmental factors. SNHL can occur following excessive exposure to intense levels of sound/noise. Finally, SNHL occurs inevitably as an outcome of the natural aging process.

Congenital and Early-Onset Hearing Loss: Genetic and Environmental/Unknown Causes

Congenital and early-onset SNHL can be caused by many factors. Contemporary consensus suggests that approximately 50% of congenital or early-onset SNHL is due to genetic (inherited) causes, and the remaining 50% is caused by environmental or unknown factors (American College of Medical Genetics, 2002). It is likely that the "unknown" cause of today will be determined to be genetic, as advances continue in the genetic mapping of hearing loss.

A factor that complicates the understanding of inherited hearing loss specifically is the fact that there are several modes of inheritance: autosomal (recessive or dominant); sex-linked (typically, on X chromosome); mitochondrial; gross chromosomal (numerical or structural); and multigenic (multiple gene locations). Knowledge of mode of inheritance is an important component of genetic counseling. (See Arnos et al., 1996, for a more detailed discussion of modes of inheritance.) Regardless of type of causation or of mode of inheritance, SNHL can appear as one feature among other physical character-istics (syndromic) or it can appear as an isolated funding (nonsyndromic).

Genetic Cause: Syndromic Presentation

Approximately 30% of all inherited hearing loss appears as part of a syndrome (Van Laer, Cryns, Smith, & Van Camp, 2003). As stated earlier, a syndrome is a group of medical or physical characteristics that occur together. At this time, over 400 syn-dromes have been identified with hearing loss as a feature (Nance, 2003). Friedman et al. (2003) provided a summary of the molecular genetic information available for 109 of these syndromes.

The syndromic nature of hearing loss with many associated abnormalities suggests that a common cause exists either in a disruption in the timing of development or in the development of tissues that have a shared importance in development. Syndromic SNHL has been historically important because of demonstrable linkages to major or-gans or to other major body systems. In any given person with a syndrome, there is vari-ability in the number of abnormalities that appear and in the severity of the abnormality, often resulting in subtypes of a classic syndrome. Pendred Syndrome in-cludes early-onset SNHL and associated thyroid dysfunction. Usher Syndrome includes early-onset SNHL and progressive retinitis pigmentosa. Waardenberg Syndrome in-cludes SNHL and pigmentation abnormalities of skin, hair, and eyes. Alport Syndrome includes SNHL and kidney dysfunction. Jervell, Lange-Nielsen Syndrome includes SNHL and cardiac problems. Several of these syndromes have been the focus of intense research in gene mapping.

Genetic Cause: Nonsyndromic Presentation

Approximately 70% of all inherited hearing loss appears in isolation—that is, not part of a syndrome—and therefore is referred to as **nonsyndromic.** Approximately 80% of nonsyndromic SNHL is attributed to autosomal recessive transmission (Griffith and Friedman, 2002); that is, neither parent manifests the hearing loss but each parent con-tributed the same recessive gene for hearing loss. Much recent research has demon-strated that mutations in the gene GJB2 (located on chromosome 13q11.12) are responsible for 50% to 80% of all autosomal recessive SNHL (Tekin et al., 2001). GJB2 is instrumental in the construction of Connexin 26, a gap junction protein that is criti-cally important in the chemical activity (primarily, potassium recycling) of the sensory cells in the cochlea, specifically in the transportation of chemical ions across cell mem-branes. SNHL is also associated with mutations in other genes (CLDN14, KCNQ4, PDS) responsible for endolymph maintenance.

Mutations in additional genes have been identified that affect the construction of proteins responsible for the structural integrity and function of the cochlea. At least three genes (TECTA, COL11A2, and OTOA) have been implicated in abnormalities of the tectorial membrane resulting in SNHL, and still other genes (for example, MYO7A, MYO15) have been identified that are important for the physical integrity of the audi-tory hair cells (Van Laer, Cryns, Smith, and Van Camp, 2003). Clearly, our knowledge about the genetics of hearing loss is expanding on a daily basis. One of the additional outcomes of the genetics research is an enhanced fundamental understanding of the molecular and biochemical processes responsible for hearing.

Environmental/Unknown Causes

For children with congenital or early-onset SNHL, etiological factors fall into four categories: noxious prenatal influences (infections, maternal drug ingestion, exposure to environmental toxins); neonatal health status and treatment; postnatal acquired infections; and unknown.

Noxious prenatal influences known to cause SNHL include a variety of prenatal infections as well as maternal ingestion of certain medications. Prenatal infections (transmitted transplacentally from mother to fetus) include: toxoplasmosis; rubella; cytomegalovirus; herpes simplex virus; and syphilis (collectively known as TORCHES). All these infections, when acquired in utero, can cause SNHL in combination with multiple, medically significant abnormalities.

Cytomegalovirus (CMV) is the most common intrauterine infection and is stated to occur in 1% of all live births (Brookhouser, 2000). Because this virus has periods of latency, it may be asymptomatic at birth, although 10–15% of these infants will eventually develop SNHL. Children who are symptomatic at birth have a greater risk of developing SNHL. CMV is probably the leading cause of late-onset and progressive SNHL in children. Early detection of the virus followed by antiviral therapy has been shown to reduce the incidence and severity of SNHL in symptomatic neonates (NIDCD, 2002).

Maternal transmission of the rubella virus during the first two trimesters of pregnancy leads to the triad of congenital conditions known as congenital rubella syndrome (CRS): SNHL; cataracts; and heart disease. Since 1969, when a vaccine was developed, the incidence of SNHL secondary to maternal rubella has decreased in the United States and in other countries employing a vaccination program. The most recent prevaccine epidemic in the United States occurred in 1964–1965; it resulted in approximately 12,000 cases of SNHL (Trybus et al, 1980). In contrast, for the period 1990–2001, 121 cases of confirmed CRS were reported to the Center for Disease Control (Zimmerman and Reef, 2002a). CRS with SNHL can still occur in nonimmunized populations, and non-U.S.-born immigrants should be considered a population at risk for rubella (Zimmerman and Reef, 2001). Rubella and CRS remain a global concern, as 48% of the world's countries do not have a rubella vaccination program, resulting in an estimated 110,000 cases of CRS annually (Zimmerman and Reef, 2002a).

Congenital syphilis is a transplacentally transmitted consequence of acquired maternal syphilis. Congenital syphilis has two phases: early and late. In early congenital syphilis, there are multisystem abnormalities such as low birth weight, enlarged liver and spleen, a characteristic rash on the palms and soles, but SNHL or ear abnormalities are generally not prominent features (Burns and Meyerhoff, 1991). In late congenital syphilis, the number and onset of symptoms is variable across patients. SNHL has been observed to occur in 25% to 38% of persons with congenital syphilis with late childhood onset (Schuknecht, 1993). The presentation of SNHL may be sudden or fluctuating and may be asymmetrical with poorer than expected speech understanding scores. Accordingly, children with late-onset, progressive, or fluctuating SNHL should have a medical evaluation including laboratory testing for syphilis. In addition to

SNHL, late congenital syphilis has other characteristics including notched teeth, interstitial keratitis (an inflammation of the corneas), and various skeletal deformities. Due to an increase in the number of reported cases of syphilis in the late 1980s to early 1990s, it is likely that there will be an comparable increase in the number of cases of late congenital syphilis with SNHL in the early part of the 21st century. Syphilis is treatable with penicillin.

In addition to maternally transmitted infections, certain medications can cross the placenta and cause SNHL and other abnormalities in the developing fetus. These include: quinine; diphenyl hydantoin (Dilantin™); and isotretinoin (Accutane™). Because the negative effects of these medications are well known, physicians have to be vigilant and precautionary when prescribing them for women who are potentially childbearing. In addition, the effects of maternal exposure to environmental toxins, such as dioxin and polychlorinated biphenyls (PCBs), have been implicated in inner ear dysfunction.

It has been long recognized that a neonate with fragile health status is at greater risk for SNHL. Specific factors implicated in the development of SNHL in the medically fragile newborn include: low birth weight; prematurity; perinatal sepsis (infection); perinatal anoxia or hypoxia (oxygen deprivation); and kernicterus secondary to hyperbilirubinemia (deposition of poorly metabolized red blood cells in the cochlea and in the auditory nerve pathway). Ironically, some treatments for the fragile neonate may increase the risk to develop SNHL. For example, certain medications may save a neonate's life but coincidentally, damage that child's inner ears—that is, some medications have ototoxic effects.

Postnatal acquired infections, specifically, infection due to bacterial meningitis, has historically been a leading cause of infant mortality and in survivors, a major cause of severe-profound SNHL. Three types of bacteria account for the majority of cases of bacterial meningitis: Haemophilus influenzae, type B (also known as Hib); Neisseria meningitidis; and Streptococcus pneumoniae. Prior to the development of a Hib vaccine in 1985, 70% of all infant meningitis was due to Hib. In the United States prior to the vaccine, there were approximately 12,000 cases of Hib meningitis annually, with approximately 1000–3000 of the survivors with severe-profound bilateral SNHL. Subsequent to the Hib vaccine, less than 300 cases of meningitis due to Hib are reported annually in the United States (Brookhouser, 2000). Regardless of type of meningitis, the incidence of postmeningitic SNHL for survivors is 15–20%.

Finally, SNHL with unknown etiology will probably be demonstrated to be genetic in origin in most cases. However, there probably are also circumstances in which unaccountable, synergistic effects lead to SNHL.

Infectious Diseases Affecting the Inner Ear

In addition to meningitis as described above, there are other infectious disease entities that can enter the body and cause SNHL. These include: acquired syphilis ("otosyphilis"); herpes zoster oticus; and measles and mumps.

Much like Hib meningitis, the effectiveness and widespread application of the MMR (measles, mumps, rubella) vaccine has dramatically reduced the incidences of these viral diseases in the United States and by extension, the likelihood that SNHL will result.

Classically, mumps was well known for causing a severe-profound, unilateral SNHL. Because mumps vaccination is used in only 38% of the countries in the world, findings of mumps-caused SNHL may occur in nonvaccinated immigrant populations (Zimmerman & Reef, 2002b). Occurrences of these diseases may occur in families and communities that refuse vaccination (for example, in home-schooled children).

Herpes zoster oticus (also known as Ramsay Hunt syndrome) is caused by the varicella zoster virus that also causes chicken pox and leads to a classic presentation of intense otalgia, unilateral SNHL, dizziness, facial palsy, and the appearance of vesicles (blisters) on the auricle (Adour, 2000). It is relatively common with an estimated annual incidence of 5 cases per 100,000 persons. Because of their intense otalgia, patients with herpes zoster oticus are often difficult to test audiometrically as they are often intolerant of earphone placement or of probes in the ear canal as is necessary for many audiology tests.

Untreated acquired syphilis has three stages: primary, secondary, and tertiary. Between the secondary and tertiary stages is usually a long stage during which symptoms and disease progression are not apparent. Symptoms of SNHL and dizziness usually appear during the tertiary stage. Syphilis that affects the auditory system at this time is called otosyphilis. The SNHL of otosyphilis is typically progressive and possibly fluctuating, bilateral but asymmetrical, and accompanied by worse than expected speech understanding performance. Similar audiometric profiles are seen for patients with Ménière's disease and also with acoustic neuroma. For this reason, otosyphilis has been called "the great imitator."

Ototoxicity and Susceptibility to Ototoxicity

Ototoxicity (literally, ear poison) refers to the capacity for certain pharmacological agents (medications and chemical substances) to cause SNHL secondary to sensory cell damage and interference with inner ear metabolism. These medications have significant positive therapeutic benefit when used for their intended purposes; unfortunately, there are other unintended and undesirable effects in their application. Specifically, ototoxic drugs affect the inner ear and can cause SNHL, balance dysfunction, and tinnitus. These changes may be permanent and severe or may reverse with cessation of the medication. Although many substances have been shown to have potentially ototoxic effects, the emphasis in this review is on the four classes of substances that are in common medical therapeutic use.

Ototoxic drugs generally fall into four categories: antineoplastic drugs (example: cis-platinum, used in chemotherapy to inhibit/reduce growth of cancer cells/tumors); aminoglycoside antibiotics (historical example: streptomycin, used in tuberculosis treatment; common example: gentamycin or amikacin, used to combat bacteria infections/sepsis); loop diuretics (example: furosemide, used to promote excretion of urine); and analgesics and antimalarials (analgesic example: products containing salicylates [aspirin], used for pain and fever reduction; antimalarial example: quinine, historically used to treat malaria, now also used for reduction of blood-related leg cramps).

Cis-platinum is stated to be the most common ototoxic agent in common clinical use (Campbell et al., 2003a). Although the occurrence of cis-platinum ototoxicity is variable across patients taking it, a review of several studies by Schweitzer (1993) revealed that the majority of persons (62%) taking cis-platinum suffered some degree of ototoxic change. As with most ototoxic effects, the SNHL following cis-platinum begins and is most severe for the higher audiometric test frequencies, with involvement and progression toward lower frequencies. The SNHL is typically irreversible and may not be manifested for a few days following the cessation of the drug. Campbell et al. (2003b, 2003c) have reported on their promising work on "otoprotective" drugs that modify or prevent the SNHL associated with cis-platinum ototoxicity. At present, these drugs include glutathione ester (Campbell et al., 2003b) and D-methionine or D-met (Campbell et al., 2003c).

Aminoglycoside antibiotics cause SNHL by inhibiting the metabolism of potassium in the auditory hair cells and by affecting the structural interconnections ("tip-links") of the outer hair cells. The incidence of SNHL or balance dysfunction due to aminoglycoside ototoxicity is estimated to be 10% (Wackym, Storper, & Newman, 2000). Depending on the specific aminoglycoside antibiotic, the effect may be more on hearing, "cochleotoxic," or on balance, "vestibulotoxic," or on both. The ototoxic effects are typically bilateral and irreversible. Unless and until otoprotective drugs are developed, the utilization and additional development of alternative medications with adequate therapeutic effect but not ototoxicity will remain a focus in minimizing SNHL associated with aminoglycoside antibiotics.

Recently, Pandya et al. (1997) confirmed that the A1555G mutation in the mitochondrial 12S ribosomal RNA was associated with aminoglycoside antibiotic ototoxicity. In other words, this genetic mutation promotes susceptibility to ototoxicity. Because mitochondial DNA is inherited solely from the mother, the inheritance pattern is matrilineal—that is, the mother passes her mitochondrial DNA all her children.

Loop diuretics typically cause reversible bilateral, high-frequency SNHL and tinnitus. Changes appear to occur in the stria vascularis. Changes may be minimized by slow administration of the medication. Often, loop diuretics are used in patients with renal compromise and often also in combination with an aminoglycoside antibiotic, so synergistic effects of the medications to the conditions need to be considered.

Finally, it is well known that high dosages of salicylates (aspirin) and quinine cause reversible, bilateral, high-frequency SNHL and tinnitus. Although the exact mechanism for their effects and reversibility are unknown at this time, it is probable that these drugs temporarily interfere with the auditory hair cell metabolism.

Sudden Onset of Hearing Loss

The National Institute on Deafness and Other Communication Disorders (2004) estimated that there are 4000 new cases of sudden-onset hearing loss annually in the United States. Sudden-onset hearing loss is usually SNHL in nature, and if the cause is unknown, is called idiopathic sudden sensorineural hearing loss (ISSHL). In the majority of these cases, the exact cause is rarely uncovered. Typically, ISSHL presents unilaterally (that is, in one ear only) and can vary in degree of severity of hearing loss and also in degree of loss of speech understanding. In many cases, the patient will also experience balance problems. Physicians typically consider three possible causes: (1) a viral infection; (2) a vascular insult, such as a blood vessel occlusion; or (3) an inner ear membrane rupture (also known as a fistula).

Because causation is rarely known, treatment for ISSHL is multimodal, involving the simultaneous administration of different medications, usually an antibiotic drug, an anti-inflammatory drug and often, antiviral therapy. The use of anti-inflammatory medications (a 10-day, tapered, corticosteroid therapy) is a standard treatment procedure (Gates, 2000) but one that must be initiated soon after the onset of hearing loss for maximum potential effectiveness. Therefore, these patients are seen on highest priority in otology/audiology clinics. The majority of patients will experience partial or possibly complete recovery; however, one-third of the patients who experience sudden sensorineural hearing loss will show no recovery. Depending on the severity of the hearing loss and the speech understanding loss, hearing aid amplification may be useful.

Ménière's Disease/Endolymphatic Hydrops

Ménière's disease refers to a characteristic group of symptoms: unilateral and, typically, low-frequency SNHL; tinnitus, usually described as "roaring"; aural fullness or pressure; and balance problems/dizziness (true vertigo: a sensation described as "spinning"). Additionally, the person with Ménière's disease usually demonstrates reduced speech understanding performance. The National Institute on Deafness and Other Communication Disorders (2004) estimated that there are approximately 615,000 individuals diagnosed with Ménière's disease and an additional 45,000 new cases are diagnosed annually in the United States.

Other disorders may present with similar symptoms, but what is distinctive about Ménière's disease is that these symptoms appear in episodes; that is, a person with Ménière's disease may go for years without an episode or symptom. When symptoms occur, they may fluctuate in presentation and/or severity. A person with Ménière's disease may manifest all the symptoms (typical Ménière's disease), or solely have auditory symptoms (cochlear Ménière's disease) or solely have balance problems/vertigo (vestibular Ménière's disease). Although Ménière's disease usually presents unilaterally, in many patients, ultimately both ears are affected. The hearing status of the affected ear may progress to be nonfunctional. The episodic, debilitating, and unpredictable episodes of vertigo are anxiety provoking in many patients.

In Ménière's disease, the actual pathology is **endolymphatic hydrops,** which loosely means excess fluid in the endolymph. The endolymph is the fluid contained in the sensory organ sac (the membranous labyrinth), which bathes both the hearing organ (in the channel known as the scala media) and the various balance organ tissues (the semicircular canals, the utricle, and the saccule). Endolymph is initially secreted by the stria vascularis in the scala media and by the dark vestibular cells in the balance organs. Endolymph does not freely circulate within these spaces but all spaces have ducts (tubes) that direct their endolymph outflow into a common endolymphatic duct, terminating in the endolymphatic sac where the endolymph is metabolically processed ("resorbed"). The consequence of endolymphatic hydrops is that excessive pressure builds up and compromises the structures, integrity, and mechanical function of the inner ear.

In endolymphatic hydrops, there are two plausible explanations for why there is excess fluid present in the endolymph. Either too much endolymph is secreted or the outflow processing/resorption through the duct system and into the endolymphatic sac is impaired. Most otologic authorities favor the latter hypothesis, malabsorption

(Paparella et al., 1991; Lambert, 2000). The underlying cause for the occurrence of endolymphatic hydrops is currently unknown. There is no cure for Ménière's disease at this time. Medical management typically includes the use of medication (example: meclizine, sold as Antivert) for short-term suppression of vertigo and a long-term salt-restricted diet (Baloh, 2000). Supportive counseling and education concerning the natural history and progression of the disease is critical in the management of persons with Ménière's (Paparella et al., 1991). Surgical treatment employing an endolymphatic shunt has been controversial in that some surgeons and centers have reported successes, while many other surgeons and centers have not replicated those successes. The effectiveness of the surgery has been difficult to isolate because persons with Ménière's disease usually get better spontaneously. Still, the unpredictable episodes of vertigo prompt many patients to seek destructive surgeries solely for the remediation of their vertigo. One such example is the surgical placement of ototoxic medication directly into the balance organs (select chemical vestibulectomy) for the express purpose of destroying the balance organ tissues in the fluctuating and malfunctioning inner ear. While this procedure achieves its goal, it often also causes total hearing loss in that ear as well, and this risk has tempered the use of this procedure.

Hearing Loss Secondary to Noise Exposure

The auditory system can be damaged by exposure to intense levels of sound. Although the effects of exposure to injurious levels of sound could theoretically be evident across the auditory mechanism, generally, most damage secondary to extreme acoustic exposure affects the inner ear, causing a high-frequency SNHL. In theory, with precaution, preparation, and use of ear protection, such as earplugs, it is arguable that this hearing loss could be prevented or minimized (Ward, 1991).

Hearing loss secondary to extreme acoustic exposure typically has two damaging components. The first type of damage is mechanical and affects primarily the stereocilia of the outer hair cells of the inner ear followed by degeneration of auditory nerve fibers. The second type of damage is biochemical, which occurs also in the inner ear and is theorized to occur because the overstimulated inner ear system exceeds its capacity to maintain appropriate chemical balances.

In general, the hearing loss that follows an acute exposure to a brief but intense sound (impulse or impact noise, for example) is referred to as **acoustic trauma**. Hearing loss attributed to habitual exposure to intense sound is referred to as **noise-induced hearing loss (NIHL)**. In either case, the initial audiometric presentation shows bilateral SNHL particularly in the higher audiometric test frequencies, with 4000 Hz usually affected more. With continued exposure to injurious levels of sound, as in NIHL, the hearing loss worsens and affects adjacent test frequencies. In both acoustic trauma and NIHL, concomitant effects include worsening speech understanding and tinnitus.

Hearing loss secondary to occupational or military noise exposure is considered a monetarily compensable disability. Usually, the individual's audiometric test results are an important factor in determining the monetary value of the compensation. Again, because NIHL can theoretically be minimized or prevented, employers and government agencies usually engage in hearing conservation programs intended to minimize hearing loss and its attendant costs.

Hearing Loss Associated with Aging (Presbycusis)

Hearing loss is common (prevalent) in older persons. It is extremely likely that everyone has an older relative or acquaintance with whom communication is difficult because that person cannot hear adequately. In one of a series of studies on older adults in Beaver Dam, Wisconsin, Cruickshanks et al. (1998) established that 46% of adults aged 48–92 years of age had hearing loss. Furthermore, the chance that a person had hearing loss significantly increased with increased age; that is, the older the person, the more likely they were to have hearing loss. Additionally, hearing loss was found to be more common in older males than in older females. In a follow-up study of the occurrence (incidence rate) of hearing loss in older adults, Cruickshanks et al. (2003) established that 21% of older adults whose initial hearing ability was categorized as without hearing loss declined sufficiently over a five-year period to be categorized as with hearing loss. In this same study, over 50% of persons who initially were categorized as with hearing loss suffered additional declines in their hearing over a five-year period. Therefore, in older persons, hearing loss is common and worsening of hearing ability is likely as a person gets older.

In a review of data available from the Administration on Aging (2004), the population of persons aged 65 and over years of age in the United States increased 11-fold in the 100 years from 1900 to 2000. In 2000, there were approximately 35 million persons aged 65 years and older; this number is projected to more than double to 71 million persons by the year 2030. Considering the prevalence of hearing loss (46%, conservatively) and the incidence rate of hearing loss (21%) in this population, it seems clear that significant challenges and opportunities lie ahead for audiologists and hearing care professionals who work with older adults.

Presbycusis (literally, old hearing) is the name for the hearing loss that occurs as a person ages. Another term seen in current scientific literature is **age-related hearing loss (ARHL)**. The aging person represents the sum of all natural aging changes (for example, decline in muscle tone and mass; changes in skin elasticity) as well as the accumulation of all diseases, toxins, and trauma suffered over the course of a lifetime. Accordingly, presbycusis is attributed to the cumulative and synergistic effects of the natural aging process with a variety of risk factors. In another Beaver Dam study, Wiley et al. (2001) attempted to isolate the contribution of the natural aging process by excluding several significant risk factors for hearing loss, and in fact, advanced age alone was found to be associated with increased likelihood of the presence of hearing loss. In addition to this age-only effect, there are several significant risk factors for hearing loss, which include: prior exposure to injurious levels of sound/noise; certain medical conditions, especially previous ear disease and ear surgery; cardiovascular disease; past pharmaceutical use, especially ototoxic drugs; and smoking. Other factors whose contributions are unclear at this time include: the influences of other physical and medical conditions (for example: diet; diabetes; high blood pressure; and other physical stressors); and genetic disposition.

Regardless of the exact cause, these changes affect all components and tissues of the auditory system. The most significant hearing-related changes involve structures in the inner ear. The sensory cells of the inner ear lack the capacity for significant repair, so degrading change and damage are irreversible. The classic description of the physical and pathological changes that occur in presbycusis comes from a series of reports, summarized in Schuknecht (1993), which correlated hearing test information to physical findings of temporal bones. Schuknecht (1993) described several types of presbycusis based on the areas in the inner ear where the greatest degradation and changes were observed. For example, sensory presbycusis is a description of inner ear changes primarily to the sensory cells (outer hair cells); strial presbycusis is a description of changes primarily to the stria vascularis; and neural presbycusis describes changes to the neural fibers that originate in the inner ear. Significantly, persons with neural presbycusis typically had poorer speech understanding abilities in life.

The typical audiometric presentation of presbycusis is a gradual onset of a slowly progressive, bilateral SNHL, with poorer hearing sensitivity in the higher frequencies and often accompanied by reduced speech understanding. In part because of the typical gradual onset of hearing loss, persons with a hearing loss due to aging are often unaware of or are reluctant to acknowledge their changing hearing. This has inevitably negative social and familial consequences.

The treatment of a person with presbycusis begins with the recognition and acceptance of the condition by the person with their willingness to take positive action to deal with it. Counseling and education for the person and significant family/others can initially focus on their problems with proposals for remedies for those problems. It is likely that an older person with hearing loss would benefit from some combination of the use of amplification devices (assistive listening devices for telephone, television; personal hearing aids), training in compensatory and coping skills, and participation in support groups, such as SHHH for social support, advocacy, and additional education.

CONDITIONS AFFECTING THE AUDITORY NERVE AND PATHWAY TO BRAIN

The nerve that begins in the inner ear and exits the bony inner ear through the internal auditory canal to travel into the brainstem of the central nervous system is known as the acoustic nerve (the VIIIth cranial nerve, sometimes shown as 8th nerve). The VIIIth cranial nerve actually consists of three discrete nerve bundles: one from the cochlea (for hearing); and two from the vestibular system (for balance). Upon entering the brainstem, the nerve bundles separate to travel to their different terminations within the nervous system. Information in the hearing nerve pathway traverses the brainstem and midbrain and continues along to the brain. Sensorineural hearing loss that is attributed to dysfunction in this nerve network is referred to as **retrocochlear** (literally, behind the cochlea) hearing loss. Retrocochlear hearing loss has two general causes: (1) tumors or other masses affecting the acoustic nerve; and (2) neurodegenerative disorders, which interfere with efficient transmission along the nerve network.

Acoustic Nerve Tumors

The generally used, but not exactly accurate, name for the most common neoplasm that affects the acoustic nerve is **acoustic neuroma**. This name is inaccurate for several reasons. First, the growth itself usually arises from one of the vestibular (balance) nerves of the VIIIth cranial nerve, not the hearing (acoustic) nerve bundle. Second, the origin of the neoplasm is not the entire nerve, but rather, the origin is from the cells that provide the covering of the nerve; these cells are known as Schwann cells, so technically, a neoplasm from the Schwann cells would be a **schwannoma**. Finally, this type of neoplasm is not a malignancy (a cancer) as "-oma" may imply; however, even the growth of benign tissue in spaces it's not designed for can and usually does cause problems. An expanding acoustic neuroma can press against adjacent structures (for example, the VIIth cranial nerve/the facial nerve: the nerve that animates the face) and compromise their function. Ultimately, an enlarging acoustic neuroma could compress the brainstem, in which case, it would seriously compromise vital life functions and thus, be lethal.

Acoustic neuromas have an incidence of 1/100,000 in the general population and they account for 10% of all intracranial neoplasms and specifically, upwards of 75% of all neoplasms in the area of the skull base known as the cerebellopontine angle (Schuknecht, 1993). Generally, the treatment of an acoustic neuroma is surgical removal or reduction. Magnetic resonance imaging (MRI), enhanced with gadolinium, is the diagnostic tool of choice for the physician. Advances and availability of MRI have resulted in the identification of very small (completely within the internal auditory canal, or intracanalicular) acoustic neuromas that in turn lead to improved outcomes with surgery. Other neoplasms in the cerebellopontine angle include meningiomas (benign neoplasms arising from meningeal tissues) and epidermoid tumors (similar to cholesteatoma, described earlier).

In most cases with acoustic neuroma and other neoplasm at the cerebellopontine angle, the clinical presentation may include a unilateral tinnitus, a progressive, unilateral/asymmetrical (that is, worse in one ear) sensorineural hearing loss, poor speech understanding, and balance dysfunction. In some cases, there may be indications of involvement of the facial nerve (for example: weakness of facial muscles) on the same side as the tumor. The cause of the typical acoustic neuroma is unknown at present.

When patients present with bilateral acoustic neuromas, the underlying cause is usually **neurofibromatosis**, type 2 (NF2), an inherited/genetically transmitted condition that causes multiple neuromas, typically on sensory nerves in the head as well as in the spinal cord. Treatment for the neoplasms caused by NF2 is surgical reduction of tumors with attempts to preserve facial nerve function and hearing. Generally, the prognosis for the retention of serviceable hearing in NF2 is poor, with or without surgery. When NF2 affects both hearing nerves, the functional connections to the brain are lost and even the use of conventional hearing aid amplification would be useless. One option is the use of an Auditory Brainstem Implant or ABI that would bypass the cochlea and the auditory nerve and serve to provide direct neural stimulation into the brainstem.

Auditory Neuropathy/Auditory Dyssynchrony

Auditory neuropathy/auditory dyssynchrony is a label for the generic condition in which the outer hair cells of the inner ear function within normal limits, but the medial primary auditory neuron segments do not (Starr et al., 1996; Berlin, Hood, & Rose, 2001). A variety of potential etiologies have been implicated in auditory neuropathy/auditory dyssynchrony, and therefore, at present, this is a challenging disorder to accurately characterize. Complicating this discussion is an evolving nomenclature (Rapin &

Gravel, 2006) seeking to correlate test findings and labels to specific pathologies and sites of pathologies in the auditory system. For example, recent advances in imaging technology have documented a condition called cochlear nerve deficiency in which auditory neuropathy is seen in persons with absent or small cochlear nerves as verified by magnetic resonance imaging (Buchman et al., 2006). It is likely that further advances in imaging studies, as well as in genetic mapping, will lead to greater clarification of auditory neuropathy/auditory dyssynchrony.

Other Nerve Conditions

A variety of medical and physical conditions can affect the auditory nerve pathway in the brainstem and brain, resulting in retrocochlear hearing loss/balance dysfunction. Generally, systemic disease or pathology of the brainstem and brain will have multiple effects, of which hearing loss/balance dysfunction may be considered relatively insignificant. Some causes of retrocochlear hearing loss/balance dysfunction have already been discussed and include: trauma to temporal bone; infectious disease (meningitis); otosyphilis; vascular disorders (example: vertebrobasilar artery insufficiency); and neurodegenerative conditions, especially demyelinating disorders that compromise transmission along the nerve pathways (example: multiple sclerosis). The audiometric presentation of the above disorders will be variable, typically asymmetrical, and often fluctuant. Audiometric procedures that are sensitive to neural transmission (namely, the auditory brainstem response test—see Chapter 7) will typically demonstrate test abnormalities.

(Central) Auditory Processing Disorders

Another disorder that is uniquely different from those just described is called a (central) auditory processing disorder [(C)APD]. (C)APD is a deficit that is manifested as some deficit in the processing of acoustic stimuli. This deficit is etiologically distinct from higher-level language and cognitive problems; however, (C)APD may coexist with deficits in other modalities. (C)APD may be observed in conjunction with an organic disease such as a lesion or tumor in the brain stem or in the cortical regions of the auditory nervous system. However, it is more commonly seen in children with normal peripheral hearing sensitivity but with neuromaturational delays or morphological disorders involving underdeveloped or misshapen cells in the auditory cortex (Musiek & Gollegly, 1988). ASHA (2005) recently prepared a position statement that defines this disorder as follows:

> (Central) auditory processing disorder [(C)APD] refers to difficulties in the processing of auditory information in the central nervous system (CNS) as demonstrated by poor performance in one or more of the following skills: sound localization and lateralization; auditory discrimination; auditory pattern recognition; temporal aspects of audition, including temporal integration, temporal discrimination (e.g., temporal gap detection), temporal ordering, and temporal masking; auditory performance in competing acoustic signals(including dichotic listening); and auditory performance with degraded acoustic signals.

Following a detailed assessment to determine the specific skills that are affected, a treatment plan is determined to assist with minimizing or overcoming the effects of the disorder. Speech-language pathologists are often involved in remediation focusing on different forms of listening training, computer-assisted therapy programs, or sound reinforcement in the classroom.

SUMMARY

A Glimpse into the Profession Revisited

In Caitlin's case, pure tone air and bone conduction audiometry revealed a 35-dB conductive hearing loss across all test frequencies, suggesting that her inner ear function was normal in each ear but that there was a problem in the outer or middle ears. Additional testing utilizing measures of acoustic immittance (tympanometry) revealed poorly functioning middle ear systems bilaterally. An examination by an otolaryngologist revealed that Caitlin had bilateral otitis media with effusion (OME) that was characterized as "glue ear." Caitlin had accumulated noninfected fluid in her middle ear cavities that thickened, resulting in poor mobility of the tympanic membrane and middle ear ossicles in each ear, with the consequence of a mild-to-moderate hearing loss. In Caitlin's case, there existed a medical remedy for her condition. Surgical placement of pressure equalizing tubes (PETs) was performed. Postoperative hearing testing revealed that Caitlin was hearing well within normal limits and now asks her parents to talk softer. This case demonstrates that nonsuppurative OME can exist without obvious medical symptoms. In Caitlin's case, the only outward manifestation of her ear pathology was hearing loss that was subtle and probably gradual in onset. Had her parents not been so observant, her ear pathology could have silently continued to progress, possibly causing significant damage to the tissues of her ear as well as adjacent structures.

CHAPTER REVIEW

- ❏ A wide variety of conditions and pathologies can affect the auditory system and, consequently, cause hearing loss. On occasion, hearing loss is a sign that a serious health problem exists that requires prompt and aggressive medical care.

- ❏ Hearing loss may be congenital (that is, present at birth), early-onset, delayed in onset, or may occur at any time during the person's lifetime.

- ❏ Hearing loss may affect one ear only (unilateral hearing loss) or both ears (bilateral hearing loss).

- ❏ Hearing loss may be due to genetic inheritance; the effects of acute or continuous trauma; or infectious disease; it even may be as a consequence of certain medications.

- ❏ Hearing loss often occurs for reasons that cannot be explained, but which may be genetic in origin or due to an interaction of genetically determined susceptibility and environmental factors.

- ❏ Finally, hearing loss occurs inevitably as an outcome of the natural aging process.

- ❏ In the majority of cases, especially with sensorineural hearing loss, there are no suitable medical remedies, and therefore, regardless of the cause, the treatment for hearing loss is counseling/education and the provision of amplification devices, such as hearing aids.

ACTIVITIES FOR DISCUSSION

❑ In the Case Study, what was the primary indication that Caitlin had a problem? What are the implications of this type of indication?

❑ What disorders primarily affect the outer and middle ears?

❑ What disorders primarily affect the inner ear?

❑ What disorders are more significant for children?

❑ What disorders are more likely to be found in adults?

REFERENCES

Administration on Aging (2004). Statistics on the aging population.

Adour, K. (2000). Inflammatory disorders of the facial nerve: Bell's palsy, Ramsay Hunt syndrome, otitis media, and Lyme disease. In R. Canalis & P. Lambert (Eds.), *The Ear: Comprehensive Otology* (pp.719–734). Philadephia: Lippincott Williams and Wilkins.

American Academy of Family Physicians (2004). Clinical practice guideline: Otitis media with effusion. 1–64.

American Academy of Family Physicians & American Academy of Pediatrics (2004). Diagnosis and management of acute otitis media, 1–36.

American College of Medical Genetics—Genetic Evaluation of Congenital Hearing Loss Expert Panel (2002). Genetics evaluation guidelines for the etiologic diagnosis of congenital hearing loss. *Genetics in Medicine,* Vol. 4, No. 3, 162–171.

American Speech-Language-Hearing Association (2005). (Central) Auditory Processing Disorders—The Role of the Audiologist [Position statement]. http://www.asha.org/members/deskref-journals/deskref/default

Arnos, K., Israel, J., Devlin, L. & Wilson, M. (1996). Genetic aspects of hearing loss in children. In F. Martin & J. Clark (Eds.), *Hearing Care in Children* (pp. 20–44). Needham Heights: Allyn and Bacon.

Ator, G., Jenkins, H., Becker, D., & Canalis, R. (2000). Acoustic neuroma and other tumors of the cerebellopontine angle. In R. Canalis & P. Lambert (Eds.), *The Ear: Comprehensive Otology* (pp. 847–867). Philadelphia: Lippincott Williams and Wilkins.

Baloh, R. (2000). Vertigo of peripheral origin. In R. Canalis & P. Lambert (Eds.), *The Ear: Comprehen-sive Otology* (pp. 647–664). Philadephia: Lippincott Williams and Wilkins.

Berlin, C., Hood, L., & Rose, K. (2001). On renaming auditory neuropathy as auditory dys-synchrony. *Audiology Today, 13,* 15–17.

Bluestone, C. (1991). Diseases and disorders of the Eustachian tube—middle ear. In M. Paparella, D. Shumrick, J. Gluckman, & W. Meyerhoff, *Otolaryngology* (3rd ed.) (pp. 1289–1315). Philadephia: Saunders.

Brookhouser, P. (2000). Nongenetic sensorineural hearing loss in children. In R. Canalis & P. Lambert (Eds.), *The Ear: Comprehensive Otology* (pp. 489–510). Philadephia: Lippincott Williams and Wilkins.

Brown, O., & Meyerhoff, W. (1991). Diseases of the tympanic membrane. In M. Paparella, D. Shumrick, J. Gluckman, & W. Meyerhoff (1991). *Otolaryngology* (3rd ed.) (pp. 1271–1288). Philadephia: Saunders.

Buchman, C., Roush, P., Teagle, H., Brown, C., Zdanski, C., & Grose, J. (2006). Auditory neuropathy characteristics in children with cochlear nerve deficiency. *Ear & Hearing, 27,* 399–408.

Burns, D., & Meyerhoff, W. (1991). Granulomatous disorders and related conditions of the ear and temporal bone. In M. Paparella, D. Shumrick, J. Gluckman, & W. Meyerhoff, (1991). *Otolaryngology* (3rd ed.) (pp. 1529–1559). Philadephia: Saunders.

Campbell, K., Larsen, D., Meech, R., Rybak, L., & Hughes, L. (2003a). Glutathione ester but not glutathione protects against cisplatin-induced ototoxicity in a rat model. *J Am Acad Audiol, 14,* 124–133.

Campbell, K., Meech, R., Rybak, L., & Hughes, L. (2003b). The effect of D-methionine on cochlear oxidative state with and without cisplatin administration: mechanisms of otoprotection. *J Am Acad Audiol, 14,* 144–156.

Campbell, K., Kelly, E., Targovnik, N., Hughes, L., Van Saders, C., Gottlieb, A., Dorr, M., & Leighton, A. (2003c). Audiologic monitoring for potential ototoxicity in a phase I clinical trial of a new glycopeptide antibiotic. *J Am Acad Audiol, 14,* 157–168.

Canalis, R., & Lambert, P. (2000a). Acute suppurative otitis media and mastoiditis. In R. Canalis & P. Lambert (Eds.), *The Ear: Comprehensive Otology* (pp. 397–408). Philadephia: Lippincott Williams and Wilkins.

Canalis, R., & Lambert, P. (2000b). Chronic otitis media and cholesteatoma. In R. Canalis & P. Lambert (Eds.), *The Ear: Comprehensive Otology* (pp. 409–431). Philadelphia: Lippincott Williams and Wilkins.

Canalis, R., Abemayor, E., & Shulman, J. (2000). Blunt and penetrating injuries to the ear and temporal bone. In R. Canalis & P. Lambert (Eds.), *The Ear: Comprehensive Otology* (pp. 785–800). Philadephia: Lippincott Williams and Wilkins.

Carhart, R. (1950). Clinical application of bone conduction. *Arch. Otol., 51,* 798–807.

Cheple, M. (1991). Hearing aids. In M. Paparella, D. Shumrick, J. Gluckman, & W. Meyerhoff. *Otolaryngology* (3rd ed.) (pp. 1017–1024). Philadephia: Saunders.

Cruickshanks, K., Tweed, T., Wiley, T., Klein, B., Klein, R., Chappell, R., Nondahl, D., & Dalton, D. (2003). The 5-year incidence and progression of hearing loss: The epidemiology of hearing loss study. *Arch Otolaryngol, 129,* 1041–1046.

Cruickshanks, K., Wiley, T., Tweed, T., Klein, B., Klein, R., Mares-Perlman, J., & Nondahl, D. (1998). Prevalence of hearing loss in older adults in Beaver Dam, Wisconsin. The Epidemiology of Hearing Loss Study. *Am J Epidemiol, 148,* 879–886.

Friedman, T., Schultz, J., Ben-Yosef, T., Pryor, S., Lagziel, A., Fisher, R., Wilcox, E., Riazuddin, S., Ahmed, Z., Belyantseva, I., & Griffith, A. (2003). Recent advances in the understanding of syndromic forms of hearing loss. *Ear & Hearing, 24,* 289–302.

Gates, G. (2000). Sudden sensorineural hearing loss. In R. Canalis & P. Lambert (Eds.), *The Ear: Comprehensive Otology* (pp. 523–536). Philadephia: Lippincott Williams and Wilkins.

Goodhill, V., Harris, I., & Canalis, R. (2000). Otosclerosis. In R. Canalis & P. Lambert (Eds.), *The Ear:*

Comprehensive Otology (pp. 467–487). Philadephia: Lippincott Williams and Wilkins.

Griffith, A., & Friedman, T. (2002). Autosomal and X-Linked Auditory Disorders. In B. Keats, A. Popper, & R. Fay (Eds.), *Genetics and Auditory Disorders* (pp. 121–227). New York: Springer-Verlag.

Handler, S., & Magardino, T. (2000). Otitis media with effusion. In R. Canalis & P. Lambert (Eds.), *The Ear: Comprehensive Otology* (pp. 383–396). Philadephia: Lippincott Williams and Wilkins.

Hashisaki, G. (2000). Complications of chronic otitis media. In R. Canalis & P. Lambert (Eds.), *The Ear: Comprehensive Otology* (pp. 433–445). Philadephia: Lippincott Williams and Wilkins.

Hough, J., & McGee, M. (1991). Otologic trauma. In M. Paparella, D. Shumrick, J. Gluckman, & W. Meyerhoff, *Otolaryngology* (3rd ed.) (pp. 1137–1160). Philadephia: Saunders.

Kemperman, M., Stinckens, C., Kumar, S., Joosten, F., Huygen, P., & Cremers, C. (2002). The branchio-oto-renal syndrome. In C. Cremers & R. Smith (Eds), *Genetic Hearing Impairment* (pp. 192–200). Basel: Karger.

Kryzer, T., & Lambert, P. (2000). Diseases of the external auditory canal. In R. Canalis, & P. Lambert (Eds.), *The Ear: Comprehensive Otology* (pp. 341–357). Philadephia: Lippincott Williams and Wilkins.

Lambert, P. (2000). History and physical examination of a patient with dizziness. In R. Canalis & P. Lambert (Eds.), *The Ear: Comprehensive Otology* (pp. 167–179). Philadephia: Lippincott Williams and Wilkins.

Lane, H. (1992). *The Mask of Benevolence.* New York: Knopf.

Maceri, D., & Lambert, P. (2000). Management of congenital aural atresia. In R. Canalis & P. Lambert (Eds.), *The Ear: Comprehensive Otology* (pp. 359–370). Philadephia: Lippincott Williams and Wilkins.

Mattox, D., Nager, G., & Levin, L. (1991). Congenital aural atresia: embryology, pathology, classification, genetics, and surgical management. In M. Paparella, D. Shumrick, J. Gluckman, & W. Meyerhoff. *Otolaryngology* (3rd ed.) (pp. 1191–1225). Philadephia: Saunders.

Musiek, F., & Baran, J. (2007). *The Auditory System.* Boston: Pearson.

Musiek, F., & Gollegly, K. (1988). Maturational considerations in the neuroauditory evaluation of children. In F. Bess (Ed.), *Hearing Impairment in Children* (pp. 231–250). Parkton: York.

Nance, W. (2003). The genetics of deafness. *Mental Retardation and Dev Dis Res Rev, 9,* 109–119.

National Institute on Deafness and Other Communication Disorders (2002). NIDCD Workshop on congenital cytomegalovirus infection and hearing loss.

National Institute on Deafness and Other Communication Disorders (2004). Statistics about hearing disorders, ear infections, and deafness.

Pandya, A., Xia, X., Radnaabazar, J., Batsuuri, J., Dangaansuren, B., Odgerel, D., Fischel-Ghodsian, N., & Nance, W. (1997). Mutation in the mitochondrial 12S rRNA gene in two families from Mongolia with matrilineal aminoglycoside ototoxicity. *J Med Genetics, 34,* 169–172.

Paparella, M., Da Costa, S., Fox, R., & Yoon, T. (1991). Ménière's disease and other labyrinthine diseases. In M. Paparella, D. Shumrick, J. Gluckman, & W. Meyerhoff, *Otolaryngology* (3rd ed.) (pp. 1689–1714). Philadephia: Saunders.

Rapin, I., & Gravel, J. (2006). Auditory neuropathy: A biologically inappropriate label unless acoustic nerve involvement is documented. *J Amer Acad Audiology, 17,* 147–150.

Ruder, R. (2000). Reconstruction of the congenitally deformed auricle. In R. Canalis & P. Lambert (Eds.), *The Ear: Comprehensive Otology.* (pp. 371–381). Philadephia: Lippincott Williams and Wilkins.

Sajjadi, H., Paparella, M., & Canalis, R. (2000). Presbycusis. In R. Canalis & P. Lambert (Eds.), *The Ear: Comprehensive Otology.* (pp. 545–557). Philadephia: Lippincott Williams and Wilkins.

Saunders, G., & Haggard, M. (1989). The clinical assessment of obscure auditory dysfunction—1. Auditory and psychological factors. *Ear & Hearing, 10,* 200–208.

Saunders, G., & Haggard, M. (1993). The influence of personality-related factors upon consultation for two different "marginal" organic pathologies with and without reports of auditory symptomatology. *Ear & Hearing, 14,* 242–248.

Schuknecht, H. (1993). *Pathology of the Ear.* Philadelphia: Waverly.

Schweitzer, V. (1993). Ototoxicity of chemotherapeutic agents. *Otolarngol Clin North America, 26,* 759–789.

Shulman, J., Lambert, P. & Goodhill, V. (2000). Acoustic trauma and noise-induced hearing loss. In R. Canalis & P. Lambert (Eds.), *The Ear:*

Comprehensive Otology (pp. 773–783). Philadephia: Lippincott Williams and Wilkins.

Smith, M., & Canalis, R. (2000). Otosyphilis and otologic manifestation of AIDS. In R. Canalis & P. Lambert (Eds.), *The Ear: Comprehensive Otology* (pp. 587–599). Philadephia: Lippincott Williams and Wilkins.

Starr, A., Picton, T., Sininger, Y., Hood, L., & Berlin C. (1996). Auditory neuropathy. *Brain, 119,* 741–753.

Storper, I., Canalis, R., & Lambert, P. (2000). Diseases of the auricle and periauricular region. In R. Canalis & P. Lambert (Eds.), *The Ear: Comprehensive Otology* (pp. 325–339). Philadephia: Lippincott Williams and Wilkins.

Tekin, M., Arnos, K., & Pandya, A. (2001). Advances in hereditary deafness. *Lancet, 358,* 1082–1090.

Toriello, H., Reardon, W. & Gorlin, R. (2004). *Hereditary Hearing Loss and its Syndromes.* New York: Oxford.

Trybus, R., Karchmer, M., Kerstetter, P., & Hicks, W. (1980). The demographics of deafness resulting from maternal rubella. *Am Ann Deaf, 125,* 977–984.

Van Laer, L., Cryns, K., Smith, R., & Van Camp, G. (2003). Nonsyndromic hearing loss. *Ear & Hearing, 24,* 275–288.

Wackym, P., Storper, I., & Newman, A. (2000). Cochlear and vestibular ototoxicity. In R. Canalis & P. Lambert (Eds.), *The Ear: Comprehensive Otology* (pp. 571–585). Philadephia: Lippincott Williams and Wilkins.

Ward, W. (1991). Noise-induced hearing damage. In M. Paparella, D. Shumrick, J. Gluckman, & W. Meyerhoff. *Otolaryngology* (3rd ed.) (pp. 1639–1652). Philadephia: Saunders.

Wiley, T., Torre, P., Cruickshanks, K., Nondahl, D., & Tweed, T. (2001). Hearing sensitivity in adults screened for selected risk factors. *J Am Acad Audiol, 12,* 337–347.

Zimmerman L., & Reef, S. (2001). Incidence of congenital rubella syndrome at a hospital serving a predominantly Hispanic population, El Paso, Texas. *Pediatrics, 107* (3), e40.

Zimmerman, L., & Reef, S. (2002a). Congenital rubella syndrome. In *Manual for the Surveillance of Vaccine-Preventable Diseases* (3rd ed.). Atlanta: Center for Disease Control and Prevention.

Zimmerman, L., & Reef, S. (2002b). Mumps. In *Manual for the Surveillance of Vaccine-Preventable Diseases.* (3rd ed.). Atlanta: Center for Disease Control and Prevention.

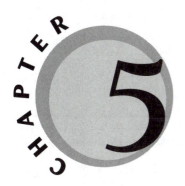

Characteristics of Hearing Impairment

Key Terms

CASE STUDY

A Glimpse into the Profession

Brian is a four-year-old who became seriously ill one night. He was rushed to the hospital and subsequently diagnosed with a severe case of bacterial meningitis. He recovered from the meningitis, but his physician indicated that a potential consequence of this serious disease can be a significant hearing loss. He was referred to the local audiologist for an evaluation. Behavioral testing was performed using special test techniques and a significant hearing loss was identified. Additional testing was performed that confirmed the validity of this finding and helped identify the type of impairment. This chapter will specifically look at how Brian's hearing loss can be characterized for identification and diagnostic purposes and to determine treatment and the long-term impact of the impairment.

DEFINING HEARING MEASUREMENT

The previous chapters have established a basic foundation for service provision to the hearing impaired by identifying the audiology providers, describing the people affected with hearing impairment, detailing the characteristics of sound and how sound is processed through the hearing mechanism, and finally, describing common diseases and conditions that affect hearing ability. Prior to discussing identification and evaluation procedures, the descriptors used to characterize hearing loss first need to be understood.

There are four basic parameters that are used to describe an individual's hearing sensitivity and/or concomitant hearing impairment. These parameters are:

Degree of hearing loss—The intensity level at which a person perceives sound; when outside the range of normal, this indicates the severity of the impairment

Configuration of hearing loss—The degree of loss across test frequencies; on a graphical display, this is the shape of the hearing loss pattern

Type of hearing loss—The characteristic that indicates the location or structure within the hearing mechanism that is causing the impairment

Symmetry of hearing loss—A comparison of the test results between the two ears

Obtaining these four key fundamental parameters is the first goal of an audiological evaluation in order to make a complete and accurate diagnosis of hearing loss. Because hearing loss is characterized based on the audiometric test results, it is necessary to understand the format by which hearing sensitivity is measured and visually displayed.

The Threshold of Hearing

As shown in Chapter 2, the complex auditory system is capable of detecting incredibly small sound pressure waves. It is also a system with a very large dynamic range. The goal of audiometric testing is to assess hearing sensitivity in response to the lowest possible sound pressure—what perceptually would be the softest sound level that is still audible. Listening to sounds that can only just be detected is referred to as **threshold of audibility**. The threshold of audibility as defined by the American National Standards Institute (ANSI) S3.20-1973 (R1986) is "The minimum effective sound pressure level of an acoustic signal producing an auditory sensation for a specified number of trials" (Yantis, 1994). The measurement of true auditory thresholds is actually based on a number of factors that include, but are not limited to, testing procedures used; whether or not the ears are tested separately or together; whether the stimulus is presented through head phones, insert earphones placed inside the ear canal, or speakers; and the alertness and perception of the individual during the testing procedure.

The ability of the human ear to differentiate small changes in the intensity of a sound is somewhat variable. Therefore, in conventional hearing testing, a threshold is approximated using a test interval of 5 dB instead of a smaller increment in order to improve the efficiency of the test results in delineating the presence or absence of a tone. The decibel values at which thresholds are established then determine the level of hearing sensitivity and subsequently the degree of hearing impairment (ASHA, 2005). Although different types of stimuli can be used to identify a hearing threshold, the most fundamental sound is a single frequency or pure tone. The simplicity of this stimulus provides a discreet measurement of several hearing thresholds across the frequency spectrum of sound.

Audiometric Zero

We have all heard the question, If a tree falls in the forest, does it make a sound even if there is no one there to hear it? This question is of interest to us because it serves to illustrate the difference between the level of actual physical sound pressure that is generated from a vibration (e.g., the tree falling), and the level at which that sound is heard by a human ear.

From the discussion in Chapter 2, it is understood that the intensity dimension of sound is measured using decibels, and that the measurement scale called **sound pressure level** is used as a reference for the physical presence of a sound, abbreviated dBSPL. However, the measurement of a given sound pressure level does not necessarily infer that the human ear can hear that sound. As indicated, the threshold of audibility is the softest level at which a sound can be detected, or the **absolute senstivity**. This sensitivity level varies as a function of sound transfer in the conductive portion of the ear as well as the equipment and psychophysical process used in testing. Figure 5.1 displays a curve of audibility thresholds across the frequency dimension plotted in sound pressure level and is referred to as minimum audible levels or the **minimal audibility curve** (Dadson & King, 1952). As seen in this figure, the threshold of audibility line is not straight or parallel to the graph indicating a need for more sound pressure at some frequencies than others for the human ear to hear the signal. Specifically, the ear tends to be more sensitive and can process sound more effectively in the mid to high frequencies and less sensitive in the low frequencies and the very high frequencies, due to the enhancement and attenuation of sound as it travels through the outer and middle ear.

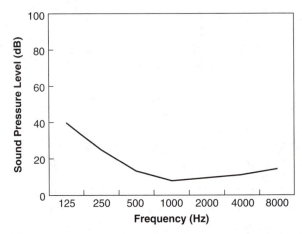

Figure 5.1   Minimal audibility curve—the average threshold of human hearing in sound pressure level as a function of frequency.

The minimal audibility curve serves as a reference of the average normal ear in which to compare the results of individuals who have some degree of hearing loss. However, for the purpose of evaluating a person's hearing sensitivity, it is somewhat cumbersome and awkward to use a curved reference on which to base test results. Therefore, a scale that references the average normal hearing thresholds, designated as **hearing level (HL)**, simplifies the process of measuring normal hearing sensitivity by converting the minimal audibility curve into a straight line called **audiometric zero**.

The definition of audiometric zero is essentially the sound pressure level that is required to reach the threshold of audibility at each frequency for the average normal hearing person. This average threshold of audibility has been determined and referenced as a standard by the American National Standards Institute (ANSI). The current standard (ANSI, 2004) designates the sound pressure level needed to obtain audiometric zero or 0 dB HL and is based on the type of equipment used. By making this conversion from the sound pressure level scale to the hearing level scale, it simplifies the process of measuring someone's hearing ability in reference to average normal hearing rather than the actual sound pressure that can be measured. Because audiometric zero is an average of normal hearing thresholds, there are some individuals who can hear sounds below 0 dB HL. Recording of test results, then, needs to allow for thresholds that may occur at −5 and −10 dB HL.

The Audiogram

As an evaluation is performed, the threshold responses from the listener are plotted onto a graph in a format that allows the examiner to characterize the results. The **audiogram** is a graphic representation of hearing test results using the dimensions of frequency and intensity and applying the hearing level scale just described (see Figure 5.2). Specific symbols are used to denote the hearing ability of the person being tested. The frequencies used to measure hearing are consistent with a musical scale measured in octaves and

Figure 5.2 An example of a standard audiogram . Note that 20 dB of intensity on the ordinate scale equals one octave on the abscissa.

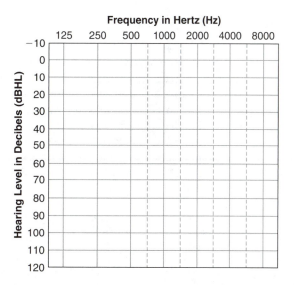

represent the range of sounds, including speech, that commonly are heard. For example, the range from the center note or middle C on the piano (256 Hz) to the next subsequent C (512 Hz) is called an octave. The specific pure tone frequencies used as stimuli in a hearing test follow this same pattern using a multiplier of two (128, 256, 512, 1024 Hz) but begin with 125 Hz, similar to the musical note one octave below middle C. Subsequent test frequencies are multiples of 125 Hz, or in other words, 250 Hz, which coincides somewhat with middle C, 500 Hz, 1000 Hz, 2000 Hz, 4000 Hz, which approximates the highest note on the piano, and 8000 Hz. It also is recommended that midoctave frequencies, 750 Hz, 1500 Hz, 3000 Hz, and 6000 Hz be used during testing when there is a difference of 20 dB or more between the thresholds of successive octave frequencies. The frequency sound dimension measured in hertz (Hz) is represented on the abscissa, or *x*-axis, of the audiogram. The dimension of sound intensity is represented along the ordinate, or *y*-axis, of this graph using the decibel scale of hearing level (dB HL). It is divided into 10-dB segments, which range from −10 dB to 120 dB HL. The upper limit of the audiogram has changed recently from 110 dB HL because of the advances in capacity of newer audiometers.

In order to maintain uniformity from one audiogram to the next, size and spacing are standardized. The distance between octave frequencies on the abscissa should equal the distance of 20 dB on the ordinate (ASHA, 1990). The audiogram is rather unusual when compared to most graphs because the zero line is drawn at the top rather than at the bottom of the graph. This unique design is used so that better hearing thresholds are shown at the top of the audiogram and as hearing worsens, the results are correspondingly displayed at a lower point on the graph.

The process of performing a hearing test requires the patient to respond to a series of pure tone signals that are presented. The intent is to identify the softest intensity level at which the person will respond or the threshold. When this level is identified, a symbol is then placed on that particular vertical frequency line corresponding to the specific intensity level.

Audiometric Symbols

Although there are different sets of symbols used for displaying hearing test results, the most common **audiometric symbols** are those recommended by the American Speech-Language-Hearing Association (1990). When sound is transmitted through the medium of air using standard headphones, speakers, or insert earphones, the term used to signify this procedure is **air conduction testing.** The symbols for standard pure tone testing of air conducted stimuli, are a red 0 for the right ear and a blue X for the left ear as indicated in Figure 5.3. The guideline of using the colors red and blue is not strictly applied because of the loss of color in most duplication.

The presentation of signals to an ear does not always result in an independent response from that ear. In other words, when a very intense signal is presented to one

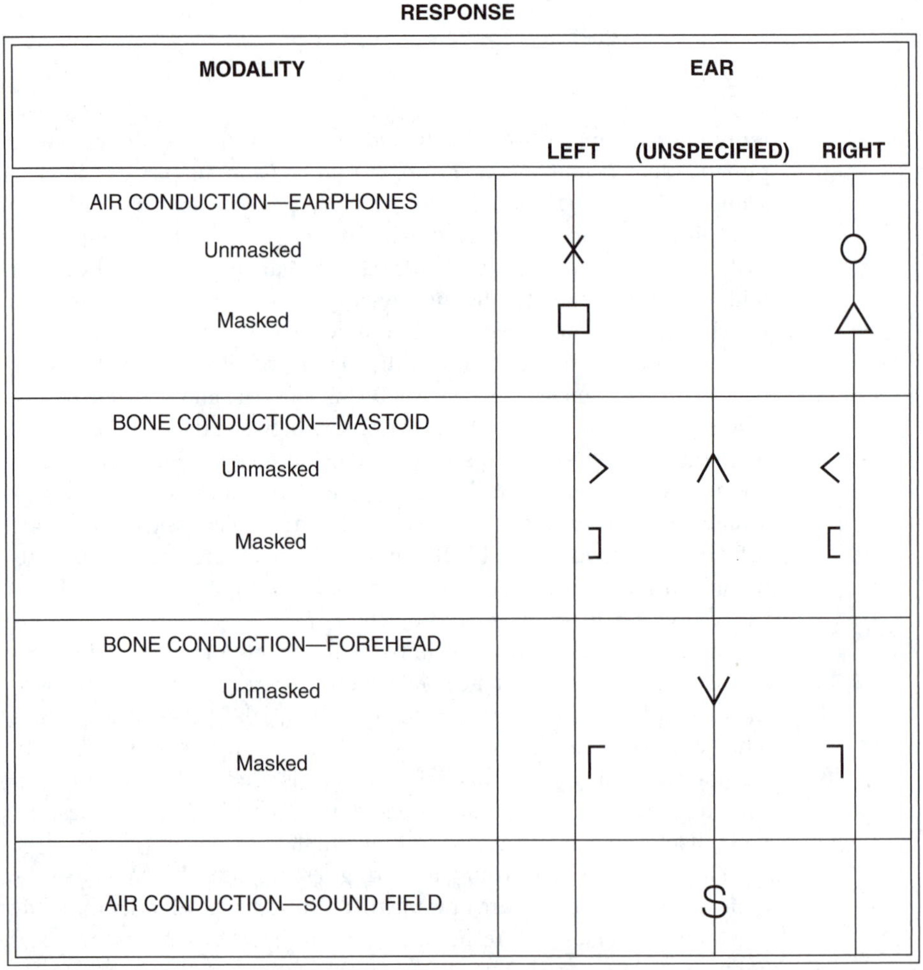

RESPONSE

MODALITY	EAR		
	LEFT	(UNSPECIFIED)	RIGHT
AIR CONDUCTION—EARPHONES Unmasked Masked	X □		O △
BONE CONDUCTION—MASTOID Unmasked Masked	>]	∧	< [
BONE CONDUCTION—FOREHEAD Unmasked Masked	⌐	V	⌐
AIR CONDUCTION—SOUND FIELD		S	

Figure 5.3   ASHA-recommended response symbols for use in pure tone audiometry

ear (the test ear) there is the possibility that the sound can be conducted by bone transmission through the head and be heard by the other ear (the non–test ear). It then becomes necessary to prevent the participation of the non–test ear so as to obtain valid results from the ear being tested. The isolation of a given ear for testing is accomplished by introducing a different signal or noise to mask the ability of the non–test ear from hearing the test signal. When this masking noise is introduced to the non–test ear, the measurement symbols for air conduction testing change to a triangle (△) for the right ear and a square (□) for the left ear in the same corresponding colors. The air conduction test results, whether masked or unmasked, are then connected for each ear using a solid line.

In addition to air conduction, audiometric testing is also performed using **bone conduction**. This uses a different sound pathway by setting the bones of the skull into vibration with a transducer called a bone vibrator. When pure tone testing is performed through the modality of bone conduction, different symbols are used. For unmasked thresholds, the "<" and ">" symbols are plotted to the side of the corresponding frequency vertical line and represent placement of the bone vibrator on each respective mastoid bone behind the pinna. The right unmasked bone conduction threshold is placed on the left side of the line and the left ear test result is placed on the right side of the line. The reason for this seemingly contradictory symbol placement stems from medical charting in which the examiner envisions the individual being tested facing them. A simple way to visualize this symbol placement is to picture the face of the examinee on the audiogram, with the right ear of the individual on the left side as the examiner views the audiogram and correspondingly the left ear on the right side.

It is important to note that a signal presented through a bone vibrator during bone conduction testing is transmitted uniformly throughout the skull regardless of the vibrator placement. Therefore, a sound presented by bone conduction to the left ear potentially can be heard by the right ear cochlea. In other words, unmasked bone conduction is non–ear specific and represents the response of the better cochlea only. The unmasked bone conduction symbols thus represent the location of the vibrator placement rather than the actual auditory response from a specific ear. This principle of sound transfer from one ear to the other by bone conduction will be discussed in a subsequent chapter. Because of the unique nature of the bone conduction of sound, a signal of sufficient intensity presented by a bone vibrator placed anywhere on the skull will reach the cochlea of each ear. For this reason, another popular bone vibrator placement is on the forehead because of its uniform ease of positioning. The forehead placement symbol is "V" for unmasked results. When masking noise is introduced to the non–test ear during bone conduction testing, the masked test results are displayed using "[" and "]" symbols for mastoid placement near each respective ear and the symbols, ⌈ and ⌉ when the forehead placement is employed.

In certain circumstances, as in a patient who is unwilling to cooperate with normal test procedures, the use of headphones or a bone vibrator may not be possible. In these cases, signals are presented through speakers, typically located in a sound-treated room. This type of process is termed **sound field testing**. Because the signal reaches both ears, results specific to each ear cannot be measured, and so an "S" symbol is used to denote this type of procedure.

In case of a profound hearing impairment, the maximum output of the audiometer is often reached and the person being tested still cannot hear the tone. The appropriate mark, right or left, masked or unmasked, is placed on the audiogram, and an arrow pointing downward is then attached to the signal denoting that there was no measurable response to sound at the audiometer's maximum intensity limit (see Figure 5.4). Although it is not included in the recommended set of symbols, an "A" is often used to represent a threshold in sound field when wearing some form of amplification such as hearing aids, signifying an "aided" response.

At the completion of air and bone conduction testing with or without masking, the many symbols along with the lack of color differentiation may become confusing when reviewing the test results. Jerger (1976) suggested the use of separate audiograms for each ear but employing the same symbols for both ears: circles for air conduction and triangles for

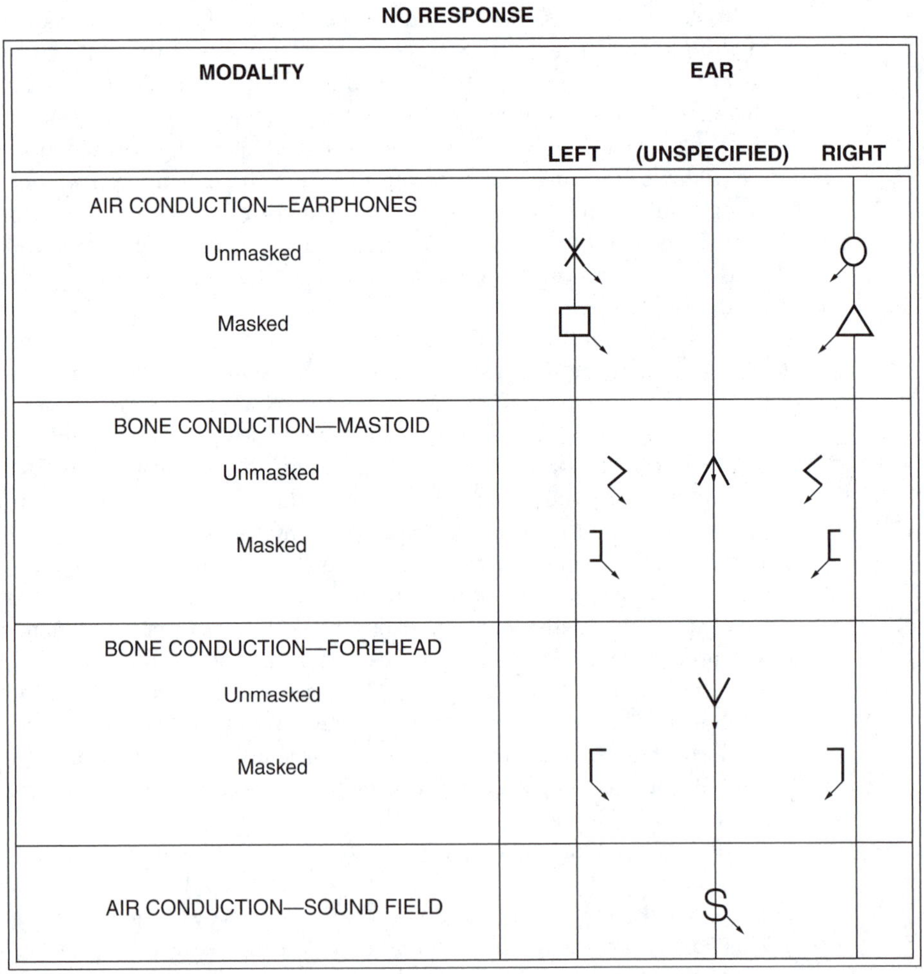

Figure 5.4   ASHA-Recommended No-Response Symbols for use in pure tone audiometry

bone conduction that are open in the unmasked condition and solid in the masked condition. Although the use of this set of symbols is not as widespread as the ASHA recommended symbols, the idea of two audiograms has become common practice.

DEGREE OF HEARING LOSS

Degree of hearing loss is a parameter that defines the severity of someone's hearing impairment, or in other words, how intense a sound must be presented before it is heard, which determines their threshold of audibility. For example, if a 1000-Hz tone is presented at 35 dB and a patient indicates hearing it, but does not respond to the same tone at a level of 30 dB, their hearing threshold would be reported as 35 dBHL. This result signifies the degree or level of intensity that is required to for a particular sound to be made audible.

The Accepted Standard

Specific descriptors have been assigned to different degrees of hearing impairment as recommended by Goodman (1965) and later modified by Clark (1981) as listed in Table 5.1. This scale of hearing impairment is commonly used in audiometric testing (Gelfand, 1997; Yantis, 1994) and is also displayed in Figure 5.5 on an audiogram.

Historically, normal hearing sensitivity has been considered −10 to 25 dB. Even today many service providers in the medical community use this range up to 25 dB as a passing result or a normal hearing diagnosis. However, research has suggested that hearing levels between 16 and 25 dB can cause a variety of problems such as the inability to detect some speech cues or signals from a distance (Northern & Downs, 1991). When persons with this level of hearing, children in particular, are placed in a difficult or demanding listening environment such as a classroom setting, they show increased difficulty in processing information as well as fatigue due to the greater effort required to hear. Thus, hearing levels in this range are considered an educationally significant hearing deficit for school-age children (Brackett, 1997;

Table 5.1 Degrees of hearing loss

Degree	dBHL
Normal Hearing	−10–15 dB
Slight or Minimal	16–25 dB
Mild	26–40 dB
Moderate	41–55 dB
Moderately Severe	56–70 dB
Severe	71–90 dB
Profound	>90 dB

Source: Clark (1981), "Uses and Abuses of Hearing Loss Classification," *ASHA, 23*

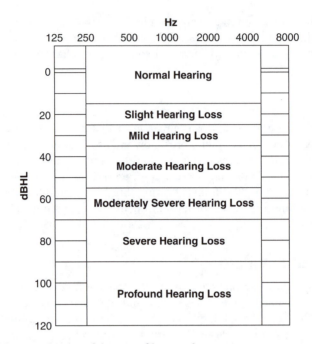

Figure 5.5   Audiogram display of degrees of hearing loss

Anderson, 1991; Blair, Peterson, & Viehweg, 1985). The current guidelines have incorporated the category of slight or minimal hearing loss with these implications in mind (Clark, 1981).

Unfortunately, many screening programs across the country still institute a threshold screening level of 25 dB despite the implications of hearing loss in the slight range. This is in part due to the noisy environment in which the testing is performed and the desire economically to minimize the number of referrals. However, if screening is performed at a level of 25 dB, and a child passes the screening, their level of hearing thresholds may still be the cause of poor educational performance. Conversely, however, a normal hearing level criteria of 25 dB may accurately reflect a proper diagnosis for an elderly individual who is confined to a nursing home. Hearing at this level may not be considered significantly diminished to warrant intervention in this case because of the reduced daily hearing demands. Therefore, the use of the slight or minimal loss classification in determining hearing handicap may require a variable interpretation based on the circumstances of the individual.

As the degree of loss worsens, the implications of the hearing impairment naturally increases. Hearing sensitivity measured between 26 and 40 dBHL is considered a mild hearing loss. With the level of conversational speech generally measured at 45 to 50 dB HL, one might surmise that speech would not necessarily be affected by this degree of loss. However, speech covers a wide range of frequencies and intensity levels. A specific speech measurement called the *audibility index,* formerly referred to as the articulation index, incorporates weighting for each frequency and level of intensity based on the amount of sound energy at each location along the spectrum in order to identify a percent value (Olsen, Hawkins, & Van Tasell, 1997). A simple method of displaying this index is by

Figure 5.6   Count-the-dot audiogram—
a simple method of calculating the
articulation index (audibility index)
Source: G. Mueller & M. Killion (1990), "An
Easy Method for Calculating the Articulation
Index," *The Hearing Journal,* 45(9)

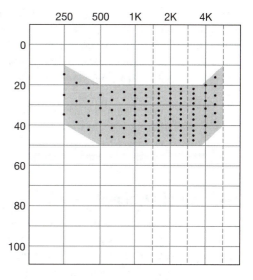

using a count-the-dot audiogram developed by Mueller & Killion (1990) in which each
dot represents 1% of speech audibility (see Figure 5.6). When this index is applied to hearing test results, an individual with a 30-dB hearing loss could miss 30 to 40% of the speech
signal depending on the environment and the distance from the signal. Thus, the label
"mild" can be misleading, particularly when considering the dramatic impact this degree
of loss can have on a child's ability to hear and develop clear speech (Flexer, 1999).

A hearing loss measured in the range of 41 to 55 dBHL is labeled as a moderate hearing loss. The effect of this degree of hearing impairment is quite dramatic because much
of conversational speech is rendered inaudible. Reception of everyday conversation as well
as the ability to hear environmental sounds is compromised, and so generally, the moderately hearing-impaired person will perceive a significant hearing loss because of its negative impact on communication. When the loss reaches 56–70 dBHL, or a moderately
severe hearing loss, the effect on the reception of everyday conversational speech can be
significant enough to render 100% of the signal inaudible. This degree of hearing loss requires some form of amplification in order to maintain normal auditory-oral communication and have regular daily human interaction without a significant amount of difficulty.

Although a severe hearing loss in the 71 to 90 dBHL range can create extreme hard-
ship on an individual's ability to perceive environmental sounds and communicate normally, there may still be adequate residual hearing to provide significant auditory benefit
with proper amplification and other auditory intervention. Generally, a person with a
servere hearing impairment using appropriate amplification has the potential to perceive
all speech sounds as well as other sounds in their surroundings.

Hearing levels that are greater than 90 dBHL constitute a profound hearing loss. This
category of loss typically coincides with the term of deafness previously described. Very
few individuals with hearing loss exhibit a total absence of hearing with no measurable
responses. Even a profound loss will retain some audibility with thresholds that are measurable within the range of audiometric assessment.

As the sensitivity of hearing on the audiogram takes shape with each measured threshold, it becomes clear that audibility can vary dramatically across the frequency spectrum.

A **pure tone average (PTA)** is a simple way to summarize the degree of hearing loss for the varied threshold levels. The PTA is a mean calculation for the thresholds at 500, 1000, and 2000 Hz. These three frequencies are known as the "speech frequencies" due to the amount of energy located in that region of the frequency spectrum (Carhart, 1971; Fletcher, 1950). The PTA calculation provides a way to specify the degree of hearing loss with a single index and can also be used to verify other test results. Its disadvantage is the inaccurate representation of the hearing loss when there are sharp variations in thresholds for each of the frequencies. In these cases, the typical three frequency PTA is not a good indicator or the degree of hearing loss and so, a PTA using the better two speech frequencies is calculated (Fletcher, 1950). This is referred to as the two-frequency or Fletcher average.

The Use of Descriptors

The commonly used descriptors for degree of loss have no direct scientific basis and can potentially be misleading. For example, a categorization of a loss in the "mild" range implies that it may not be significant enough to cause concern when, in fact, this degree of loss can result in a significant disabling condition. A study conducted by Haggard & Primus (1999), evaluated the perceptions of adults to different degrees of hearing loss. A simulated representation of slight, mild, and moderate hearing losses were presented to parents of school-age children who were asked to determine both an approximate percentage of hearing loss as well as descriptors that best describe the hearing loss. The results revealed an average perceived percentage of hearing loss of 46% for a slight loss, 64% for a mild loss, and 82% for a moderate hearing loss. In addition, the most common descriptors out of 17 choices, used to describe a slight simulated hearing loss, were "difficult" and "handicapping." For a mild hearing loss the most common descriptors chosen were "serious" and "handicapping," and for a moderate hearing loss, the descriptors most selected were "severe" and "extreme." These results are quite alarming considering the standard classifications that are in common use today. The conclusions of this study suggested that these terms tend to underrate the significance of the impairment. Thus, caution should be exercised in making an exact interpretation of the potentially disabling effect of a hearing impairment based solely on the words chosen to describe it.

AAOO and Other Classifications

Another method to characterize the degree of a hearing loss is to use a percentage score, a classification that is most easily understood. Unfortunately, percentages and decibels are not substitutes for each other; a 50 dBHL loss does not denote a 50% loss. Yet, the concept of "percentage of loss" is compelling. A formula was developed and modified by the American Academy of Otolaryngology and the American Council of Otolaryngology (AAO/ACO, 1979) that calculates an average of several frequencies and derives a percentage of hearing loss. This scheme is based on the amount of speech information in those frequencies. The calculations assume that normal hearing would result in a 0% hearing loss score. In this case, the "low fence" (0% of loss) is at 25 dBHL. The point at which a person would have a 100% loss is the "high fence." The high fence is set at 92 dBHL, suggesting that hearing in this range results in 100% loss. This formula was modified slightly by Sataloff, Sataloff, & Vassallo (1980) and the calculations are as follows:

1. Determine the average hearing loss from the threshold responses of the four frequencies, 500, 1000, 2000, and 3000 Hz, tested for each ear.
2. Subtract 25 dB.
3. Multiply the remaining number by 1.5%. This gives the percentage of hearing impairment for each ear.

To calculate an overall percentage for both ears, continue with the next step:

4. Multiply the percentage of hearing impairment in the better ear by five and add this figure to the percentage of hearing impairment of the poorer ear, then divide this total by six. The resulting number is the hearing impairment percentage for both ears combined.

The problems that arise from using this type of formula to determine percentage are significant. The use of a percentage does not take into account the characteristic of configuration as the hearing loss varies from frequency to frequency. The formula also assumes that 25 dBHL constitutes normal hearing rather than a slight hearing impairment. The resulting score of 0% for a slight hearing loss is quite a contrast to the perception of 46% hearing loss discussed previously (Haggard & Primus, 1999). Kryter (1998) recommends that the low fence be changed to 15 dBHL to reflect a 0% score at that level.

For hearing thresholds measured at high-intensity levels, the current formula suggests that a person with a 92-dB hearing loss would have a 100% hearing impairment. At this level of hearing loss, there is dramatic variability in performance and perception of disability. In one case, an individual who is profoundly hearing-impaired may be able to take advantage of the remaining residual hearing through amplification to function quite well. However, Kryter (1998) suggests that if the ability to hear everyday sentences is the determinant for a percentage of hearing handicap prior to intervention, then the maximum percentage score of hearing loss should be set at a much lower intensity level. He recommends a high fence of 75 dB because shouted speech presented to a person with this average level of hearing loss would be inaudible. A linear function between these two fences would then require a multiplier of 1.67 rather than 1.5 to calculate an accurate percentage score. Presently, these recommended changes to the formula have not been adopted and the percentage format does not appear to be used routinely by audiologists to establish the degree of hearing loss.

CONFIGURATION OF HEARING LOSS

The underlying assumption of hearing loss that a layperson might envision is that of a particular degree of loss affecting the frequency spectrum equally. In reality, the cause of hearing loss are variable in their effects, damaging certain portions of the hearing mechanism and leaving other portions unaffected. The hearing results on a given audiogram can exhibit normal hearing sensitivity at one frequency and a profound hearing loss at another. Because of this variability, the value of obtaining frequency specific information is further exemplified and reveals the critical importance of the configuration characteristic when describing hearing sensitivity.

Characteristics of Configuration

The configuration of hearing loss can be determined by quantifying the degree of loss at each given frequency and viewing the overall shape of the results as plotted on an audiogram. For example, if a moderate hearing loss of 45 dBHL is measured at every frequency tested, the results would display a flat configuration on the audiogram. However, if the hearing loss were of a mild nature at 30 dB in the low frequencies but gradually worsened to a moderate hearing loss of 50 dB in the high frequencies, then the results would show a sloping configuration on the audiogram. By convention, configuration is usually described from left to right on the audiogram. Because the majority of variations in shape occur in the high frequencies, descriptions of the sharpness of the slope are used to characterize most configurations, such as sloping, steeply sloping, and precipitous hearing loss. In some cases, the hearing loss will be greater in the low frequencies, resulting in a rising configuration. Other classifications include hearing loss restricted to either the high or low frequencies, and trough-, saucer-, or notch-shaped configurations. When a profound hearing loss is identified with hearing thresholds only in the low frequencies, the configuration is often described as a corner audiogram. Table 5.2 gives a general description of the various configurations typically seen. Examples of these hearing loss configurations are also shown in Figure 5.7. A visual inspection of the audiograms illustrates the dramatic variation of thresholds for each individual with hearing loss.

Table 5.2   Summary of hearing loss configuration

Configuration	Description
Flat	The degree of hearing loss does not vary more than 20 dB across all frequencies.
Sloping	A gradual downward shift in the degree of loss of 5–10 dB for each successive octave frequency with high frequencies at least 20 dB poorer than low frequencies.
Steeply Sloping	A significant downward shift in the degree of loss of 10–15 dB for each successive octave frequency with high frequencies at least 40 dB poorer than low frequencies.
Precipitous	A shift of at least 20 dB for successive octave frequencies from low frequencies to high frequencies.
Rising	A shift in hearing loss to better thresholds in the higher frequencies of at least 20 dB.
High- or Low-Frequency	The hearing loss is restricted to a specific region in the high- or low-frequency range.
Trough or Saucer	At least a 20 dB or greater loss in the midfrequencies than at 250 or 8000 Hz.
Notch	Significantly poorer hearing at one frequency as compared to adjacent frequencies.
Corner Audiogram	A severe to profound hearing loss with no measurable hearing in the higher frequencies, and hearing measured only in the bottom left corner of the audiogram.

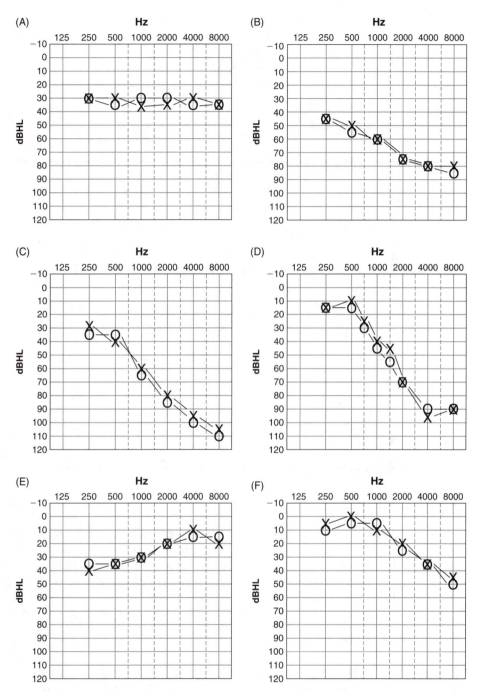

Figure 5.7 Audiogram depiction of different hearing loss configurations: (A) flat, (B) sloping, (C) steeply sloping, (D) precipitous, (E) rising, (F) high-frequency, (G) low-frequency, (H) saucer, (I) notch, and (J) corner audiogram. (Continued)

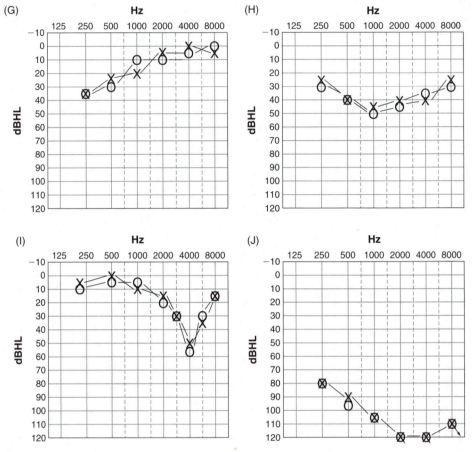

Figure 5.7   (Continued)

Symmetry of Hearing Loss

Depending on the underlying cause of a hearing loss, each ear may be affected the same or differently. In cases when the loss is symmetrical between the two ears, the term *bilateral* is often used to describe the impairment. Identical hearing thresholds for both ears is quite rare, so even variations of 5 or 10 dBHL between ears is still considered to be symmetrical as long as the respective results are generally interweaving across the frequency range. If the loss is significantly different between ears, or asymmetrical, each ear is usually described separately.

TYPE OR LOCATION OF HEARING LOSS

Type of hearing loss describes the location in the auditory pathway in which the underlying cause of the loss can be found. This particular characteristic is very important to identify because of the variable effect cause can have on auditory processing ability and the prognosis for intervention. For example, impacted cerumen in the outer ear will result in a significantly different effect on auditory processing and subsequent treatment than will damage to the inner hair cells of the cochlea. The four general categories used to classify type are called conductive, sensorineural, mixed, and nonorganic hearing loss. The identification of hearing loss type is a critical component in the diagnostic process as it influences the selection of appropriate intervention strategies, referrals, and prognosis for improving or overcoming an impairment.

Conductive Hearing Loss

A **conductive hearing loss** is defined as a disorder that involves the structures in the ear that are responsible for conducting sound to the cochlea. As a general rule, a conductive loss is a reduction of the intensity of an incoming air-conducted signal by an obstruction, abnormality, or disease in the outer or middle ear. Typical examples of conductive hearing loss consist of an obstruction in the ear canal such as impacted cerumen, some form of otitis media, a perforation of the tympanic membrane, or disorders affecting the ossicular chain, to name a few. Although conductive hearing loss is typically temporary, it can worsen and lead to a permanent condition if left untreated. In addition to a permanent hearing loss, a conductive pathology can also result in serious consequences involving surrounding structures such as paralysis of the facial nerve or bacterial meningitis. Because of these consequential effects, a rapid diagnosis and expeditious referral for treatment of the underlying condition further typifies the need for proper diagnosis of hearing loss type.

Sensorineural Hearing Loss

As the name of this type of loss implies, sensorineural hearing impairment is involved with both the cochlear function of sensory reception and the function of the auditory nerve. In most cases, sensorineural hearing impairment is due to a cochlear abnormality from damage to the inner or outer hair cell sensory receptors or other structures in the cochlea, which in turn results in a decrease in the clarity of the auditory signal. However, sensorineural hearing impairment could also be caused by problems with auditory nerve fibers, in the auditory nerve (cranial nerve VIII) or centrally in the audiotory central nervous system, extending through the brain stem to the cerebral cortex. It is difficult to differentiate these causes from a cochlear-based loss simply from the results obtained form a routine audiological evaluation, although audiologists do have other special tests in their testing arsenal to facilitate the differentiation of these variable losses. Generally, the auditory pathway from the cochlea to the brain is considered the sensorineural mechanism. Because of its location, this type of loss is usually permanent in nature and most often untreatable medically or surgically.

Although sensorineural hearing loss may have auditory thresholds that are similar in intensity level or configuration to a conductive hearing loss, the real consequence of this impairment occurs at higher levels of audibility. When processing auditory speech sounds, a person with a sensorineural hearing loss will have greater difficulty maintaining the clarity of the signal due to the reduced fine-tuning ability of the damaged sensory receptors. Examples of the underlying causes of sensorineural hearing loss include exposure to noise, presbycusis (hearing loss due to age), ototoxicity, and hearing loss from other congenital and familial causes. The most common course of intervention for sensorineural hearing loss is the fitting of hearing aids, followed by other forms of aural rehabilitation therapy.

Mixed Hearing Loss

A hearing loss that is determined to have both a conductive component and a sensorineural component is called a **mixed hearing loss.** This type of loss results from a diagnosed impairment in the cochlea compounded by the presence of a disorder in the outer or middle ear. The causes of a mixed hearing loss are quite varied and may occur from a particular disease that affects both the outer or middle ear and inner ear. A mixed hearing loss may also be temporarily caused by the presence of a wax obstruction or from otitis media, for example, coupled with a longstanding sensorineural loss. Figure 5.8 illustrates the

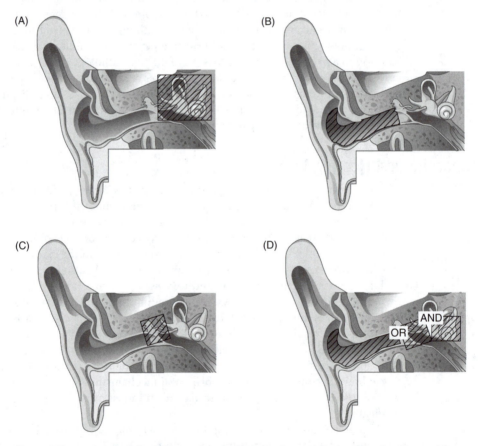

Figure 5.8 Location of the different types of hearing loss as depicted by the diagonal lines on each display of the ear: (A) Sensorineural hearing loss affecting the inner ear, (B) conductive hearing loss affecting the outer ear, (C) conductive hearing loss affecting the middle ear, (D) mixed hearing loss affecting the outer or middle ear combined with a sensorineural hearing loss in the inner ear.

relationship between the different types of hearing loss and the location of the disease or disorder in the ear. The manner in which type of hearing loss is displayed on an audiogram by comparing the air conduction and bone conduction results, is explained as part of test interpretation in the next chapter.

Nonorganic Hearing Loss

In almost all cases of hearing diagnosis, the type of hearing loss can be classified into one of the above three categories previously described. However, there are occasionally some cases when there is an unreliable suggestion of hearing loss without linkage to any underlying cause or organic pathology. This type of loss is termed a **functional** or nonorganic **hearing loss**. Functional hearing loss is often the feigning or exaggeration of a hearing impairment, usually for some ulterior purpose, such as social attention or monetary compensation. In rare cases, a nonorganic hearing loss may have a more serious underlying psychological cause. This type of psychogenic hearing disorder is termed **hysterical deafness** or **conversion deafness** and is a physical manifestation as a result of severe anxiety or emotional trauma. Regardless of the reason for the nonorganic hearing loss, it is critical that the presence of a false result is recognized and special procedures used to obtain accurate hearing levels in these cases (see Chapter 9 for further discussion).

AUDITORY PERCEPTION

As suggested by the different underlying disease processes of a conductive hearing loss compared to sensorineural hearing loss, degree and configuration do not always provide a complete picture of how well input signals are being received at the cortical level of the auditory pathway. The results displayed on an audiogram characterize threshold sensitivity but do not necessarily portray a person's ability to recognize and interpret the signal. For example, two patients diagnosed with the same degree, configuration, and type of hearing loss may have vastly different levels of auditory perception and correspondingly, different degrees of hearing disability.

Although pure tones are the primary signals used to evaluate hearing sensitivity, many individuals who choose to have their hearing evaluated do so because they experience difficulty hearing and understanding speech. Rather than a measure of audibility, a person's auditory perception is a measure of how well a sound is being received and processed. In other words, the terms *hearing audibility* or *sensitivity* relate to our general "hearing ability," whereas the terms *perception* or *recognition* describe "understanding what we hear."

In order to more comprehensively evaluate a patient's hearing perception, testing using speech as a signal is also incorporated into an audiometric evaluation. The most common form of auditory perception measurement is a word recognition score that is determined by presenting a list of words and calculating a percentage of correct responses (to be discussed in the next chapter). The audiometric threshold data on the audiogram, combined with a measure of auditory perception in the form of speech testing, provide a comprehensive description of the hearing evaluation results and the specific characteristics of a hearing loss.

SUMMARY

A Glimpse into the Profession Revisited

Now that we have established the descriptors that are typically used to characterize a hearing loss, let's return to the Case Study of Brian. The initial behavioral testing was performed with fair to good reliability based on Brian's age. As shown in Figure 5.9, Brian was diagnosed with a severe to profound, gradually sloping hearing loss that was bilateral and symmetrical. The type of hearing loss is somewhat difficult to determine in this particular case based solely on the audiogram because of the limitations of the bone conduction testing equipment. The measurement of hearing by bone conduction resulted in no responses at moderate levels as indicated by the down arrows attached to the symbols. Because there is severe to profound loss by air conduction, a conductive component could still exist, which would result in a mixed hearing loss. However, an otoscopic evaluation visualizing the ear canals indicated clear canals and intact tympanic membranes. Additional special middle ear testing determined an absence of any potential middle ear pathology. Therefore, it is very likely that this is a sensorineural hearing loss instead of a mixed loss.

Because of the severity of this particular hearing loss, the ability to receive and process speech signals is a critical factor with regard to the challenges this impairment will have on Brian's life. The prognosis for adequate speech recognition with a severe to profound hearing loss may be questionable. An additional delay in intervention would impose unnecessary negative complications. Fortunately, because of the quick identification following the onset of the hearing loss, immediate intervention with amplification will increase his chances for continued good speech and language development.

Figure 5.9   Audiometric test results for Brian, depicting a severe to profound sloping hearing loss that is presumably sensorineural with no responses to bone conduction testing.

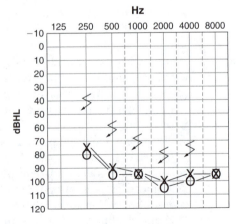

CHAPTER REVIEW

❏ The sense of hearing is a basic human function and is a critical component in our ability to communicate. When defining a hearing loss, several characteristics are used to make an accurate determination and diagnosis.

❏ The measurement of hearing sensitivity is defined by the level at which a sound is first detected or the threshold of audibility. The results of a hearing assessment are displayed graphically on an audiogram using specific symbols for each ear and for type of transducer used.

❏ The degree of hearing loss is the first and most important parameter that quantifies hearing sensitivity and a variety of descriptors are used to create this classification. A scoring percentage has been an alternative method of describing hearing loss in some medical settings. However, certain terms or scoring methods may not accurately reflect the implications of an impairment.

❏ The shape of the hearing loss as a function of frequency defines another parameter called configuration of loss that helps characterize a person's hearing ability. Certain configurations and differences between ears may have dramatic implications for perceiving and processing specific frequencies and complex sounds such as speech.

❏ The type of hearing loss is a third way in which an individual's hearing sensitivity can be quantified. This parameter is based on the underlying cause or location of the disease process causing the hearing loss. By determining the location of the cause of the hearing impairment, a proper diagnosis and correct intervention strategy can be implemented.

❏ Finally, the ability to perceive and interpret sound can also impact a person's degree of hearing disability. In addition to the measures of pure tone threshold sensitivity as displayed on the audiogram, the measurement of auditory perception using speech as a signal is an important component of a hearing evaluation to accurately characterize a hearing impairment.

ACTIVITIES FOR DISCUSSION

1. In the Case Study, should a cochlear implant be considered for Brian as the proper treatment, or should sign language be considered as an alternative form of communication?

2. Many professionals in certain parts of the country use a different symbol system on audiograms than that recommended by ASHA—circles for air conduction in both ears and triangles for bone conduction in both ears. When masking is used, the symbols are filled in. Do you think this is a better system? If so, how could the symbol system be converted?

3. Because the current terms used to describe the degree of a hearing loss may not be accurate representations, what other descriptors or methods could be used to characterize the degree of loss?

4. Based on our understanding of the disorders of the ear as discussed in Chapter 4, why would two patients with identical audiograms have vastly different auditory perception with different word recognition results?

REFERENCES

American Academy of Otolaryngology and American Council of Otolaryngology. (1979). Guide for the evaluation of hearing handicap. *Journal of the American Medical Association, 241*(19), 2055–2059.

American National Standards Institute (ANSI). (2004). *American National Standard specification for audiometers.* ANSI S3.6-2004.

American National Standards Institute. (1986). *American National Standard psychoacoustical terminology.* ANSI S3.20-1973 (R1986), New York.

American Speech-Language-Hearing Association. (2005). *Guidelines for manual pure-tone threshold audiometry.* Rockville, MD: Author. (Online), http://www.asha.org/members/deskref-journal/deskref/default

American Speech-Language-Hearing Association. (1990). Guidelines for audiometric symbols. *ASHA, 32*(Suppl.2), 25–30.

Anderson, K. L. (1991). Hearing conservation in the public schools revisited. In C. Flexer (Ed.), *Current audiologic issues in the educational management of children with hearing loss. Seminars in Hearing, 12,* 340–364.

Blair, J. C., Peterson, M. E., & Viehweg, S. H. (1985). The effects of mild sensorineural hearing loss on academic performance among young school-age children. *Volta Review.*

Brackett, D. (1997). Intervention for children with hearing impairment in general education settings. *Language, Speech and Hearing Services in Schools, 28,* 355–361.

Carhart, R. (1971). Observations on the relations between thresholds for pure tones and for speech. *Journal of Speech and Hearing Disorders, 36,* 476–483.

Clark, J. G. (1981). Uses and abuses of hearing loss classification. *ASHA, 23,* 493–500.

Dadson, R. S., & King, J. H. (1952). A determination of the normal threshold of hearing and its relation to the standardization of audiometers. *Journal of Laryngology and Otology., 46,* 366–378.

Fletcher, H. (1950). A method of calculating hearing loss for speech from an audiogram. *Acta Otolaryngologica, 90*(suppl.), 26–37.

Flexer, C. (1999). *Facilitating hearing and listening in young children* (2nd ed.). San Diego: Singular.

Gelfand, S. A. (1997). *Essentials of audiology.* New York: Thieme.

Goodman, A. (1965). Reference zero levels for pure-tone audiometer. *ASHA, 7,* 262–263.

Haggard, R. S., & Primus, M. A. (1999). Parental perceptions of hearing loss classification in children. *American Journal of Audiology, 8*(2), 83–92.

Jerger, J. (1976). A proposed audiometric symbol system for scholarly publications. *Archives of Otolaryngology, 102,* 33–36.

Kryter, K. D. (1998). Evaluation of hearing handicap. *Journal of the American Academy of Audiology, 9*(2), 141–146.

Mueller, G., & Killion, M. (1990). An easy method for calculating the articulation index. *The Hearing Journal, 45*(9), 14–17.

Northern, J. L., & Downs, M. P. (1991). *Hearing in children* (4th ed.). Baltimore: Williams & Wilkins.

Olsen, W., Hawkins, D., & Van Tasell, D. (1997). Representations of the long-term spectra of speech. *Ear and Hearing, 8*(45), 1003–1085.

Sataloff, J., Sataloff, R. T., & Vassallo, L. A. (1980). *Hearing Loss* (2nd ed.). Philadelphia: Lippincott.

Yantis, P. Y. (1994). Puretone air-conduction threshold testing. In J. Katz (Ed.), *Handbook of clinical audiology* (4th ed., pp. 97–108). Baltimore: Williams & Wilkins.

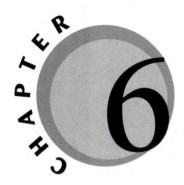

6

Behavioral Audiometric Evaluation

Key Terms

CASE STUDY

A Glimpse into the Profession

John is a 63-year-old seen by his local audiologist for a complete audiologic evaluation. The referral for this evaluation came from two sources: a hearing test obtained at his place of employment, a paper products manufacturer, with the results indicating a significant hearing loss; and complaints from John's wife about the constant need to repeat herself. John is finally willing to recognize his increased hearing difficulty and has chosen to have it evaluated. An initial query by the audiologist revealed a long-standing history of noise exposure in his work environment as well as a variety of recreational noises caused from hunting and jet skiing. There is no significant history of hearing loss in his family and John has not had any recent ear pathology nor ear surgery. John did report the presence of constant ringing sounds in both ears to which he has become accustomed and generally ignores. A visual inspection of his ear canals revealed a clear view of intact tympanic membranes. A complete audiologic evaluation was performed in order to identify the characteristics of his hearing loss and to determine appropriate treatment. This chapter will review the equipment and procedures used to conduct John's hearing evaluation as well as the process of interpreting the results.

INTRODUCTION TO HEARING ASSESSMENT

The process of assessing hearing begins with the suspicion by a friend or family member, a physician, an educator, another professional, or the individual themselves, that a hearing loss exists. This suspicion is followed by a referral for an audiologic evaluation or the identification of a problem through the failure to pass some type of hearing screening procedure. Before an actual hearing test is performed, there are several initial steps that take place including the completion of a case history, a visual inspection of the ear canals, and some preliminary gross measures of function and sensitivity that need to be performed as the introductory foundation to hearing assessment.

Referral Sources

There are several reasons why a person is seen for an audiologic evaluation and several sources from which a person might be referred in order to determine the existence of a hearing impairment. The first obvious approach would be through a **self-referral**. Individuals may notice that they are having increased difficulty understanding speech and find themselves continually requesting people to repeat themselves in conversational settings. They also may notice the need to increase the volume level of the television or radio to a level higher than what others prefer. This increased difficulty may carry over to telephone use or in work settings communicating with coworkers or the public. Based on these observed difficulties, an individual may refer themselves for a hearing evaluation to confirm or rule out a hearing loss.

Many times a referral may come from a spouse or other family member who notices the hearing difficulty much sooner than the person with the loss. The **parent** or **family referral** sometimes can be difficult because of a person's unwillingness to accept the advice or suggestion of a family member. This type of referral often occurs only after the family is insistent that something be done to resolve the increasing communication problems in the home. The recognition of a potential problem and referral by the parents of a small child is particularly important for early identification of hearing loss. Unfortunately, the presence of a hearing loss, particularly if mild in its degree, is often wrongly attributed to listening problems or an attention deficit. In other cases, individuals with hearing loss may effectively use alternative strategies and visual cues to compensate for the apparent hearing loss in an attempt to minimize its impact.

If a direct referral by the person with the potential loss or a family member does not occur for whatever reason, another avenue through which a person would receive audiological services is from a **professional referral**. Typically, a physician, a school nurse, a speech-language pathologist, or others working in medical or school settings are professionals who make this type of referral. However, the reason for the referral varies and is not always limited to the simple purpose of identifying a hearing loss. For example, a child may be referred by a pediatrician to confirm a recent diagnosis of otitis media and determine the impact the disease has on hearing. Another child referral may come from a speech-language pathologist for the purpose of ruling out hearing loss as the cause of a diagnosed speech and language delay. An otolaryngologist may refer a patient who is experiencing symptoms of dizziness or tinnitus in order to determine its relationship to hearing sensitivity and the status of the hearing mechanism. A primary care physician may have performed a hearing screening in his office and is referring a patient for a complete evaluation. Thus, the type of referral source or the reason for the referral will influence the approach in which the audiologist takes in the testing procedure. In addition to the direct and professional referrals, **hearing screening** programs for newborns and for children in school settings are other avenues through which the presence of a potential hearing loss can be identified and a referral made. Screening programs will be discussed further in Chapter 8.

The diagnosis of hearing impairment by the audiologist includes both a specific description of hearing loss characteristics and a determination of which portion of the ear is causing the impairment. In contrast, a medical diagnosis of a disease or pathology that may be the underlying cause of the hearing loss is made by a primary care physician or an otolaryngologist. The approach to diagnosing a hearing impairment is similar to that used in any other typical medical setting and begins with a case history followed by a series of assessment tools that constitute a comprehensive audiological test battery.

The Patient Inquiry

When one seeks medical assistance for any health problem, there are commonly four general questions to which a person seeks answers as part of the medical evaluation. This same sequence of questions can also be applied to an individual complaining of hearing problems. The first and foremost is a confirmation that a problem, in fact, does exist; in other words, "Is there a problem?" Often, the answer to this question may be obvious just by communicating with the patient or from subjective reporting by a spouse or family member. It also can be answered through a simple screening procedure with pass/fail criteria. Once a problem has been identified, a second question emerges, "How serious is the problem?" Answering this question involves a more in-depth evaluation process measuring hearing thresholds and determining the degree and configuration of the hearing loss. The third question typically asked is, "What is the underlying cause or location of the problem?" This analysis involves another series of tests to help determine the type and/or cause of the hearing loss. Finally, the fourth common question is, "What type of treatment will reduce or overcome the problem?" At the conclusion of a complete hearing evaluation, the intent is to ameliorate the problem through some form of intervention such as medical treatment with the use of pharmaceuticals, surgery, or possibly the simple procedure of cerumen removal. If these intervention approaches are not possible, then hopefully the hearing impairment can be overcome or minimized through amplification and rehabilitation. Throughout the evaluative process, an audiologist or any other health care professional should maintain an awareness of these four questions and the desire of the patient to have them answered. As the assessment procedure unfolds, from the case history to the completion of audiometric testing, satisfactory answers to these questions can be identified.

Case History

As with any other health care assessment, a **case history** is always the best place to begin. This pretest interview is typically comprised of a series of questions that provide information to allow the professional to focus attention on the concerns and complaints of the patient. The questions are also designed to identify possible serious medical conditions that would require an immediate referral to a physician or other professional. Although the format of an audiological case history varies from clinic to clinic, it is comprised fundamentally of five basic categories of questions as follows:

Hearing History

Information regarding hearing difficulty in different listening environments helps assist in determining the severity of the loss and how much it is affecting communication ability and general quality of life. Specific questions include: The length of time the hearing loss has been noticed; whether it occurred suddenly or has there been a gradual deterioration over time; specific environments and circumstances in which the hearing loss is most noticeable; and whether the difficulty is noticeable in one or both ears.

Medical History

Unlike a normal case history that would be taken by a primary care physician or specialist that is specific to general health, the medical portion of an audiological history focuses on the disorders related to the ear. The questions include: A recent history of ear infections; any medical or surgical treatment received to overcome a preexisting disease process in the ear(s); use of medication for the same purpose; any form of dizziness associated with hearing loss; or the presence and significance of tinnitus.

Noise History

This category of the case history includes questions involving employment history and any exposure to noise during that employment; noise exposure during service in the military; exposure to noise through recreation using motorized equipment such as motorcycles or jet skis; or exposure to noise through hobbies or work at home using a lawn mower, air blower, or woodworking tools.

Family History

The fourth category attempts to address questions regarding hereditary factors that potentially underlie a hearing problem. These questions need to be specifically worded so as to separate family members with hearing loss likely caused from noise exposure or the normal aging process from those whose hearing loss is from some type of genetic cause. In other words, if a parent of a patient developed a hearing loss at the age of 70, the effect of the hearing loss is likely due to aging rather than hereditary factors as compared to a patient with a family member who has had a severe hearing loss since birth.

Rehabilitation/Academic History

The final area of a case history is comprised of questions that address the issue of receiving any intervention for hearing loss that already has been diagnosed. For example, questions might include inquiry about hearing aid experience, or in the case of children, any auditory habilitation that has been provided. As part of this line of questioning, additional information could be obtained regarding the impact of the hearing loss on academic performance and the type of services, such as speech and language therapy, that have been provided.

A sample case history form that summarizes the categories of questions just described is shown in Figure 6.1. The organization of this particular form is designed to

---

Case History Form

Name _____   Date of Service _____

I. Purpose for Visit

❑ Hearing Loss   ❑ Tinnitus   ❑ Dizziness

❑ Physician/School Referral   ❑ Re-evaluation   ❑ Other_____

II. Hearing History   (Severity, Situations of Difficulty, Time Period, Symmetry)

III. Medical History
A. Pathology and Treatment (ME Pathology, Drainage or Pain, Surgeries, Current Medications, General Health)

B. Tinnitus (Duration, Severity, Symmetry, Type, Effects)

C. Vertigo (Duration, Severity, Incidence, Effects)

IV. Occupational/Noise History (Industrial, Military, Recreat., Duration, Degree, Prevention)

V. Family History (Hearing Loss Before Age 50, Relationship, Type)

VI. Rehab./Academic History
(Previous HA Use, AR Tx, Sp. & Lang., Previous Intervention, Classroom Placement)

Figure 6.1   A sample of a summary case history form

Child Case History Form

Name: _____   Date: _____

1. For what reason was this hearing test arranged? _____

2. Has your child ever had a hearing test?	Yes	No
3. Do you have any concerns about your child's hearing?	Yes	No
4. Does your child seem to hear better on some days than others?	Yes	No
5. Does anyone in the family (sisters, brothers, aunts, grandparents, etc.) have a handicap or problem with language, learning, hearing, speech, etc.?	Yes	No
6. Were there any complications during pregnancy or delivery?	Yes	No

7. Were any of the following present after your child's birth or during the first two months?

Stayed in hospital after mother	Prematurity
Birth weight less than 5 lb	Poor weight gain
Did not respond to sounds or people	Appeared yellow
Was in an incubator or isolette	Infections at birth
Difficulty breathing	Physical deformities
High fever	

8. What is your child's general health?	Good	Average	Poor
9. Is your child taking any medication now?		Yes	No
10. Has your child ever been hospitalized?		Yes	No
11. Has your child experienced ear infections or other ear disorders?		Yes	No
12. Has your child had any ear surgery?		Yes	No

13. What illnesses has your child had?

High fever	Dizziness
Convulsions	Pneumonia
Measles	Heart problems
Head or ear injury	Rheumatic fever
Encephalitis	Allergies
Meningitis	Asthma
Tonsillitis	Other: _____

14. Has your child ever received speech therapy?	Yes	No
15. Do you have any concerns about your child's speech and language?	Yes	No
16. Do you have any concerns about your child's physical or mental development?	Yes	No
17. If your child attends school, has he or she repeated any grades?	Yes	No
18. Do you believe your child has any learning problems?	Yes	No

19. What questions would you like to have answered as a result of today's hearing test?

_____

_____

Figure 6.2   A sample of a pediatric case history form

present the five general categories and allow the examiner to ask specific probing questions in each area. Figure 6.2 is a sample child case history form with itemized questions from the ASHA Guidelines for the Audiologic Assessment of Children From Birth to 5 Years of Age (ASHA, 2004).

Otoscopy

Following a thorough case history, the first step in an audiologic evaluation is to assess the status of the outer ear by visually inspecting the ear canal by a procedure called **otoscopy**. This procedure is performed using an **otoscope**, which is a handheld device comprised of

Figure 6.3   A handheld otoscope
Source: Courtesy of Welch Allyn, Inc.

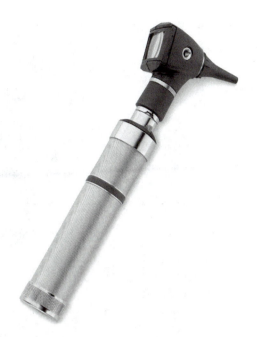

a light source, a magnifier, and a sterile or disposable speculum that allows for insertion into the ear canal (see Figure 6.3). The ear canal can then be inspected for any cerumen buildup, foreign objects, growths, or inflammation of the skin lining. The tympanic membrane can also be visualized to identify any perforations, inflammation, or abnormalities.

The purpose of otoscopy performed by an audiologist is not to diagnose a pathological condition. That type of medical diagnosis is part of a physician's scope of practice. However, if an obvious abnormality or disease process is noted during the inspection, such as draining ears, inflammation, bleeding, skin abrasions, noticeable pain or discomfort, or an apparent tympanic membrane perforation, a referral should be made for a medical assessment prior to or following the audiologic evaluation depending on the severity of the abnormality. The primary purpose for otoscopy as part of this evaluation then is to ensure that the ear canal is clear and the tympanic membrane can be visualized in order to proceed with the testing.

If there is an excessive amount of wax sufficient to interfere with test results, the audiologist may choose to remove it or refer for cerumen management by a physician. In cases where there is some wax buildup but an opening to the tympanic membrane is still apparent, the partial blockage likely will not affect the test results and testing can be performed and the cerumen can be removed at a later time.

New technological advances in medicine have resulted in the development of the video otoscope. This device combines a standard otoscope or similar device, with a video camera and a color monitor (see Figure 6.4). Rather than viewing the ear canal and tympanic membrane through a regular eyepiece, the structures are displayed on a video monitor. This device provides a closer inspection of the ear for the examiner and allows the patient or others to view the image as well.

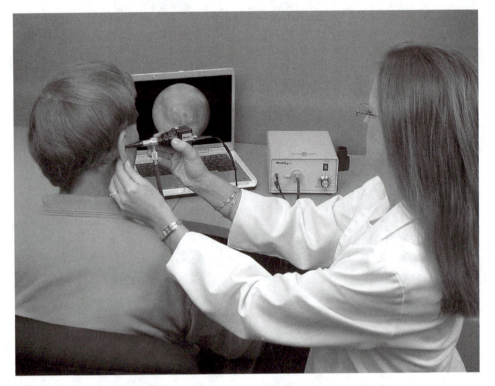

Figure 6.4 A video otoscope
Source: Courtesy of MedRx, Inc.

Nonelectronic Measures of Hearing

A cartoon taped to the sound booth in our clinic shows a patient sitting waiting to be seen by his physician. The nurse is indicating by the caption that the doctor is now going to give him a hearing test, and behind the patient is the doctor ready to crash two cymbals together. Although this is an obvious exaggeration of a hearing test for comic effect, prior to the advent of electronic instruments, there were a variety of gross testing procedures used to obtain some indication of a person's hearing ability. These tests came in the form of simple methods such as the coin-click test, rubbing fingers together near the patient's ear, clapping behind the patient, and so forth.

A variety of **noise makers** such as rattles, shakers, and bells have also been used in an attempt to identify hearing ability. Today, some of these different noise makers still have certain value in obtaining a basic measure of a person's hearing ability (e.g., orientation to the signal). They are used occasionally with individuals who are unable to give precise behavioral responses, such as infants, toddlers, or patients with multiple disabling conditions. These groups of individuals will often respond better to a variety of noises from toys rather than precisely calibrated pure tone signals. However, it is important to note that these are gross measures and give only an informal indication of hearing status.

A series of tests using tuning forks were developed in the middle nineteenth and early twentieth centuries in an effort to refine the testing procedures from the gross measures indicated above. Tuning fork tests are not commonly used by audiologists today, but continue to be an informal measure performed by some otolaryngologists (Harrell, 2002; Hinchcliffe, 1988; Miltenburg, 1994) to differentiate type of hearing loss and obtain a preliminary indication of the existence of a conductive component as well as the symmetry between ears.

Another simple measure of hearing sensitivity that can provide a preliminary reference for future testing is general conversational observation. During a case history, the ability of the patient to communicate at levels of normal conversation suggests that a severe hearing loss may be ruled out. On the other hand, a patient who continually has difficulty conversing and requires repetition at louder levels may be a likely indicator that a more significant hearing loss exists. These simple observations can facilitate the hearing evaluation by providing a preliminary indication of the individual's hearing ability and allowing the audiologist to determine the most appropriate approach in performing the evaluation.

THE AUDIOMETER

Types

The present method of determining hearing sensitivity is with the use of an electronic device called an audiometer. The introduction of the audiometer at the beginning of the twentieth century provided a more precise way of evaluating hearing sensitivity. An audiometer produces a variety of pure tones differentiated by frequency, presented over a range of intensity levels. It also produces different noise signals and serves to regulate speech when presented via a microphone or compact disc player.

Clinical versus Portable Audiometers

There are several types of audiometers manufactured that vary depending on the specific setting in which the testing will be performed. For example, a **clinical audiometer** is a desktop design that typically provides all the capability needed for an audiologist to perform most audiometric testing (see Figure 6.5). It typically consists of two channels, which permits two different signals to be presented to each ear separately.

Another commonly used type is a **portable audiometer** as shown in Figure 6.6. As the name implies, this audiometer allows portability to perform testing in almost any quiet environment for screening in schools, testing in industry, or evaluation in nursing facilities. This type of audiometer comes in several models from styles that perform just simple screening or pure tone testing to more sophisticated models that have enough capability to complete a thorough audiological evaluation.

Manual versus Automatic Audiometers

Another way to differentiate audiometer type is based on manual or automatic operation. When an examiner is controlling the presentation of a signal, it is considered to be manual operation of the audiometer. This is the most common form in clinical and

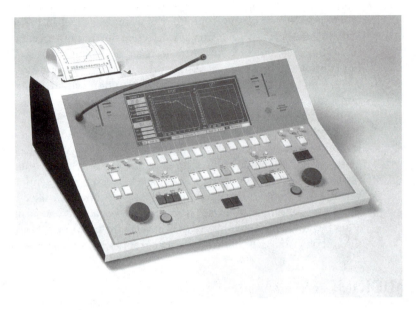

Figure 6.5 A clinical audiometer
Source: Courtesy of Interacoustics.

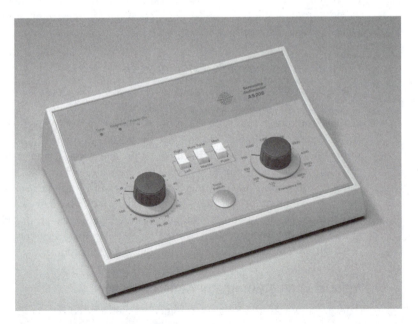

Figure 6.6 A portable screening audiometer
Source: Courtesy of Interacoustics.

portable audiometers. An automatic audiometer is usually computerized and is programmed to present signals based on a specific response from the person being tested. After a signal is presented, the person will respond by depressing a response switch or button if the signal is heard. The audiometer will then change the presentation level of the next signal based on whether or not a response was made. Automatic audiometers are commonly installed in mobile testing vans that are driven to industrial facilities or schools and set up so that many individuals can be tested simultaneously. However, a disadvantage to this type of test procedure is the loss of direct control by the examiner.

Components

There are several components that are common to all types of audiometers and necessary for their operation. The specifications of each audiometer are determined by the American National Standards Institute and are based on the particular type and function of the audiometer (ANSI S3.6, 2004a). Refer to the schematic representation of a portable screening audiometer in Figure 6.7 for identification of the following primary components.

Oscillator/Frequency Selector

The pure tone oscillator generates the pure tones in varying frequencies. These frequencies are at octave and midoctave points of 125, 250, 500, 750, 1000, 1500, 2000, 3000, 4000, 6000, and 8000 Hz. There are some clinical audiometers that will extend

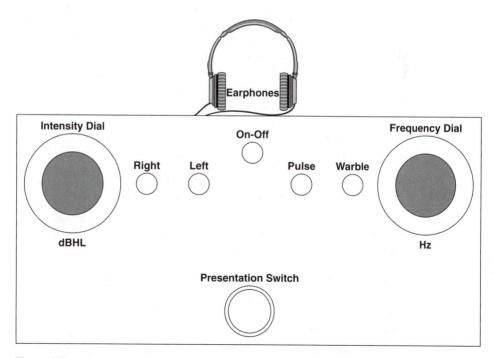

Figure 6.7   Schematic representation of the primary components of a portable screening audiometer

beyond these frequencies to higher levels. The oscillator is a component that is internal to the equipment and not visible on the operating panel. However, there is typically a dial or push button to control the frequency of the pure tone signal, which is called a frequency selector dial or switch.

Intensity Dial

The intensity or attenuator dial selects the level of intensity that is being presented, with a typical range of −10 dBHL to a maximum level of 120 dBHL. In some clinical audiometers this extends to 120 dBHL. At the lower frequencies of 125 Hz and 250 Hz, and at the highest frequencies of 6000 Hz and 8000 Hz, many audiometers have a lower intensity limit because of the amount of acoustic energy required to generate those particular types of signals. The maximum levels at these particular frequencies may be as low as 75–90 dBHL. The interval step most common on the intensity dial is a 5-dB increment consistent with conventional measurement of hearing thresholds.

The Presentation Switch

Each audiometer has a switch or push button that allows the examiner to present the signal to the patient. The length to which this button is manually depressed will dictate the duration of the signal being presented. The term *interrupter switch* is sometimes used because this same switch will allow the examiner to reverse its operation so that the signal presentation can be turned on indefinitely, and only when the button is depressed is the signal interrupted. This reverse operation is often used when conducting speech audiometry and the signal is continuously presented, eliminating the awkward necessity of constantly depressing the presentation switch.

Output Transducers

The electronic components that convert, or transduce, energy from one form to another are called *output transducers*. For example, a speaker is a transducer that converts an amplified electrical signal to an acoustic signal. There are a variety of transducers that can be selected to route the signal to either ear of the patient.

A common type of output transducer used today is the TDH 39, TDH 49, or TDH 50 standard headphones or **supra-aural earphones**. This type of transducer allows for the easiest placement on the patient and is clearly the most efficient means to perform screening or hearing threshold testing with a portable audiometer. An example of common supra-aural earphones is shown in Figure 6.8.

In recent years, a new type of transducer has been introduced for testing called **insert earphones**. This type of transducer (see Figure 6.9) sends the signal from a square housing as shown, through a long piece of tubing, which is inserted into the ear canal using a soft foam or rubber tip. Although less efficient for quick screening, there are some distinct advantages to this type of transducer in the clinical setting. Sometimes, the cartilaginous tissue surrounding the opening of the ear canal will collapse from the pressure of the headband of supra-aural earphones. In these cases, the actual process of testing hearing can cause hearing loss, compromising the accuracy of the test results. Insert

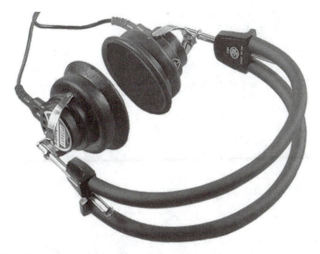

Figure 6.8   TDH-50 supra-aural earphones
Source: Courtesy of Interacoustics.

earphones eliminate the problems associated with testing individuals who have collapsed ear canals. Using headphones also presents a concern about hygiene as their use is shifted from patient to patient; this problem is resolved by using the foam or rubber disposable tips. Another reason for the use of insert earphones is the greater efficiency they provide when it becomes necessary to conduct masking procedures, which will be discussed later in the chapter.

Figure 6.9   Insert earphones
Source: Courtesy of Aearo Technologies.
E-A-RTONE® (and/or E-A-RLINK®) is a
trademark licensed to Aearo Technologies.

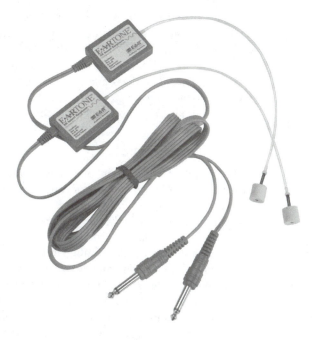

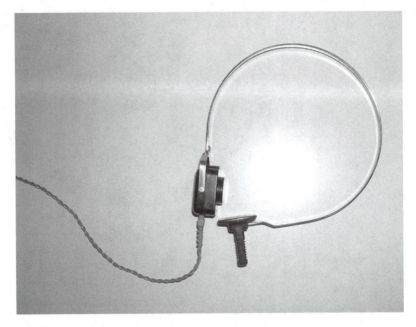

Figure 6.10   A bone vibrator

Another type of transducer that is part of the output transducer classification of components is the **bone vibrator** or oscillator. This is a small black vibrator with a headband, shown in Figure 6.10, from which signals are sent via vibrations of the oscillator directly by bone conduction to the inner ear. The bone vibrator is typically placed on the mastoid bone behind either ear or on the forehead.

Speakers are another type of transducer used in audiometric evaluations to test infants and small children when they are unwilling to allow earphone use. In other testing procedures, speakers are used when evaluating the performance of an individual who wears hearing aids to verify benefit. A major limitation when using speakers is the inability to obtain testing data for each ear independently.

Input Signal Selector

The remaining components of an audiometer serve a secondary function, but increase the flexibility of tests being performed and facilitate an audiometer's ease of operation.

The input signal selector is a set of switches used to select a signal to be sent to the output transducer, whether it be a pure tone, a speech signal, noise, or a signal coming from an outside source such as a cassette or compact disc player. In clinical audiometers, this component is often a separate series of controls. In portable audiometers, it is incorporated into the frequency selector switch. The presentation of pure tones can also be altered in various ways. For example, an examiner can use a pulsing sequence when presenting a pure tone or use the option of modulating the frequency of the pure tone, which creates a unique sound called a warble tone. This type of variation is often used when testing an individual who is difficult to test or has a short attention span and needs an alteration of the signal to maintain their attention. Another reason to vary the signal from its standard continuous tone is for patients who experience tinnitus and are having difficulty differentiating between the test tone and the internal ringing in their ear(s).

Additional Components

In clinical audiometers, there are a variety of secondary components that assist the audiologist in the testing process. These components generally are designed to monitor the signal presentation and include a volume unit (VU) meter to verify the intensity level of a speech signal and a talk-over button that will allow the examiner to communicate with the patient without altering test setup. Some components are also available to track the patient's response—a speaker or headset for the examiner to listen for the patient's responses, and a light indicator to monitor responses to stimuli when a response switch or button is used by the patient.

Calibration

Audiometric test results can only be considered an accurate measure of a person's hearing sensitivity if the audiometer being used is properly calibrated. In other words, if the intensity level of a signal that is heard is not consistent with the level indicated by the audiometer, the results will be invalid. Precise **calibration** is essential for accuracy in testing and is regulated by specific ANSI standards (2004a). It is typically performed annually by an audiologist or technician who specializes in calibration procedures. Figure 6.11 shows a sound

Figure 6.11 Sound level meter, audiometric analyzer, and artificial ear equipment used to perform calibration of an audiometer
Source: Courtesy of PCB Piezotronics, Inc., Larson Davis division.

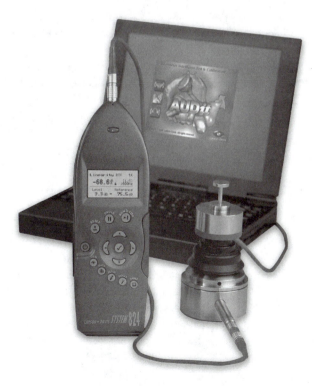

level meter and other equipment used to measure output signals from an audiometer and calibrate the accuracy of the sound presentation.

In addition to an exhaustive annual calibration, audiometers should be checked by the examiner prior to use. A daily listening check can verify the operation of an audiometer to determine that the frequency and intensity of an outgoing signal is consistent with what is indicated on the measurement dials. Test frequencies can be checked by listening for distortion or intermittent responses in the signal. Obviously without the use of sophisticated equipment, exact intensity levels cannot be determined. However, if the examiner has previously been tested and has a record of his or her own hearing thresholds, a simple self-administered hearing test can rule out any serious problems with the intensity of the signal. As intensity is varied using the intensity dial, it is also important that each incremental change approximates that change in intensity level and that increases and decreases in intensity are generally linear.

With regular use, the cords from an audiometer to the earphones might become damaged, causing an intermittent response. Also, the intrusion of dirt and dust into the various switches and dials may cause noise or distortion in the signal as well. Careful examination of these components need to be conducted to ensure that the signal is not compromised. It is much easier to take five minutes to perform a daily listening check than it is to be forced to retest five children because the left earphone was not properly plugged into the audiometer.

PURE TONE AUDIOMETRY

The human ear has the capability of hearing and processing a variety complex sounds through different pathways to the brain. For this reason, it is necessary to use several different types of tests to identify and diagnose hearing impairment. Using the dimensions of sound, namely intensity and frequency, we can measure the level at which an individual can begin to hear across a broad frequency spectrum. When pure tones are presented through the normal auditory pathway beginning with the outer ear using headphones or insert earphones, the pathway of air conduction is being used. This is the most fundamental test to measure hearing ability and the basis for standard hearing screening and audiometric testing.

The Test Environment

A major portion of audiometric testing occurs at extremely low levels in order to measure the threshold of audibility. Therefore, an unusually quiet environment is essential to perform a hearing test. Typically, when a screening procedure is performed in a school or hospital setting, a quiet exam room is necessary to minimize the interference of competing noise. Because hearing screening tends to be performed at a slightly higher intensity level than the actual minimal hearing level needed to measure thresholds, it is feasible to do this in a regular quiet room. Supra-aural earphones or insert earphones also provide some additional sound attenuation to obtain reasonably accurate hearing levels when testing. However, a complete evaluation not only involves the measurement of thresholds with earphones, it may also include testing with the use of a bone vibrator or speakers when the ears are

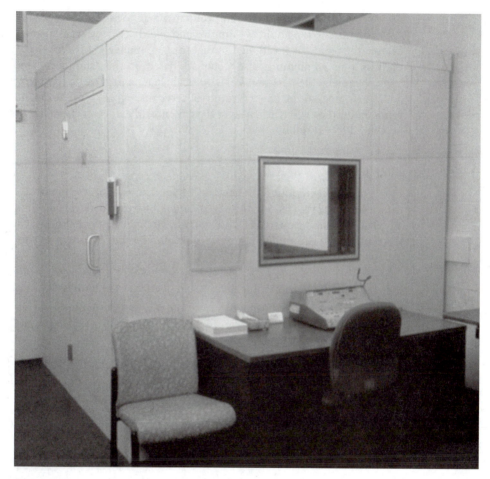

Figure 6.12   A sound-treated test booth
Source: Courtesy of IAC America.

unoccluded. It is then essential that the environmental noises are further attenuated with some type of soundproofing. In most audiology clinics, a **sound-treated test booth** is used to provide the needed sound attenuation to perform a complete audiological test battery. Figure 6.12 is a display of an audiometric sound booth with typical characteristics such as metal panels on the walls and multiple pane windows, carpet on the floor, and an attenuated ventilation system. Maximum permissible ambient noise levels for sound-treated audiological test rooms are established in the ANSI S3.1-1999 standard (ANSI, 2003).

Test Preparation

Now that correct operation of the audiometer and an adequate test environment have been established, the testing process can begin. The first step in obtaining accurate hearing thresholds is to position the patient properly for testing. The accuracy of hearing test results is contingent upon the ability of patients to focus on the procedure and to isolate their response to the auditory stimulus and avoid other external distractions. It is critical that the patient is positioned so that they are unable to observe the examiner during the test, thus eliminating false responses based on the examiner's hand or eye movements. A preferable position is at a 90-degree angle in relation to the examiner and the audiometer so that the patient cannot observe the signal presentation, but the examiner can monitor the overall alertness of the patient and detect any facial expressions that can be helpful in interpreting responses.

Instructions

Pure tone testing requires a behavioral response and so unlike many other medical procedures, measuring hearing thresholds includes participation from the patient. Generally patients are cooperative and will provide reliable responses when given clear instructions. ASHA guidelines (2005) recommend that instructions should include the following:

- Indicate the purpose of the test—that is, to find the faintest tone that can be heard
- Emphasize that it is necessary to sit quietly, without talking, during the test
- Indicate that the participant is to respond whenever the tone is heard, no matter how faint it may be
- Describe the need to respond overtly as soon as the tone comes on and to respond overtly immediately when the tone goes off
- Indicate that each ear is to be tested separately with tones of different pitches
- Describe inappropriate behaviors such as drinking, eating, smoking, chewing, or any behavior that may interfere with the test
- Provide an opportunity for any questions the listener may have

The instructions to a patient are very important and will influence the accuracy to the test results. The following is a sample of instructions given to a patient:

We will now conduct a test to measure your hearing ability. I will place these earphone tips in (headphones over) your ears. You will hear a series of tones that will be very faint. Please listen carefully and raise your hand (or press the switch) whenever you hear a tone, and then put your hand back down and wait for the next tone. We will test each ear separately. Please sit quietly during the test so that you will be able to hear the tones. Do you have any questions?

Response to the tone can either be with a raised hand, the pressing of a response switch that is provided, or verbally with a simple "yes." The choice of response mode will be based on the capabilities of the patient and selected by the audiologist to obtain the most accurate test results. If hand raising or a response button is used, patients will often keep their hand raised or the button depressed even after the tone is no longer present. So the meaning of an overt response when the tone goes off is to instruct the patient to remember to lower their hand or release the switch and ready themselves for the next pure tone signal.

Earphone Placement

Proper supra-aural earphone placement is important to ensure the validity and accuracy of the test results. Patients should be instructed to remove hats, headbands, glasses, or earrings that might interfere with the earphone placement. A simple technique that can be used to consistently place the rubber cushions of the earphones directly over the ear canals is to push up the headband to its maximum position and grasp the cushions so that the fingers are protruding slightly inward from the cushions. Facing the patient, the earphones are placed over the ears while feeling for the back edge of the pinnas with the fingers which will position the center of the earphone diaphragm directly over or close to the opening of the ear canal. Once the earphones are placed, the headband can then be lowered to the top of the head to retain the proper placement. Insert earphones should be placed comfortably deep in the ear canal, monitoring for any interference from cerumen at the tip of the insertion. Figures 6.13 and 6.14 are examples of headphone and insert earphone placement, respectively.

Testing Methods

Early clinical procedures in determining thresholds with the use of an audiometer were quite varied and affected the validity and reliability of the test results (Tyler & Wood, 1980; Harris, 1979; Hirsch, 1952; Carhart & Jerger, 1959; Reger, 1950;

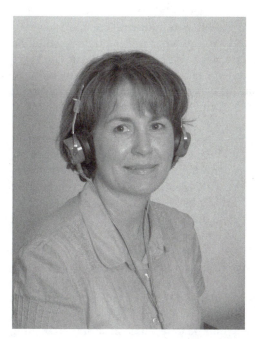

Figure 6.13   A picture of properly placed supra-aural earphones for air conduction testing

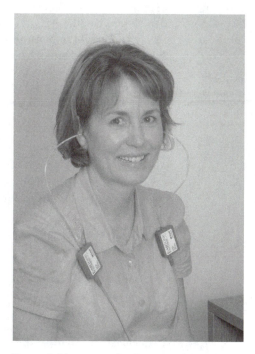

Figure 6.14   A picture of properly placed insert earphones for air conduction testing

Hughson & Westlake, 1944). The complexity and variability of these procedures demanded the need for a formalized approach to audiometric testing. The first clinical procedure, formally adopted in 1944, was developed by Hughson and Westlake, in which an ascending method was used. This procedure essentially increased the intensity of the tone until it was made audible at which time the patient would respond. The procedure was repeated until a response was obtained at least three times.

Modifications to this technique were suggested by Reger (1950) and Carhart and Jerger (1959) and have been traditionally known as the **modified Hughson-Westlake** method. This procedure was adopted by ASHA (1978) and has become standardized as the preferred method for clinical assessment (ASHA, 2005; ANSI, 2004b). The following is a general outline of the steps recommended for testing.

Order and Type of Signal Presentation

Although there is not a specific rule for which ear to begin testing, if information is available regarding the differences between ears, the better ear should be tested first. Thresholds results from the better ear can be useful for additional testing when masking is required to correctly test the poorer ear. Continuous or pulsed pure tone signals should be used. A recent study by Burk and Wiley (2004) has shown that the use of pulsed tones will increase a test participant's awareness of the stimuli.

The initial test frequency is 1000 Hz because it is the center frequency on the audiogram and easy to perceive. Following 1000 Hz, the test frequency sequence, in order, should be 2000 Hz, 4000 Hz, 8000 Hz, and then 1000 Hz is retested, to confirm test reliability. If the retest threshold at 1000 Hz differs from the first test, the lower of the two thresholds may be accepted, and at least one other test frequency should be retested. The retest of 1000 Hz is not necessary when testing the second ear. The lower frequencies, 500 Hz and 250 Hz, are then tested. Generally 125 Hz is not included in the standard audiological testing procedure. However, for individuals with severe to profound hearing losses, it is often useful to identify hearing thresholds at this lowest frequency.

Once the standard octave frequencies have been tested, a threshold measure at midoctave frequencies of 750 Hz, 1500 Hz, 3000 Hz, and 6000 Hz may be necessary for several reasons. When there is a 20-dB or greater difference between successive octave frequencies, it is useful to identify the slope of the hearing loss by determining the threshold at that midoctave. For example, if test results at 1000 Hz reveal a threshold of 30 dBHL and 2000 Hz shows testing results of 60 dBHL, the degree of loss measured at 1500 Hz between 30 dBHL to 60 dBHL can be quite significant with regard to the implications of the hearing loss.

Another reason for testing midoctave frequencies is for the purpose of identifying the effect of noise exposure in the high frequencies as part of monitoring in hearing loss prevention programs (USDoL, 1983). The testing standard in industrial work settings requires the testing of 3000 and 6000 Hz because of the impact of noise on those frequencies. In addition, midoctave frequency information can be helpful in improving the precision of fitting some technologically advanced hearing aids.

Familiarization

Once instructions are given and the first test frequency is selected, the testing procedures begin with a preparatory phase to familiarize the patient with the test signal. This phase begins with the presentation of a tone at a comfortable level that is audible to the patient, typically 30 dBHL. If no response occurs, present the tone at 50 dBHL. If there is still no response, increase the intensity successively in 10-dB increments until there is a response. After the patient responds positively to the presentation of the tone, a descending technique is used with a signal reduction in 10-dB intervals until the patient no longer responds.

Threshold Determination

The next phase of this method utilizes a simple "down 10, up 5" rule to determine the specific threshold. When the person responds to a tone, the examiner drops the intensity level down 10 dB until there is no response and then the signal is increased by 5 dB until a response is obtained. ASHA (2005) guidelines define threshold as "the lowest decibel hearing level at which responses occur in at least one half of a series of ascending trials, with a minimum of two responses required out of three presentations at a single level." The lowest level is then marked on the audiogram with the appropriate symbol indicating the threshold of hearing at that frequency. The procedure is then repeated for each of the successive frequencies for that ear, and then the other ear is tested in the same manner. A schematic representation of both the familiarization and threshold determination phases of this procedure is demonstrated in Figure 6.15.

Figure 6.15 A schematic of the modified Hughson-Westlake technique for hearing testing including the familiarization phase and the "down 10, up 5" sequence of the threshold search phase.

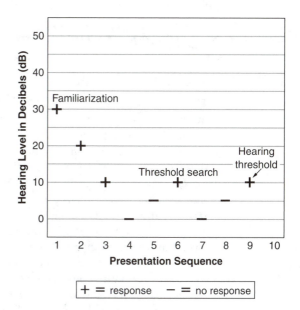

Figure 6.16 An audiogram depicting thresholds within the normal range of hearing for both ears

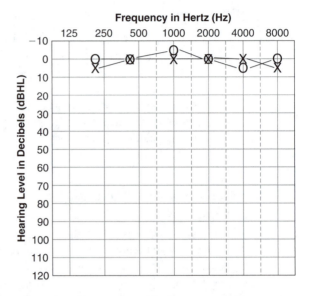

When this testing method is initiated using standard headphones or insert earphones as described earlier, a tone presented through the complete hearing mechanism from the ear canal through the auditory nervous system is called an air conduction threshold. As the air conduction thresholds are noted on the audiogram, a graphic representation of an individual's hearing sensitivity emerges. The resulting air conduction thresholds on the audiogram are an accurate representation of threshold of audibility across the frequency spectrum. An illustration of pure tone air conduction test results within the normal hearing range is shown in Figure 6.16.

BONE CONDUCTION TESTING

Pathways of Sound Transmission

The ear processes sound through two distinct pathways. The normal process of hearing in our day-to-day listening—just described as fundamental to audiometric testing—is the air conduction pathway as shown with an earphone in Figure 6.17A. It is important to note that sound transmitted by the air conduction pathway travels through all portions of ear, from the outer ear canal to the tympanic membrane, carrying sound to the ossicles and moving the fluid of the inner ear to stimulate the sensory receptors, which transduce the signal to nerve impulses transmitted to the auditory nervous system. The second pathway is a rather complex process of transmitting sound by bone conduction. This transmission occurs when an acoustic wave is presented at a sufficiently loud level through a headphone or insert earphone to set the bones of the skull into vibration; this then transmits the sound not only to the inner ear or cochlea of the test ear, but also to the cochlea of the non–test ear (see Figure 6.17B). In this way, the non–test ear can erroneously participate in the test and will need to be masked in order to eliminate its participation (this will be discussed later).

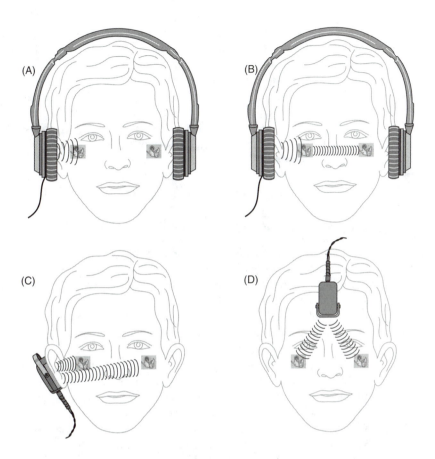

Figure 6.17 Illustration of air conduction and bone conduction pathways of sound transmission: (A) air conduction using supra-aural earphone, (B) air conduction of a higher-intensity sound that crosses over by bone conduction to the cochlea of the non–test ear, (C) bone conduction with mastoid bone vibrator placement, (D) bone conduction with forehead bone vibrator placement. Note that the bone conducted sound is transmitted to both cochleas simultaneously regardless of bone vibrator placement.

Bone conducted sound transmission also occurs when sound is actually generated by a bone vibrator placed on the skull that vibrates the bone and directly transmits the sound through this same process. This second way is utilized in audiometric testing procedures to directly measure and identify the sensitivity of the inner ear. Again, note that the sound is transmitted to both cochleas and special masking procedures are required to isolate each ear to obtain accurate test results. Two locations for bone vibrator placement and the transmission of a bone conducted sound are shown in Figures 6.17C and 6.17D. The more popular of the two placement sites, used by the vast majority of audiologists, is to position the vibrator on the prominence of the mastoid process behind the pinna (Martin, Champlin, & Chambers, 1998). The primary reason for this preferred placement is because the sensitivity to a bone conducted signal is greatest at the mastoid and because it is in close proximity to the test ear. A major disadvantage of using the mastoid for bone conduction testing is the inconsistency of placement due to the rounded surface of the mastoid process, which can cause the vibrator to move suddenly during testing. Obstruction from hair that is caught up between the skin and the vibrator also may affect the accuracy of the test results.

The second placement of the bone vibrator is on the forehead. The primary advantage of the forehead placement is the consistency from test to test because of the flat surface area and a secure fit to the head. However, despite its consistent test reliability, it is a less-sensitive measure by as much as 10 dB, which requires more vibration and further limits the maximum intensity levels in which bone conduction testing can be conducted. Because of this variability between placement sites, the examiner cannot switch from one placement to another without proper calibration of the audiometer.

Bone Conduction Testing Procedures

The purpose of measuring hearing through the transmission of a bone conducted sound is to determine the integrity of the inner ear and auditory pathway. In other words, it is a technique that specifically measures **sensorineural sensitivity**. The ability to measure the sensitivity of the inner ear creates the opportunity, by a process of elimination, to determine the type of hearing impairment that is present. By performing bone conduction testing, the underlying cause or location of the hearing impairment can be determined.

The test procedures to measure hearing sensitivity by bone conduction are very similar to the methods used to obtain air conduction threshold testing, although a different transducer is used. A bone vibrator is placed on the skull and the emitted tones vibrate the skull to stimulate the cochlea directly. Because it cannot be determined which ear is being tested due to the direct transmission of the signal to both cochleas, the decision of which ear to test first is unimportant. Once the patient is instructed and the bone vibrator is placed on the head, the same method to obtain air conduction thresholds is used. The appropriate unmasked bone conduction symbols are then placed accordingly on the audiogram. Figure 6.18 displays an audiogram with a mild flat hearing loss as

Figure 6.18 An audiogram illustrating a mild, flat hearing loss bilaterally. Masking procedures will need to be applied to determine bone conduction thresholds for each ear.

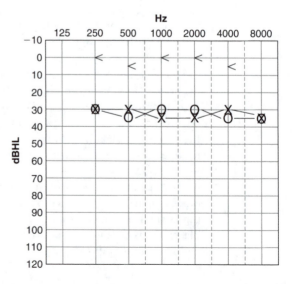

indicated by the air conduction thresholds. Unmasked bone conduction thresholds with the bone vibrator placement on the right mastoid indicate normal sensorineural sensitivity for at least one ear. However, despite the right side placement, the sound was transmitted to both cochleas and so the ear that responded to the stimulus cannot yet be determined.

MASKING

The principle of sound transmission by bone conduction is very valuable in the evaluation and diagnostic process. It provides information to help determine the type of hearing loss, whether it is conductive, sensorineural, or mixed, by comparing it to the air conduction test results. However, this phenomenon can have a confounding variable. When a sufficiently intense test signal is presented by air conduction testing, it can cross over to the ear not being tested by virtue of bone conduction as shown in Figure 6.17B. This cross hearing or **crossover effect** can make it difficult in the testing process when trying to isolate a particular ear and determine both hearing sensitivity and sensorineural sensitivity. It cannot be determined whether the patient is responding to a tone in the test ear or whether they are responding to the tone that is being heard in the non–test ear because of the crossover effect. This effect occurs even more frequently during bone conduction testing because of the immediate transfer of sound to both ears at low-intensity levels. Therefore, a method was developed as part of testing to eliminate this crossover of sound and isolate each ear being tested. This principle is called **masking** and has been a topic of extensive research and discussion in the field of audiology (Katz & Lezynski, 2002; Sanders & Hall, 1999; Yacullo, 1996). The American National Standards Institute (ANSI S3.6-1989) defines masking, in part, as follows: "The process by which the threshold of audibility for one sound is raised by the presence of another (masking sound)." The clinical purpose for using masking in audiological testing is essentially to rule out participation of the non–test ear by introducing a masking sound into that ear.

Noise Used for Masking

There are several types of noise that have been used to eliminate cross hearing. Historically white noise, which is a random representation of all frequencies of equal intensity, has been used as a masking signal; it creates a noisy sound similar to the static in between stations on a radio. Other types of masking noise have been found to be more effective in providing the same masking effect with greater efficiency. Today, the common type of masking noise used when testing pure tones is called narrow band noise. This noise is characterized by a particular bandwidth of sound that surrounds the frequency being tested. The bandwidth is determined by calculating the most accurate and efficient noise spectrum needed to sufficiently mask out the test tone from crossing over to the non–test ear. Speech-weighted noise is similar to white noise in that it represents a broadband of sound, but it is shaped to mirror the spectrum of speech and is used when masking is necessary to eliminate participation of the non–test ear during speech audiometry.

Masking During Air Conduction Testing

One of the most important concepts to understand in the evaluative process is that of **interaural attenuation.** Because of the crossover effect, sound transmitted by either air conduction or bone conduction will be directed to both ears by bone conduction when it is sufficiently loud. Interaural attenuation is described as the amount of reduction in intensity that occurs as a signal crosses through the head from one ear to the other. Interaural means "between ears," and attenuation means "reduction in intensity."

An example of this principle is as follows: Let us assume that an individual's hearing threshold is 0 dBHL in the right ear and 100 dBHL in the left ear at 1000 Hz. The tone is presented to the impaired left ear until the patient responds. Because the sound will cross over to the normal right ear once a certain intensity level is reached, say 50 dB, this patient will respond at that level. Because the hearing impairment is actually 100 dBHL, we know that the 50 dBHL response is because the sound has crossed over and was heard in the right ear. Thus, the interaural attenuation at 1000 Hz is 50 dB for this particular patient. In this case, if there is a 50-dB or greater difference between the two ears, some type of interference or masking noise must be introduced to the right ear to rule out its participation in order to obtain an accurate threshold in the left ear.

A complication of this principle is that the level of interaural attenuation will vary as a function of transducer being used, the stimulus frequency that is presented, and the individual being tested. Some historical studies that were conducted using supra-aural earphones to determine interaural attenuation levels showed significant variability in results between frequencies as well as within each study from person to person at a given frequency by as much as 40 to 80 dB (Snyder, 1973; Coles & Priede, 1968; Chaiklin, 1967; Liden, Nilsson, & Anderson, 1959). Because each individual's interaural attenuation is different, it is not possible to determine the actual level at which crossover occurs during testing. It is necessary, therefore, to employ the lowest level of interaural attenuation as the minimum possible value at which sound can cross over to the non-test ear for each frequency using supra-aural earphones (Yacullo, 1996; Studebaker, 1967). This value varies between 40 dB and 50 dB depending upon the frequency being tested (Katz & Lezynski, 2002; Goldstein & Newman, 1994), so a conservative approach would be to use an interaural attenuation value of 40 dB. The use of insert earphones offers better interaural attenuation particularly in the low frequencies (Sklare & Denenberg, 1987; Killion, Wilber, & Gudmundsen, 1985). Recommended minimum interaural attenuation values for insert earphones is 75 dB at 1000 Hz and below, and 50 dB at frequencies above 1000 Hz (Yacullo, 1996).

Applying interaural attenuation levels for supra-aural earphones, let us assume an individual is being tested for the first time. The test results show a threshold of 10 dBHL in the right ear. The left ear is then tested and the person responds at 50 to 60 dBHL as shown in Figure 6.19. Because the minimum interaural attenuation is not known for this individual, we must suspect that the 50-dB threshold obtained in the left ear could possibly be a crossover effect and that the right ear is responding to the tone. Therefore, because the difference between the thresholds of the two ears is the same or greater than the minimum interaural attenuation of 40 dB, masking must be introduced to rule out participation of the right ear. On the other hand, if the response in the left ear was 40 dBHL, the difference between the two ears would only be 30 dB and the minimum

Figure 6.19 An audiogram representing normal hearing in the right ear and presumably a moderate to moderately severe hearing loss in the left ear. However, there is a 40 dB or greater difference between the thresholds of the two ears suggesting a possible crossover effect. The left ear thresholds could be a "shadow curve" of the right ear. Masking noise introduced to the right ear is necessary to determine the true hearing thresholds in the left ear.

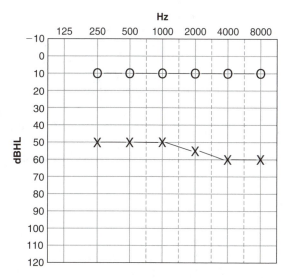

interaural attenuation level would not have been reached, resulting in a true hearing threshold for the left ear. As shown in Figure 6.20, once masking noise was introduced to the right ear, the true threshold for the left ear emerged, suggesting that the initial unmasked result originated from a right ear response.

Figure 6.20 After applying masking noise to the right ear, correct masked air conduction thresholds are measured for the left ear, indicating a moderately severe to severe sloping hearing loss.

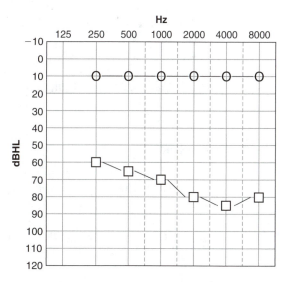

Masking During Bone Conduction Testing

The principle of interaural attenuation has a much more frequent application during bone conduction testing. Interaural attenuation by bone conduction is essentially 0 dB. This is due to the fact that when a bone vibrator is placed on the mastoid process or the

Figure 6.21 An audiogram displaying a mild flat bilateral conductive hearing loss. Note that masking for bone conduction was necessary in order to obtain accurate results for both ears.

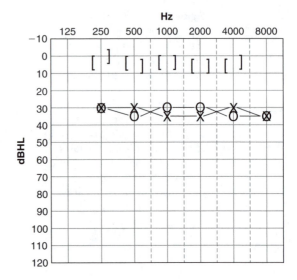

forehead, the signal essentially goes to both cochleas simultaneously as shown in Figures 6.17C and 6.17D. For example, an individual has been tested and air conduction thresholds of 30 dB are measured in both ears. Bone conduction testing is then performed with the bone vibrator placed on the right mastoid bone. The patient responds by bone conduction at a level of 0 dBHL (see Figure 6.18). It cannot be determined whether the 0-dB threshold is a result of a response from the right cochlea or the left cochlea even though the bone vibrator placement is on the right side. Therefore, it is necessary to introduce masking noise into the left ear to rule out its participation and accurately assess the sensorineural sensitivity in the right ear. The same procedure would then need to be applied to the left ear with masking noise presented to the right ear in order to measure the bone conduction thresholds of the left ear as well (see Figure 6.21).

Rules of Masking

There are some very straightforward rules that can be used to determine when masking is needed. The rule for masking when performing air conduction testing, as modified from Goldstein and Newman (1994), is as follows:

> If the difference between the air conduction threshold of the test ear and the air conduction or bone conduction threshold of the non–test ear equals or exceeds the minimum level of interaural attenuation, then masking must be used. (p. 117)

With further study of this principle, the rule is fairly simple in its application. Because the minimum interaural attenuation varies as a function of the frequency and the transducer used, masking principles can become somewhat complicated. So, if the minimum level of 40 dB is applied to all frequencies, a simplified definition for when to mask is as follows:

If there is a 40 dB or greater difference between the air conduction threshold of the test ear and the air conduction or bone conduction threshold of the non–test ear when using supra-aural earphones, masking must be used.

The use of 40 dB comes from the fact that this is the lowest level that interaural attenuation has been measured at certain frequencies with certain transducers. By applying this level it can safely be assumed that proper elimination of the non–test ear has occurred even though masking noise may be employed sooner than necessary. Thus, if an audiologist or audiometrist were to obtain results with a 40-dB or greater difference between ears at a particular frequency, the threshold for the poorer ear is inconclusive because of the possibility of crossover until masking noise is presented to the better ear.

As previously indicated, the interaural attenuation by bone conduction is 0 dB. For this reason, masking must be applied quite routinely when doing bone conduction testing. The masking rule is based on the difference between the air conduction thresholds and the bone conduction thresholds, or the *air-bone gap*. A significant air-bone gap is defined as the difference between thresholds that is greater than 10 dB. Therefore, a rule that can be applied to determine when masking is necessary during bone conduction testing is:

When the air conduction threshold of the test ear and the bone conduction threshold of that same ear differ by more than 10 dB (or a significant air-bone gap), use masking. (Goldstein & Newman, 1994, p. 117)

There are some professionals who propose that masking procedures should always be used in the non–test ear when performing bone conduction testing. The suggestion that masking is not necessary for all bone conduction testing is illustrated in the following example. If air conduction testing is performed on an individual with the results indicating thresholds at 50 dBHL in both ears, and an unmasked bone conduction threshold is also measured at 50 dBHL, an air-bone gap is not present. Because the bone conduction threshold is unmasked, it is not known which ear responded to the tone, but logically the better cochlea will hear the tone first. However, the poorer cochlea could not be any worse because the air conduction threshold is at the same level and a measure of the sensorineural portion of the ear could not have a poorer threshold than the entire ear as measured by the air conduction result. By a process of elimination, it can be concluded that the bone conduction thresholds of both ears are the same and masking is not needed to differentiate the thresholds in each ear. In a busy clinical practice, it is often necessary to use methods that are the most efficient without compromising the accuracy. The rule of using masking when testing bone conduction in every case is not a very efficient use of time considering that, in many bilateral sensorineural cases, unmasked bone thresholds provide enough information to diagnose the type of hearing loss.

If bone conduction testing identifies thresholds at an intensity level that is lower than the air conduction thresholds, it is called a negative air-bone gap. Because bone conduction involves different ways or modes of sound transmission, the relationship between air conduction and bone conduction is not entirely clear. It is possible, therefore, that the response to a bone conducted sound could result in a poorer threshold than a sound transmitted through earphones (Barry, 1994). Errors may also occur because the bone vibrator is not calibrated accurately, or the patient has an obstruction such as hair between the bone vibrator and the skin, or there is inconsistency in the patient's responses.

When the bone oscillator vibrates at high-intensity levels particularly in the low frequencies, the stimulation can become tactile rather than auditory. In cases of severe hearing loss, a patient may respond by bone conduction at lower levels because of this tactile sensation of feeling rather than actually hearing the tone. If an audiogram exhibits a predominately sensorineural hearing loss for most frequencies but shows an air-bone gap when bone conduction thresholds are measured at 40 to 50 dBHL in the lower frequencies, it is possible that these responses are vibrotactile and the hearing loss is likely sensorineural in nature.

The procedures that describe how masking should be introduced is a complicated process and beyond the scope and focus of this textbook. Suffice it to say, the principle of interaural attenuation and the need for masking is an integral part of the audiology evaluation process and should never be compromised. By applying the masking rules as indicated above, an accurate determination can be made regarding the test results and whether or not additional testing and masking needs to be performed.

TEST INTERPRETATION

Diagnosing Hearing Loss

Once the pure tone results have been determined for both air conduction and bone conduction procedures, the hearing loss can be interpreted and diagnosed. The format used to interpret the audiometric results is based on the characteristics of hearing loss described in Chapter 5. Upon viewing the audiogram, the parameters of degree of hearing loss, configuration of hearing loss, and type of hearing loss can be applied to the results. In addition, the results need to be interpreted with regard to the differences and similarities between the two ears. Generally, if there is symmetry between the two ears they are characterized and described simultaneously. However, if there is a significant deviation from one ear to the other, it is simpler to describe them separately. The basic purpose for characterizing the hearing loss in this manner is to provide a summary for diagnostic clarification when reporting the information to the patient, the family, or other professionals. The sequence in which parameters are used to describe the summary results may vary from professional to professional. But a typical way of interpreting an audiogram is indicated in the descriptions of the audiograms in Figure 6.22. The characteristic of type or cause of hearing loss is not included in these particular figures and will be added later.

Audiogram A in Figure 6.22 would be described as a *mild flat bilateral hearing loss*. This description and or diagnosis indicates that the thresholds occur in the mild hearing loss range with regard to degree, that they do not vary across the frequency with regard to configuration, and that there is symmetry between the two ears. The second example of audiometric results is shown in audiogram B, characterizing a *mild to moderate sloping hearing loss bilaterally*. When the degree of loss varies across the audiogram,

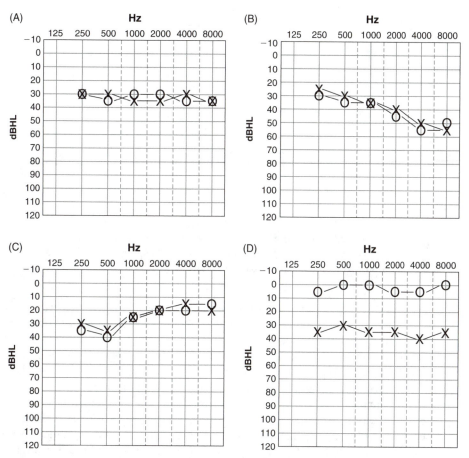

Figure 6.22 Audiograms displaying the audiometric characteristics, degree, configuration, and symmetry: (A) a mild flat bilateral hearing loss, (B) mild to moderate sloping hearing loss bilaterally, (C) mild to slight rising hearing loss bilaterally, (D) normal hearing in the right ear and a mild flat hearing loss in the left ear. The type of hearing loss has not been determined because bone conduction testing has yet to be administered.

the description is usually from low frequencies to high frequencies or left to right. The configuration is described as sloping because of the 5- to 10-dB variation from frequency to frequency. Audiogram C illustrates a *mild to slight rising bilateral hearing loss* following the same left to right format of reporting. The description of the audiogram D would be separated for each ear because of the asymmetry as shown. Beginning with the right ear, the audiogram would be characterized as *hearing within normal limits for the right ear and a mild flat hearing loss in the left ear.*

In Figure 6.23, audiogram A shows a greater change in the degree of loss with a configuration described as *a mild to severe steeply sloping hearing loss bilaterally.* The example exhibited on audiogram B indicates a *bilateral severe to profound sloping hearing loss.*

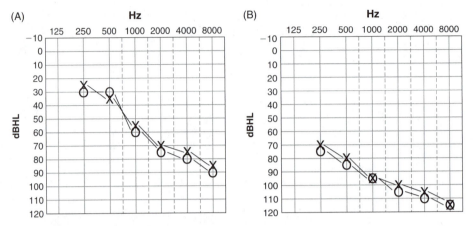

Figure 6.23 Audiograms displaying the audiometric characteristics, degree, configuration, and symmetry for a (A) mild to severe steeply sloping bilateral hearing loss, and (B) severe to profound sloping hearing loss bilaterally.

In many cases, the audiogram interpretation does not follow classic categorization as seen in the audiograms just described. In cases that exhibit dramatic changes in the degree of hearing loss, the format of interpretation needs to be modified accordingly. For example, in Figure 6.24, the description for audiogram A is *normal hearing sensitivity through 1000 Hz with a precipitous drop to a profound high-frequency hearing loss bilaterally*. Audiogram B in Figure 6.24 shows another example that is difficult to describe in the usual format. A description would be a *profound low-frequency hearing loss showing a corner audiogram with no measurable hearing above 1000 Hz in both ears*.

Generally it is assumed that prior to audiogram interpretation, the test results have been completed and appropriate masking has been utilized. However, as shown in audiogram C, the test results indicate *normal hearing sensitivity in the right ear but a moderate hearing loss in the left ear with unmasked air conduction thresholds*. When the masking rule of a 40 dB or greater difference between the two ears is applied, it is clear to see that the results for the right ear are inconclusive because there may be a crossover effect with the left ear responding to the stimulus. Once masking has been applied, the results would be displayed using masking symbols as shown in audiogram D indicating, in fact, true thresholds at the level of a *moderately severe to severe hearing loss* in the left ear.

Diagnosing Type of Loss

Now that the basic foundation of audiogram interpretation has been described with regard to degree, configuration, and symmetry of hearing loss, the bone conduction thresholds can be added to include another major puzzle piece of this interpretive process. Before applying the bone conduction results, however, it is important to understand how comparisons of the air conduction and bone conduction thresholds determine the type of hearing loss.

As indicated previously, when performing air conduction thresholds with either supra-aural or insert earphones, the sound is transferred through all portions of the ear from

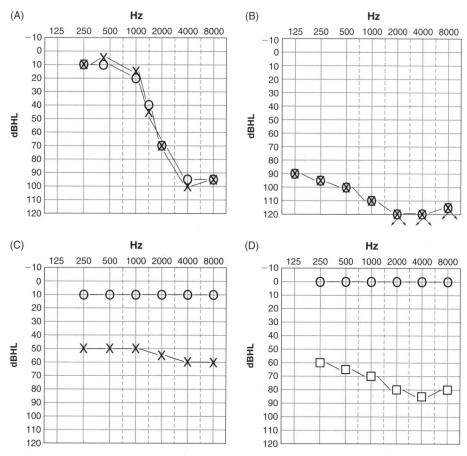

Figure 6.24 Audiograms displaying the audiometric characteristics, degree, configuration, and symmetry for (A) a normal hearing sensitivity through 1000 Hz with a precipitous drop to a profound high-frequency hearing loss bilaterally, and (B) profound low-frequency hearing loss showing a corner audiogram with no measurable hearing above 1000 Hz in both ears. Audiogram C represents normal hearing in the right ear and unmasked thresholds in the left ear that are inconclusive because of potential crossover effect. Audiogram D is the same patient using masking procedures, which results in accurate thresholds in the moderately severe to severe hearing loss range for the left ear.

the outer ear up through the central auditory pathway in order for the patient to respond. Thus we are measuring the entire auditory system. When a signal is presented by bone conduction using either mastoid or forehead placement, the signal is transmitted by bone directly to the inner ear, bypassing the conductive system of the outer and the middle ear. Therefore, bone conduction is measuring the sensorineural component of the system.

When the air conduction thresholds or response from the entire ear is compared to the bone conduction thresholds or the sensorineural portion of the ear, the difference in results is essentially the portion of the ear that remains, or the conductive component of the ear. This is illustrated in the following examples.

Example 1:

Threshold		Testing Procedure
30 dB	=	Air Conduction (The Entire System)
0 dB	=	Bone Conduction (Sensorineural Component)
30 dB	=	The Difference (Conductive Component or Air Bone Gap)

In Example 1, there is a 30-dB hearing loss at a given frequency by air conduction and a 0-dB threshold by bone conduction, which is the sensorineural component. The difference then between the entire system and the sensorineural component is 30 dB, which is interpreted as a conductive hearing loss.

Example 2:

Threshold		Testing Procedure
45 dB	=	Air Conduction (The Entire System)
45 dB	=	Bone Conduction (Sensorineural Component)
0 dB	=	The Difference (Conductive Component or Air-Bone Gap)

In Example 2, the air conduction thresholds are measured at 45 dBHL and the bone conduction results also reveal thresholds of 45 dBHL. The difference, therefore, is 0 dB, indicating the absence of an air-bone gap and resulting in a sensorineural hearing loss.

Example 3:

Threshold		Testing Procedure
65 dB	=	Air Conduction (The Entire System)
30 dB	=	Bone Conduction (Sensorineural Component)
35 dB	=	The Difference (Conductive Component or Air-Bone Gap)

Example 3 reveals thresholds by air conduction at 65 dB and thresholds by bone conduction at 30 dB. The difference between these two measurement results is an air-bone gap of 35 dBHL. In this particular case, a portion of this hearing loss is caused from a disorder in the sensorineural system and a portion of it is caused by a problem in the outer or middle ear of the conductive system, resulting in a mixed hearing loss.

The above illustrations can now be applied to an audiogram to complete the diagnostic picture by including type of hearing loss. The earlier discussion of bone conduction testing depicted a *mild flat conductive hearing loss bilaterally* (Figure 6.21). This result is determined by air conduction thresholds or the entire system measured at 30–35 dBHL and the bone conduction thresholds or sensorineural component measured generally at 0–5 dBHL. The difference or the air-bone gap is 30 dB indicating a conductive hearing loss. Note that because there was a significant air-bone gap, masking procedures were employed to obtain accurate bone conduction thresholds for each ear. Figure 6.25 displays several audiograms with completed air and bone conduction test results. Audiogram A shows a *mild to moderately severe sloping sensorineural hearing loss*. The interpretation of this audiogram is determined by noting that the air conduction and bone conduction thresholds

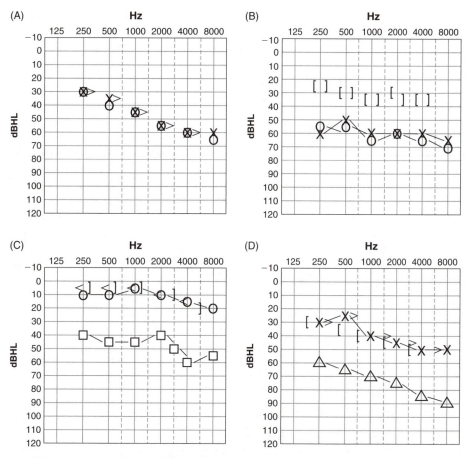

Figure 6.25 Audiograms displaying the audiometric characteristics, degree, configuration, type, and symmetry for a (A) mild to moderately severe sloping sensorineural hearing loss bilaterally, (B) moderately severe flat mixed bilateral hearing loss, (C) normal hearing in the right ear and a moderate to moderately severe conductive hearing loss in the left ear as indicated by the large air-bone gap (note the slight sensorineural component at 4000 Hz in the left ear), and (D) mild to moderate sloping sensorineural hearing loss in the left ear and a moderately severe to severe sloping mixed hearing loss in the right ear.

are essentially identical with no air-bone gap which results in a sensorineural hearing loss. A closer look at audiogram A reveals that the bone conduction thresholds are only shown for the right ear. Recall that the unmasked bone conduction threshold comes from the better ear and the threshold in the poorer ear cannot be worse than the air conduction thresholds, indicating that it can only be at the same level. The interpretation is a sensorineural hearing loss in both ears even though there is only one set of unmasked bone conduction thresholds. A representation of a *bilateral moderately severe flat mixed hearing loss* is displayed in audiogram B. The sensorineural portion of the hearing loss is the area above the bone conduction thresholds and the conductive component is between the air and bone results, or the air-bone gap. Audiogram C depicts *normal hearing sensitivity* in the right and a *unilateral conductive hearing loss of a moderate degree* in the left ear. An unusual audiogram (D) depicting both a sensorineural loss and a mixed loss is shown with the resulting interpretation being a *mild to moderate sloping sensorineural hearing loss in the left ear* and a *moderately severe to severe mixed hearing loss in the right ear*. A possible cause of this result might be an existing symmetrical sensorineural hearing loss in both ears compounded by impacted cerumen creating a greater loss in the right ear.

SPEECH AUDIOMETRY

The audiologic evaluation to this point has focused on measurements of hearing sensitivity in response to pure tones. As discussed previously, the pure tone signal provides a simple sound that is easily identifiable and provides frequency-specific information to determine the degree and configuration of a hearing impairment. However, the signal that is of greatest interest in determining the extent of hearing disability is speech. In conjunction with the pure tone air conduction and bone conduction audiometry, speech audiometry is an essential part of an audiological test battery. The ability to use speech in daily conversation will reveal more accurately the handicapping condition of a given hearing loss. Because of the complex nature of a speech signal, it can also be used to diagnose processing ability and the way in which various disorders affect it, particularly at higher levels along the auditory pathway. Speech measures often provide a more reliable result and can help verify the accuracy of the pure tone results. The assessment tools used in speech audiometry are designed to ascertain a person's ability to perceive speech and determine the disabling effects of a hearing loss and the prognosis for success with intervention.

Speech Threshold Measures

Speech Recognition Thresholds

The **speech recognition threshold (SRT)**, synonymous with speech reception threshold, is a routine part of the audiology test battery and has three basic purposes:

- As the name implies, the SRT is a threshold measure for speech.
- The pure tone test results can be verified by comparing the SRT to the pure tone average of the speech frequencies.
- The SRT is a reference level for further speech testing.

Specifically defined, "the speech recognition threshold is the minimum hearing level for speech at which an individual can recognize 50% of the speech material" (ASHA, 1988). Because this test is a threshold measure, it is logical then that the words used are the most easily identifiable. These preferred materials are called *spondees* or *spondaic words*—compound words with equal stress on each syllable (e.g., hotdog, baseball, airplane, toothbrush), and are homogenous with respect to audibility. The most common spondee list used to measure the SRT is the Central Institute for the Deaf (CID) Auditory Test W-1.

Although several different approaches have been recommended for determining the SRT (ASHA, 1988; Martin Dowdy, 1986; Tillman & Olsen, 1973; Chaiklin & Ventry, 1964), there is no set standard or procedure, only guidelines and recommendations

(Brandy, 2002). Each method suggests either a descending, ascending, or ascending/descending method with 5-dB steps in some approaches and 2-dB steps in others, all of which yield similar results. Ultimately, the intent of each procedure is to determine the lowest level that at least 50% of the responses are correct.

Speech Detection Thresholds

The **speech detection threshold** (SDT) is a measure that requires a patient to respond merely to the audibility of a speech signal rather than identifying a specific word. It is defined as the "minimum hearing level for speech at which an individual can just discern the presence of a speech material 50% of the time" (ASHA, 1988). Although the SDT (also referred to as the *speech awareness threshold,* or SAT) is not a standard procedure in routine audiological assessment, it is a valuable tool when the SRT is unobtainable. The evaluation of groups with special needs (e.g., nonverbal developmentally disabled adults, infants and small children, and some patients with profound hearing loss) necessitates the use of the SDT due to their inability to recognize words and respond appropriately as part of the SRT procedure.

The SDT is determined by presenting any speech signal—familiar words, running speech, or speech babble—at an intensity level that is estimated to be above the person's hearing level, using the same procedure recommended for pure tone testing (ASHA, 1988).

Word Recognition Testing

Now that a threshold for speech has been established, a true indicator of how well a person processes sound is discovered by presenting a stimulus at a comfortably loud level with all the necessary speech cues audible to the listener. **Word recognition testing**, formerly referred to as speech discrimination, is uniquely different from all previous measures because the speech stimulus is presented at a suprathreshold level in order for the patient to recognize and process the signal through the auditory system. Therefore, it is a measure of how well a person understands based on a percentage score rather than a threshold measure.

Word Lists

In the process of performing word recognition testing, it is important to use a stimulus that has a high level of reliability and repeatability to obtain an accurate measure of auditory processing. Historically and at present, word recognition testing utilizes word lists containing 50 items that are phonetically balanced (PB) with respect to the frequency of occurrence of these particular phonemes in everyday English language (Brandy, 2002). By using these PB word lists in the audiological evaluation, a percent-correct score is calculated and the ability for an individual to understand speech in that ear can be ascertained. The most prevalent word lists used today include the CID Auditory Test W-22 (Hirsh et al., 1952), which is a series of four lists of 50 words that are commonly used in spoken language; The Northwestern University Auditory Test number six (NU-6) with a similar format of four lists with 50 words that were modified and recorded by Tillman & Carhart (1966); and the Maryland CNC word lists (Causey et al., 1984) that are currently used in Veterans Affairs hospitals and clinics. For a complete treatment of these and other recognition tests, see Brandy (2002).

Test Procedures

Word recognition testing requires that several parameters be selected prior to starting the test procedures. If these parameters are selected improperly, the results of the testing and the measure of speech recognition could be significantly compromised.

1. *Presentation level.*   An accurate measure of auditory processing can be determined only when the signal is sufficiently loud so that the words are easily heard. Because the intensity of speech varies by about 30 dB from the loudest sound /a/, to the softest sound /th/, the suprathreshold level should be at least 30 dB above threshold so that all the speech sounds are audible. For example, if the results of testing reveal an SRT of 40 dBHL, then the presentation level would be set at 70 dBHL, or 30 dB above threshold. Although levels of 30–40 dB above the SRT are commonly used, the intent of the test is to obtain the maximum score possible, regardless of presentation level. It may be necessary to increase the level in cases where there is a steeply sloping configuration in order to ensure that the higher-frequency speech sounds are audible. In contrast, a patient with a more severe hearing loss may not tolerate a presentation level that is 30 to 40 dB above threshold because of loudness discomfort. In this case, the presentation level will need to be adjusted down so that it would be comfortable for the patient, but set at the upper limit of their most comfortable level. It is important to recognize that a softer level may compromise the accuracy of the results and may not yield a maximum speech recognition score.

Another factor influencing presentation level is seen in rare cases of sensorineural hearing loss that are caused by a retrocochlear disorder. As the intensity level increases when testing these patients, the test scores will actually become poorer. When this type of disorder is suspected, it may be necessary to conduct the test at different intensity levels to measure the changes in performance and determine the need for additional diagnostic testing.

On occasion, word recognition testing will be conducted at a level of normal conversation which is measured at 50 dBHL (Cox & Moore, 1988). The test score provides an estimate of a person's word recognition ability in everyday listening situations. The result of this test for a person with a significant hearing loss will likely be quite poor because many speech sounds are inaudible at that level. The value of performing the test, knowing that it may yield a poor score, is to assist with counseling patients and their families who may not fully comprehend or are unwilling to accept the significance of the hearing loss and its impact on communication.

2. *Recorded versus monitored live-voice.*   The word lists previously discussed have been recorded and are commercially available for use in word recognition testing. By using the recorded word list either on a cassette tape or compact disc, the consistency from test to test is greatly improved (Brandy, 1966; Carhart, 1965). Another method to use when performing speech testing is monitored live-voice. This refers to the use of a microphone attached to the audiometer with a volume unit (VU) meter to monitor the level of the signal as the words are being presented. Speech is a very dynamic signal and the intensity level can be difficult to control. The use of the VU meter will allow the examiner to monitor her or his voice to maintain consistency as each word is presented. In a busy audiology clinic, this procedure increases the speed and flexibility of testing because the presentation is controlled by the examiner. The disadvantage to using monitored live-voice is the variability in voices from examiner to examiner and in particular, male to female. Thus, the efficiency of this technique can be offset by the compromise made in the

accuracy of the results. However, the majority of audiologists use monitored live-voice (Wiley et al., 1995), despite recommendations to the contrary. Although some studies have reported good reliability with carefully monitored presentations by live-voice (Beattie et al., 1978; Creston et al., 1966), the preferred approach is to use a recorded word list especially in cases when the results will determine some form of compensation or legal action.

3. *Carrier phrase.*   The presentation of each word is usually preceded by a phrase such as "say the word . . ." or "you will say . . . ." The purpose for this phrase is to ready the patient in preparation to hear the test word. The Maryland CNC recordings embed the test word within the phrase in this manner, "say . . . again," in order to simulate the effect of coarticulation in running speech (Causey et al., 1984). Although it is not necessary to use a carrier phrase when measuring an SRT, studies have shown that its absence during word recognition testing may result in poorer scores (Gelfand, 1975; Gladstone & Siegenthaler, 1971).

Now that the basic parameters have been established by selecting the level of presentation and a recording of an appropriate word list, the testing can be performed. Word lists are presented, maintaining a consistent intensity level, to each ear and the percentage scores are recorded. The end test results provide an indicator of the auditory processing ability of the individual. This information can then be used to assist in the differential diagnosis of hearing impairment, and in cases of cochlear loss, the prognosis for aural rehabilitation. Figure 6.26 displays the results of two audiologic evaluations

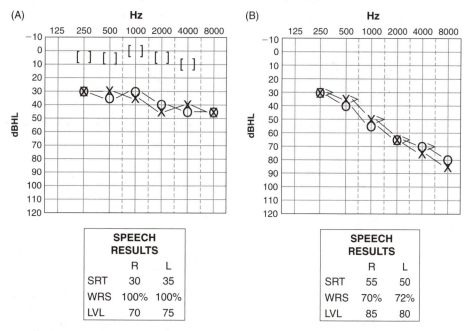

Figure 6.26   Audiograms illustrating the audiometric evaluation results for two cases: (A) mild flat bilateral conductive hearing loss with consistent speech recognition thresholds and excellent word recognition ability (100%) measured at levels of 70 and 75 dBHL, and (B) mild to severe steeply sloping sensorineural hearing loss with speech recognition thresholds that are consistent with the pure tone averages, and fair word recognition ability when measured at intensity levels of 85 and 80 dBHL.

including air conduction, bone conduction, and speech audiometry results. Note the correlation between the pure tone findings and the speech recognition thresholds, and the level at which word recognition testing was performed with the resulting test scores.

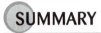 SUMMARY

A Glimpse into the Profession Revisited

The case of John was introduced at the beginning of the chapter. As you may recall, he is being seen for a complete audiometric evaluation to determine the reasons for hearing difficulty in a variety of situations. Air conduction and bone conduction testing were performed as well as speech audiometry to evaluate John's hearing sensitivity. Before reading the next section, or the figure caption, review the audiogram in Figure 6.27, and try to make a diagnosis and interpretation of the test results.

The test findings of John's hearing evaluation can be characterized as a slight to severe precipitous hearing loss bilaterally. Bone conduction testing resulted in similar thresholds, which revealed the absence of an air-bone gap, indicating a sensorineural hearing loss. Speech recognition thresholds were consistent with the pure tone results and word recognition ability was measured at 82% and 84% for the right and left ears, respectively. The test results were explained to John and based on the findings, it was recommended that he be fitted with hearing aids binaurally to compensate for and assist in overcoming his significant hearing loss.

Figure 6.27 Audiometric test results for John, revealing a slight to severe precipitous sensorineural hearing loss bilaterally. Speech recognition thresholds were measured at 20 dBHL, consistent with the PTA-2 average. Word recognition testing was administered at 70 dBHL with the scores indicating good performance in both ears.

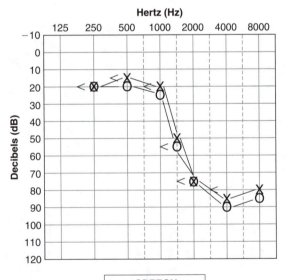

CHAPTER REVIEW

❑ This chapter has discussed the components and administration of an audiometric evaluation to assess the status of an individual's hearing ability.

❑ The identification of hearing impairment typically occurs from an appropriate professional, family, or self-referral and/or the detection of a problem through a screening program.

❑ Once individuals have been determined to be at risk for hearing loss, they are candidates for a complete audiological assessment. This evaluation typically begins with a thorough case history with questions specific to hearing. The history is followed by a visual examination of the ear canals using an otoscope. The case history and otoscopic examination create an appropriate foundation for the audiometric evaluation procedures.

❑ Components of the evaluation include a measure of hearing sensitivity through air conduction and bone conduction pathways. Using a calibrated audiometer in a quiet test environment such as a sound-treated booth, a person's hearing ability can be assessed and a diagnosis of hearing impairment can be determined. This is accomplished by presenting a series of pure tone stimuli and measuring the lowest level or threshold of audibility for the person being examined.

❑ The standard procedure used to accomplish an audiometric evaluation is a recommended technique that includes familiarization of the test stimulus and then a search phase to identify hearing thresholds. The thresholds are then plotted on an audiogram for interpretation.

❑ Test results can be interpreted by characterizing the hearing loss with specific terms such as degree, configuration, and symmetry. The process of interpretation also involves a comparison of the air conduction and bone conduction results in order to determine the type of hearing loss and to differentiate between a conductive, sensorineural, or mixed impairment.

❑ Occasionally, the signal presentation can be at a high-intensity level sufficient to cross over and be heard by the non–test ear. When this situation occurs, a masking noise is introduced to that ear in order to eliminate its participation in the test process. Masking procedures allow for a separate and independent diagnosis of hearing sensitivity in each ear.

❑ A final component to an evaluation is the measure of speech perception. A threshold measure of speech is followed by an assessment of speech processing using word recognition testing. These results can help determine the implications of the hearing loss with regard to auditory processing ability and gauge the prognosis of intervention.

ACTIVITIES FOR DISCUSSION

1. In the Case Study, how long do you think John has had a hearing loss? Was it progressive? What do you suppose is the underlying cause of the loss, or is there more than one cause?

2. In many cases there is a delay in referring someone for an audiological evaluation, whether it be a professional, the family, or self-referral. What are the reasons for this delay?

3. Why is a pure tone the primary test signal in audiometric evaluations and are there other types of stimuli that provide different or better information?

4. Because we must determine in every case the possibility of a stimulus crossing over to the non–test ear, why isn't masking used routinely for every evaluation?

REFERENCES

American National Standards Institute. (2004a). *Specifications for audiometers* (ANSI S3.6-2004). New York: Author.

American National Standards Institute. (2004b). *Methods for manual pure-tone threshold audiometry* (ANSI S3.21-357 2004), New York: Author.

American National Standards Institute. (2003). *Maximum permissible ambient noise levels for audiometric test rooms* (ANSI S3.1-1999; rev. ed.). New York: Author.

American Speech-Language-Hearing Association. (2005). *Guidelines for manual pure-tone threshold audiometry.* [Online]. http://www.asha.org/members/deskref-journal/deskref/default

American Speech-Language-Hearing Association. (2004). *Guidelines for the audiologic assessment of children from birth to 5 years of age* [Online]. http://www.asha.org/members/deskref-journals/deskref/default

American Speech-Language-Hearing Association. (1988). Guidelines for determining threshold level for speech. *ASHA*, 85–89.

American Speech-Language-Hearing Association. (1978). Guidelines for manual pure tone audiometry, *ASHA*, 20, 297–301.

Barry, S. J. (1994). Can bone conduction thresholds really be poorer than air? *American Journal of Audiology*, 3(3), 21–22.

Beattie, R. C., Forrester, P. W., & Ruby, B. K. (1977). Reliability of the Tillman-Olsen procedure for determination of spondee threshold using recorded and live voice presentations. *Journal of the American Auditory Society*, 2, 159–162.

Brandy, W. T. (2002). Speech audiometry. In J. Katz (Ed.), *Handbook of clinical audiology* (5th ed., 96–110). Baltimore: Williams & Wilkins.

Brandy, W. T. (1966). Reliability of vouce tests of speech discrimination. *Journal of Speech and Hearing Research*, 9, 461–465.

Burk, M. H., & Wiley, T. L. (2004). Continuous versus pulsed tones in audiometry, *American Journal of Audiology*, 13(1), 54–61.

Carhart, R. (1965). Problems in the measurement of speech discrimination. *Archives of Otolaryngology*, 82, 253–260.

Carhart, R., & Jerger, J. F. (1959). Preferred method for clinical determination of pure-tone thresholds. *Journal of Speech and Hearing Disorders*, 24, 330–345.

Causey, G. D., Hood, L. J., Hermanson, C. L., & Bowling, L. S. (1984). The Maryland CNC test: normative studies. *Audiology*, 23, 552–568.

Chaiklin, J. B. (1967). Interaural attenuation and cross-hearing in air-conduction audiometry. *Journal of Auditory Research*, 7, 413–424.

Chaiklin, J. B., & Ventry, I. M. (1964). Spondee threshold measurement: a comparison of 2- and 5-dB steps. *Journal of Speech and Hearing Disorders*, 29, 47–59.

Coles, R. R. A., & Priede, V. M. (1968). Problems in cross-hearing and masking. Institution of Sound and Vibration Research, *Annual Report*, 26, England.

Cox, R. M., & Moore, J. N. (1988). Composite speech spectrum for hearing aid gain prescriptions. *Journal of Speech and Hearing Research*, 31, 102–107.

Creston, J. E., Gillespie, M., & Krohn, C. (1966). Speech audiometry: tape vs. live-voice. *Archives of Otolaryngology*, 83, 14–17.

Gelfand, S. A. (1975). Use of the carrier phrase in live voice speech discrimination testing. *Journal of Auditory Research*, 15, 107–110.

Gladstone, V. S., & Siegenthaler, B. M. (1971). Carrier phrase and speech intelligibility score. *Journal of Auditory Research*, 11, 101–103.

Goldstein, B. A., & Newman, C. W. (1994). Clinical masking: A decision-making process. In J. Katz (Ed.), *Handbook of clinical audiology* (4th ed., pp. 109–131). Baltimore: Williams & Wilkins.

Harrell, R.W. (2002). Puretone evaluation. In J. Katz (Ed.) *Handbook of Clinical Audiology*. 5th ed. Lippincott, Williams & Wilkins, pp. 71–93.

Harris, J. D. (1979). Optimum threshold crossings and time window validation in threshold pure-tone audiometry. *Journal of the Acoustical Society of America, 66,* 1545–1547.

Hinchcliffe, (1988). Tuning fork tests. *British Journal of Audiology,* May.

Hirsh, I. J. (1952). *Measurement of hearing.* New York: McGraw-Hill.

Hirsh, L., Davis, H., Silverman, S., Reynolds, E., Eldert, E., & Benson, R. (1952). Development of materials for speech audiometry. *Journal of Speech and Hearing Disorders, 17,* 321–337

Hughson, W., & Westlake, H. D. (1944). Manual for program outline for rehabilitation of aural casualties both military and civilian. *Transactions of the American Academy of Ophthalmology and Otolaryngology, 48*(Suppl.), 1–15.

Katz, J., & Lezynski, J. (2002). Clinical masking. In J. Katz (Ed.), *Handbook of clinical audiology* (5th ed., pp. 124–141). Baltimore: Williams & Wilkins.

Killion, M. C., Wilber, L. A., & Gudmundsen, G. I. (1985). Insert earphones for more interaural attenuation. *Hearing Instruments, 36,* 34–36.

Liden, G., Nilsson, G., & Anderson, H. (1959). Masking in clinical audiometry. *Acta Otolaryngologica, 50,* 125–136.

Martin, F. N., Champlin, C. A., & Chambers, J. A. (1998). Seventh survey of audiometric practices in the United States. *Journal of the American Academy of Audiology, 9,* 95–104.

Martin, F. N., & Dowdy, L. K. (1986). A modified spondee threshold procedure. *Journal of Auditory, Research, 26,* 115–119.

Miltenburg, (1994). The validity of tuning fork tests in diagnosing hearing loss. *Journal of Otolaryngology,* August.

Reger, S. N. (1950). Standardization of pure-tone audiometer testing technique. *Laryngoscope, 60,* 161–185.

Sanders, J. W., & Hall, J. W. (1999). Clinical masking. In F. Musiek & W. Rintelmann (Eds.), *Contemporary perspectives in hearing assessment* (pp. 67–87). Boston: Allyn & Bacon.

Sklare, D. A., & Denenberg, L. J. (1987). Technical note: Interaural attenuation for Tubephone insert earphones. *Ear and Hearing, 8,* 298–300.

Snyder, J. M. (1973). Interaural attenuation characteristics in audiometry. *Laryngoscope, 83,* 1847–1855.

Studebaker, C. A. (1967). Clinical masking of the non–test ear. *Journal of Speech and Hearing Disorders, 32,* 360–367.

Tillman, T. W., & Olsen, W. O. (1973). Speech audiometry. In J. Jerger (Ed.), *Modern developments in audiology* (pp. 37–74). New York: Academic Press.

Tillman, T. W., & Carhart, R. (1966). *An expanded test for speech discrimination utilizing CNC monosyllabic words.* Northwestern University Auditory Test No. 6. Technical report no. SAM-TR-66-55. San Antonio, TX: USAF School of Aerospace Medicine, Brooks Air Force Base.

Tyler, E. S., & Wood, E. J. (1980). A comparison of manual methods for measuring hearing thresholds. *Audiology, 19*(390), 316–329.

United States Department of Labor (USDoL). (1983). Occupational noise exposure: hearing conservation amendment: Final rule, *Federal Register, 48,* 9738–9785.

Wiley, T. L., Stoppenbach, D. T., Feldhake, L. J., Moss, K. A., & Thordardottir, E. T. (1995). Audiologic practices: What is popular versus what is supported by evidence. *American Journal of Audiology, 4*(1), 26–34.

Yacullo, W. S. (1996) *Clinical masking procedures.* Boston: Allyn & Bacon.

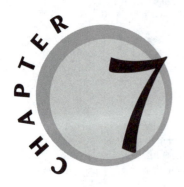

Physiologic Tests of the Auditory System

Peter J. Ivory

Key Terms

CASE STUDY

A Glimpse into the Profession

Jonas is a newborn who is immediately recognized as having a significant malformation of his right ear, along with an extremely narrow external right ear canal. These conditions are typically associated with additional malformation of the middle ear. The obvious physical differences in Jonas' right ear have not escaped the notice of his physicians or parents and these differences create many questions, distractions, and anxiety for the new parents. They ask, Does our child hear? He's a newborn—how can you test his hearing? Can he hear in his right ear? Do we need to do anything about it?

Overview of Physiologic Tests of the Auditory System

The process of assessing a person's hearing sensitivity has been discussed in Chapters 5 and 6. A group of tests incorporating estimates of hearing threshold for tones and for speech via air conduction and for tones via bone conduction, and as well, a measure of word recognition, have been in clinical use for more than 60 years. It is apparent then that these behavioral tests are sufficient to answer many clinical questions about a person's hearing. However, a key ingredient in the successful completion of all these tests is the requirement for a behavioral response from the patient—for example, a hand raise to acknowledge that a tone was heard or the repetition of a word. Some patients—young children, for example—simply may not have developed the appropriate cognitive, social, or speech skills needed to complete the required behavioral task. Other patients may not understand the instructions and task required of them. Still others may be unwilling to cooperate completely or may attempt to feign hearing loss for undetermined reasons. Therefore, a sole reliance on behavioral tests would leave many patients and their families with unanswered questions regarding their hearing.

There is, however, another way hearing can be estimated and that is by utilizing **physiologic procedures**. These procedures measure a physical response from some aspect of the person's auditory system during or following the presentation of an acoustic stimulus. Strictly speaking, these tests of the auditory system are not tests of hearing; rather, they are measures of the responses of physical structures that are needed in order for the experience we call "hearing" to occur. These tests are extremely useful because they can be completed on patients who may be incapable or unwilling to perform behavioral testing. Although they are not tests of hearing, they provide powerful data that can be used to infer the status of hearing in a patient. In addition, physiologic tests

Table 7.1 Comparison of Behavioral versus Physiologic Tests

Behavioral	Physiologic
Test of hearing	Test of the physical response of some part of the auditory system
Active participation	Passive cooperation
Patient has to understand task	No understanding of task required
Simple/inexpensive equipment	Complicated/expensive equipment
Subjective data	Objective data, but often requiring subjective interpretation

have been adapted for use in both screening and diagnostic applications. Professional practice guidelines in audiology specify the inclusion of physiologic tests in the audiologic assessment of children (American Speech-Language-Hearing Association, 2004). See Table 7.1 for a comparison of behavioral and physiological tests.

In order from outer to inner, **acoustic immittance measures** assess the function of the outer and middle ears, with implications for the inner ear, auditory nerve, and lower auditory brain stem. **Otoacoustic emission (OAE)** testing measures the function of the inner ear when a normal outer and middle ear are present. Finally, the **auditory brainstem response (ABR)** test measures the electrical signal as it travels along the auditory nerve. The ABR is a particularly useful test because all four parts of a normal ear can be included in the assessment. This chapter addresses these physiological tests.

ACOUSTIC IMMITTANCE MEASURES

Overview of Acoustic Immittance

In Chapters 5 and 6, the effective use of air conduction and bone conduction measures and comparisons was described such that problems in the conductive hearing mechanism (outer and middle ears) could be identified; this type of problem is classified as conductive hearing loss. So, one might ask, Why would we need another test that gives similar diagnostic information? There are several answers to this question. First, as stated earlier, acoustic immittance measures do not require a behavioral response from the patient; thus, these measures expand the amount of information that can be obtained from infants, children, and other difficult to test patients. Second, and perhaps more important, a medically significant middle ear disorder could be present without a clinically significant air-bone gap on pure tone audiometric findings. Findings on acoustic immittance tests may be the only indication of middle ear disease or dysfunction. Third, acoustic immittance measures often differentiate several middle ear diseases and conditions that may manifest similar test results with air conduction and bone conduction testing. In clinical work, the combination of acoustic immittance findings and standard audiometric results provides a complete, quick, and cost-effective assessment of a person's auditory system in most cases. Finally, acoustic immittance tests yield unique data—that is, data that cannot be obtained in any other way at this time.

A second question that arises in discussion of acoustic immittance measures is, What information does it provide? Acoustic immittance measures are useful in the assessment of:

1. The eardrum and middle ear function, especially in determining the presence of disease or dysfunction
2. The integrity of the auditory pathway and in determining and differentiating a cochlear from a retrocochlear lesion
3. The confirmation of pure tone audiometric test results regarding both type of hearing loss and degree of hearing sensitivity
4. Facial nerve (cranial nerve VII) integrity, on efferent pathway of acoustic reflex arc

Because acoustic immittance measures are so valuable in serving these functions, they have become a routine part of the audiological evaluation in most practice settings. Because it has been demonstrated that acoustic immittance measures are more effective than pure tone audiometry in determining whether an individual has a middle ear disorder needing medical treatment, acoustic immittance measures are considered a fundamental component of any hearing assessment program for school-age children (AAA, 1997; ASHA, 1997).

Principles of Acoustic Immittance Measures

Since the introduction and widespread adoption of acoustic immittance measures in the United States in the early 1970s, there have been significant changes in instrumentation and terminology that, at times, have created confusion in students and clinicians alike. Basically, examiners using acoustic immittance measures are interested in commenting on the efficiency of the outer and middle ears to "conduct" acoustic energy from the environment to the inner ear, that is, whether energy flows easily or not. This conduction process (notably, involving the tympanic membrane and the ossicles) has a significant mechanical component; therefore, examiners typically are tempted to couch acoustic immittance findings in purely mechanical terms, although this is not accurate (Wiley & Stoppenbach, 2002). The measurement of acoustic immittance in the ear is based on scientific principles grounded in the disciplines of acoustical, electrical, and mechanical engineering. An overview of the basic principles is presented below but the reader who is interested in the science and background details surrounding acoustic immittance measures should refer to the exemplary treatments by Wiley and Fowler (1997) and Fowler and Shanks (2002).

Acoustic immittance measures are ways to assess the flow of energy into the conductive hearing mechanism. When acoustic energy arrives at the conductive mechanism, fundamentally, one of two things can happen to it. Energy can flow into the conductive mechanism and into the inner ear: the specific term **admittance** refers to energy flow into a system. Alternatively, there can be opposition to the flow of energy into a system: the specific term **impedance** refers to the opposition of energy flow into a system. Contemporary devices utilize admittance technology to complete acoustic immittance measures, but early devices utilized impedance technologies to complete these tests. Fortunately for clinicians, these two terms are reciprocals of each other: if a system has high admittance, it has to have relatively low impedance; conversely, if a system has high impedance, it has to have relatively low admittance. The nonspecific term **immittance** refers to a measure of energy flow whether that measure is admittance-based or whether it is impedance-based. In the most simplified and probably most utilized acoustic immittance procedure (namely, single-frequency, single-component tympanometry), the clinical conclusions drawn from the test are similar regardless of whether the acoustic immittance measure was obtained with admittance technology or with impedance technology, this despite inherent differences in the underlying technologies, terminology, and units of measure.

The value of acoustic immittance measures, it seems, has not been in exploiting its underlying complexity or for that matter, in appreciating the details of its scientific groundings. Rather, it is probably the case that many users of acoustic immittance data are more interested in the practical application with clinical correlation to audiometry and other findings and in comparison to a large normative database. Physical evidence of abnormally poor energy flow into a middle ear system is compelling evidence because this may suggest the presence of a condition that may cause progressive and widespread damage with associated hearing loss or, at the very least, corroborates behavioral audiometric findings.

Instrumentation

A contemporary electroacoustic immittance meter, sometimes referred to as a middle ear analyzer, is the instrumentation that is typically used to perform immittance measurements (see Figure 7.1).

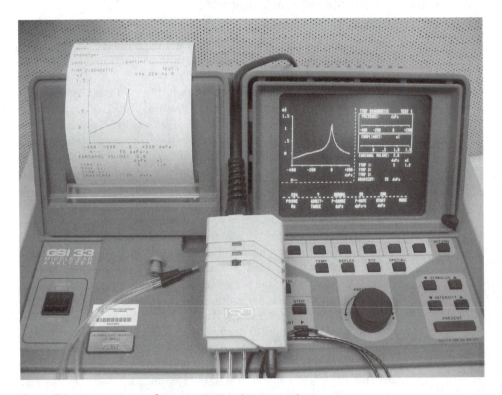

Figure 7.1 Equipment used in acoustic immittance testing
Source: Courtesy of VIASYS Healthcare

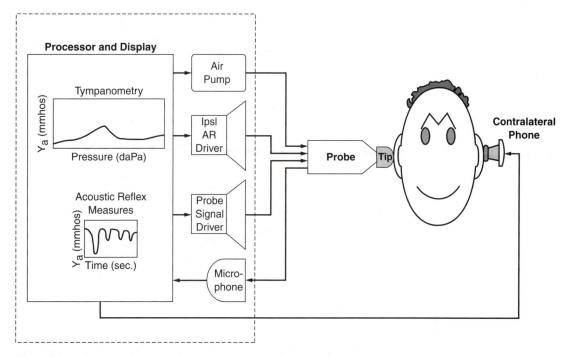

Figure 7.2   Schematic diagram of a generic acoustic immittance measurement system

Source: Reprinted with permission from T. Wiley & D. Stoppenbach (2002), Basic principles of acoustic immittance measures, chapter in J. Katz (Ed.), *Handbook of Clinical Audiology* (5th ed.). Philadephia: Lippincott Williams and Wilkins

A schematic of the components of this testing equipment is diagramed in Figure 7.2. In addition to the sound generating and measuring parts, the immittance device has a processor that converts acoustic measures obtained from the ear canal into units of acoustic admittance. Acoustic immittance devices must meet current performance and calibration standards within the tolerances specified in the national standards document (ANSI S3.39-1987).

Acoustic immittance measures of the ear begin with placing a probe tip into the ear canal. This probe tip is housed in a flexible rubber or plastic cuff that must fit snugly in the patient's ear canal to create an airtight (hermetic) seal, thus permitting instrumental changes in the air pressure of the ear canal. The cuff surrounds a casing that in turn houses three tubes. The first tube is connected to a loudspeaker driven by a device that creates an acoustic signal (hereafter referred to as the probe tone) that is delivered into the patient's ear canal. Most acoustic admittance devices permit the examiner to choose from among several frequencies for the probe tone. The default probe tone frequency in many devices is 226 Hz (in older devices, 220 Hz). This is the conventional frequency for adult tympanometry. A higher-frequency (1000 Hz) probe tone is better suited for tympanometry in infants.

A second tube enclosed in the probe tip is connected to a microphone that picks up the acoustic energy in the ear canal. This energy is a combination of the output of the instrument's loudspeaker (the probe tone) and the probe tone's interaction with the ear canal and eardrum, and indirectly, the ossicles and other parts of the middle ear. It is important to note that all actual measurements (by the microphone) are in decibels (SPL), but that these dBSPL values are converted by the internal processor into units of acoustic admittance (millimhos or mmhos). This happens because at 226 Hz, there is a known and predictable relationship between dBSPL, volume, and acoustic admittance. The data can then be used to infer the status of the outer and middle ears. Implicit to this process is the understanding that the physical structures of the ear canal, tympanic membrane, and ossicles will interact in a predictable way in both a normal condition and in conditions in which their mechanics are altered.

In general, there are two states possible: (1) a "normal" state, with good energy flow; and (2) an altered state, with poorer energy flow. Typically but not necessarily, when in the altered state, the mechanical system is not as flexible as it would be in the "normal" state; this lack of flexibility could also be considered as an increase in stiffness of the system. When mechanical systems become stiffer, energy tends to reflect away from them. In the ear canal, then, when the tympanic membrane and ossicles are stiffer, they reflect more of the acoustic energy that was emitted by the loudspeaker in the probe tip, which in turn results in an increase of energy (original signal now plus reflected signal) at the microphone. The processor is constantly monitoring both the output signal (at the loudspeaker) and the signal at the microphone. Technically, the processor is reading the voltage required to maintain a constant dBSPL in the ear canal. When more dBSPL is picked up at the microphone than was emitted at the loudspeaker, that additional energy came from somewhere—in this case, from poor mechanical function, with increased stiffness, more reflected signal, and therefore, more energy read at the microphone.

The third component is a tube within the probe tip that is connected to an air pressure pump with a pressure meter called a manometer. This device allows for air pressure change in the ear canal either by pumping more air into the ear canal (creating a positive pressure relative to ambient room pressure) or by sucking the air out of the ear canal (creating a negative pressure relative to ambient room pressure). The units of measure of pressure are given in decaPascals (daPa). These three basic components form the basis for the first of the two acoustic immittance measures, namely, tympanometry, which will be discussed in detail below.

In addition to these three basic components, one more component is needed to complete the second acoustic immittance measure, namely, **acoustic reflex testing**. This is a device to create, control, and deliver a high-intensity acoustic stimulus into the patient's ear canal, which in a normal ear will elicit the reflexive response of a momentary tightening of the ossicular chain and tympanic membrane. Typically, a tone is used as the reflex-activating stimulus and therefore is referred to as the activating tone. Please note that during acoustic reflex testing, two different tones are delivered into the patient's ear canal: the probe tone (226 Hz at an intensity under the control of the instrument); and the activating tone (adjustable in both frequency and intensity, under the control of the examiner).

In acoustic reflex testing, the stimulus tone may be delivered to the ear canal with the probe tip assembly in it (this is called an **ipsilateral**, or same side, acoustic reflex test) or by delivering the stimulus tone to the ear canal opposite the ear with the probe tip assembly (this is called a **contralateral**, or opposite side, acoustic reflex test). Other components that make up the acoustic immittance device are the various controls to alter the protocol for the testing, a video display, and a paper strip chart to print out the results. Some systems incorporate wireless technology to transmit acoustic immittance data to a computer where it may be digitally stored for later incorporation into a report or other printout.

Tympanometry

In general terms, **tympanometry** is a technique that provides a quantitative estimation of the efficiency of energy flow into the conductive hearing mechanism. Energy flow into this system is optimized under two circumstances: first, when the air pressures in the external ear canal and the middle ear cavity are approximately equal; and second, when all structures in the outer and middle ears are free of pathology or conditions of difference.

The determination of the air pressure in the two cavities of the conductive mechanism is an important aspect in quantifying the function of the system. In an absolute sense, the air pressure in the external ear canal will vary according to the ambient atmospheric pressure; however, this is not clinically important. In contrast, the air pressure of the middle ear cavity will vary depending on the status of both the eustachian tube and of the middle ear itself. Knowledge of this pressure is clinically important, and so this air pressure must be estimated.

Pathologies or conditions of difference in the middle ear and its structures fundamentally affect these structures' ability to perform normally in the transmission of energy. Because the middle ear is a mechanical system incorporating movement, pathologies or conditions of difference that affect it by compromising its ability to move cause an inefficiency in energy flow into this system.

Strictly speaking, tympanometry is the measurement of the efficiency of energy flow into the middle ear system as air pressure is varied in the external ear canal. The graph of tympanometric data is called a **tympanogram** (see Figure 7.3); it plots energy flow in units of acoustic admittance (mmhos) on the ordinate versus pressure changes in daPa on the abscissa. The first clinically available tympanometric devices were predominantly manual in test execution, requiring the examiner to make several settings and adjustments throughout the procedure. In contrast, contemporary tympanometry devices are highly automatized, so tympanometric data collection is typically quick and easy, especially with devices that are marketed as screening devices. Understanding and accommodation for abnormal test performance typically requires more sophistication in test execution and instrumentation. As with other equipment, there are published calibration and performance standards (ANSI S3.39-1987).

In contemporary tympanometry testing, first the probe tip assembly is fitted with a cuff to snugly fit into the ear canal. Upon placement of the cuffed probe tip assembly in the ear canal, the tympanometry procedure is initiated, usually by pressing a single button. If the cuff is adequate in sealing the ear canal, the **tympanometer** then automatically and systematically changes the air pressure in the ear canal over a range of positive through negative air pressures while simultaneously measuring the acoustic admittance at all these pressure settings. This procedure yields the tympanogram, as well as several individual items of data. The first item of interest is equivalent ear canal volume.

Figure 7.3   Example of a normal tympanogram obtained from an adult male using a GSI 33 middle ear analyzer. In this example, equivalent ear canal volume was 2.0 ml, tympanometric peak was at 5 daPa, overall admittance (Y_{tm}) was 1.2 ml, and tympanometric width (here labeled as gradient) was 55 daPa.

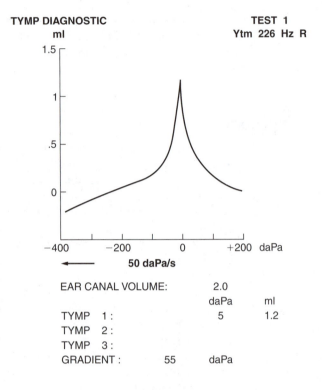

TYMP DIAGNOSTIC   TEST 1
ml   Ytm 226 Hz R

EAR CANAL VOLUME:		2.0	
		daPa	ml
TYMP 1 :		5	1.2
TYMP 2 :			
TYMP 3 :			
GRADIENT :		55	daPa

Equivalent Ear Canal Volume

The term *equivalent* is used to indicate that the value in discussion is an approximation of the actual value of interest. It's a way to acknowledge that the actual thing is not being measured, but what is being measured corresponds so closely to the actual thing that we can substitute our measurement for the thing of interest. *Equivalent ear canal volume* refers to an estimation of the volume that exists between the probe tip and the tympanic membrane (Wiley & Fowler, 1997) and is based on the knowledge that, under a standard test condition, and using a probe tone of 226 Hz, 1 cm³ of volume has an acoustic admittance value of 1 acoustic mmho. In deriving equivalent ear canal volume, the typical standard condition is the introduction of 200 daPa (a positive pressure) into the ear canal and the measure of acoustic admittance at that point is converted into a unit of volume (cubic centimeter) or alternatively with most contemporary devices, in units of milliliters (ml).

The estimation of equivalent ear canal volume will vary according to the size of an individual's ear canal as well as the insertion depth of the probe tip. Ear canal size generally varies according to age and gender. The estimation of equivalent ear canal volume can be useful when the derived value is compared to existing databases specific for age and gender (see Shanks, Stelmachowicz, Beauchaine, & Shulte, 1992 and Roup, Wiley, Safady, & Stoppenbach, 1998). If the normal range for an adult male ear canal volume varies from approximately 0.5 ml to 1.5 ml, when testing a preschooler, for example, it would be expected that the ear canal volume would more closely approximate 0.5 ml; whereas an elderly male adult may exhibit an ear canal volume closer to 1.5 ml.

An abnormally low equivalent ear canal volume may indicate a significant occlusion in the ear canal or a test artifact in which the examiner inserted the probe tip into the soft tissue of the ear canal instead of into the air of the ear canal. Conversely, an abnormally high equivalent ear canal volume suggests that a volume greater than just the ear canal exists and this may be an indication of a perforation in the tympanic membrane, as the enlarged volume reading includes both the volume of the ear canal as well as the volume of the middle ear spaces.

Peak Compensated Static Acoustic Admittance

In tympanometry, acoustic admittance is measured as pressure is changed. The term *peak compensated static acoustic admittance* (Y_{tm}) is used to indicate the maximum acoustic admittance at the one single pressure value at which it occurred (the static value). The inclusion of "peak compensated" simply indicates that the value of the ear canal volume was subtracted from the maximum admittance calculation. As with equivalent ear canal volume, the theoretical usefulness of Y_{tm} occurs when a derived value is compared to existing databases and clinical correlations. Y_{tm} is also given in units of volume or in milliliters. Generally, there are three categories of Y_{tm}: within normal limits; reduced; and excessive. The absolute values for each of these categories varies across age groups (infant, child, and adult).

There are examples of middle ear pathology when Y_{tm} is not in the range of normal. For example, in cases of otitis media, the presence of fluid in the middle ear cavities compromises the movement of the tympanic membrane. The end result will be a reduced Y_{tm}. Excessive Y_{tm} may be observed in a case of ossicular discontinuity where there is a break in the ossicular chain causing hypermobility of the middle ear system. However, in general, Y_{tm} has the least diagnostic value due to overlap of values from normal and pathologic ears (Fowler & Shanks, 2002). Both reduced and excessive Y_{tm} values may or may not indicate true middle ear pathology. Therefore, just because these results occur, they should not be misconstrued as pathology being present.

Tympanogram Peak Pressure

Tympanometric peak pressure (TPP) is the pressure given in daPa at which the peak of the tympanogram occurs (Wiley & Stoppenbach, 2002) and is an indirect estimation of the pressure in the middle ear cavity. TPP is an estimate of the air pressure at which acoustic admittance is maximum, and therefore is the pressure at which energy flows best into the conductive mechanism (Fowler & Shanks, 2002). Normal TPP is 0 daPa. In theory, abnormal TPP can occur with either a positive (greater than 0 daPa) or negative (less than 0 daPa) value.

Generally, there are no true middle ear pathologies that cause positive TPP readings, although a positively valued TPP can be viewed following various ways of inducing positive air pressure up the eustachian tubes. A common clinical procedure used to induce positive air pressure flow is known as the Valsalva maneuver (close mouth, pinch nostrils tight, and attempt to blow air out; because there's nowhere to go, the air is forced up the eustachian tubes).

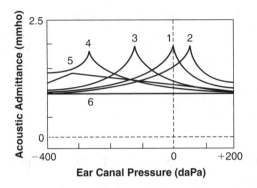

Figure 7.4 Depiction of expected changes in tympanograms throughout an episode of otitis media with effusion. At (1), the tympanogram is within normal limits, with a slight positive pressure change at (2). There is subsequent development of negative pressure at (3) and (4), with a decrease in overall admittance at (5), and ultimately a flattening of the tympanogram at (6).

Source: Reprinted with permission from C. Fowler & J. Shanks (2002), Tympanometry, chapter in J. Katz (Ed.), *Handbook of Clinical Audiology* (5th ed.). Philadelphia: Lippincott Williams and Wilkins

Negatively valued TPPs are typically indicative of some degree of eustachian tube dysfunction and are often seen as both precursors to otitis media and in resolution out of otitis media (see Figure 7.4). Negatively valued TPPs also include ears with no true pathology, and this overlap has minimized the quantitative and predictive significance of the TPP.

Tympanogram Width

All the preceding data are individual measurements aimed at quantifying specific aspects of tympanometric performance. But because the tympanogram is a line on a graph, words to describe the shape of this line have long been part of tympanometry. One approach to the quantification of tympanometric shape is to use *tympanometric width* (TW), which is a calculation of the width of the tympanogram in the region of its peak; it is given in daPa. TW is obtained by calculating half of the Y_{tm}, and then drawing a horizontal line across the entire tympanogram at this value; this horizontal line should intersect the tympanogram at two points (see Figure 7.5). The distance in daPa between these two points is the TW. As with several of the other measures, TW is useful when compared to normative populations. A normal tympanogram has a relatively sharp shape in the region of the peak that corresponds quantitatively with a TW that is less than 110 daPa in adults. The presence of significant middle ear pathology, especially otitis media with effusion, diminishes or eliminates the sharpness of this peak with a resulting larger (wider) TW. In children, abnormal TW ranges from greater than 200 daPa depending on age and previous ear infection history (ASHA, 1997). Tympanometric gradient is another approach that has been used to quantify the shape of the tympanogram, but unlike tympanometric width, which is calculated in daPa, gradient is calculated in units of acoustic admittance.

Figure 7.5 Example of tympanogram depicting calculation of tympanometric width

Source: Reprinted with permission from T. Wiley & D. Stoppenbach (2002), Basic principles of acoustic immittance measures, chapter in J. Katz (Ed.), *Handbook of Clinical Audiology* (5th ed.). Philadelphia: Lippincott Williams and Wilkins

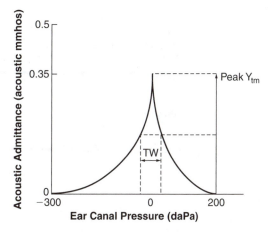

Tympanogram Description

As discussed, there are three major quantitative domains that are captured in a single tympanogram: the Y_{tm}, the TPP, and the TW. Obviously, the calculation and coordination of the numeric data available from tympanometry is challenging. It is probably the case that the description of a tympanogram that simply states these three quantitative results is probably the least prone to error and variability in interpretation, at least to knowledgeable users and consumers of tympanometry. For students of tympanometry, one approach to tympanogram description is to consider that each of the three quantitative domains has three possible categorical outcomes: a domain-specific less than normal; within normal limits, and a domain-specific greater than normal. For Y_{tm}, these outcomes are: reduced; within normal limits; and excessive. For TPP, these outcomes are: pressure negative relative to 0 daPa; within normal limits; and pressure positive relative to 0 daPa. For TW, these outcomes are: narrow (less than 50 daPa); within normal limits; and wide (greater than 110 daPa). Because each of the three domains has three outcomes, in theory, there would be $3 \times 3 \times 3$ (or 27) possible tympanograms. In clinical application, there are no common significant positive TPP outcomes, so the clinically relevant possible number of categorical tympanograms reduces slightly to $3 \times 2 \times 3$ (or 18). These outcomes are summarized in Table 7.2.

A classification system, such as the simple system just described, seeks to take the main clinical findings and create categories or types of results. In the 30-plus years that tympanometry has been utilized in the United States, several classification systems have been described in the literature. The classification system that seems to have the most widespread use is the ABC-typing system originally described by Liden et al. (1970). In this classification system as it is generally clinically used, the TPP, the Y_{tm}, and a nonquantifiable description of the shape of the tympanogram are used to define three main categories of tympanograms: A; B; C; and two subcategories of the A tympanogram, namely A_S (read as "A, sub-S") and A_D (read as "A, sub-D"). These five general types of tympanograms are shown in Figure 7.6. While popular, classification systems have the implicit peril that valuable information quantified in tympanometry is not considered.

Table 7.2 Hypothetical 226-Hz tympanograms based on descriptions of three tympanometric quantities: peak compensated static acoustic admittance (Y_{tm}); tympanometric peak pressure (TPP); and tympanometric width (TW). *Note:* Tympanograms with positive TPP are not included as these are not consistent with pathology and would be unlikely findings.

Y_{tm}	TPP	TW	Example Pathology *or Comment*
Reduced			
	Negative	Wide or no peak	Otitis media with effusion (OME)
		WNL	Eustachian tube dysfunction (ETD); OME
		Narrow	ETD
	WNL	Wide or no peak	Ossicular fixation; OME
		WNL	Ossicular fixation
		Narrow	Ossicular fixation
WNL			
	Negative	Wide or no peak	OME
		WNL	ETD; OME
		Narrow	ETD
	WNL	Wide or no peak	*Unlikely finding—possible artifact*
		WNL	Normal finding
		Narrow	Normal finding
Excessive			
	Negative	Wide or no peak	*Unlikely finding—possible artifact*
		WNL	ETD
		Narrow	Healed perforation
	WNL	Wide or no peak	*Unlikely finding—possible artifact*
		WNL	Tympanosclerosis; disarticulated ossicles
		Narrow	Tympanosclerosis; disarticulated ossicles

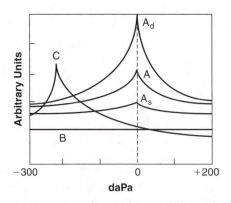

Figure 7.6 Line drawings of five tympanograms labeled according to the Jerger-Liden classification scheme: Type A is within normal limits, type A_d is peaked with high admittance, type A_s is peaked with low admittance, type B is flat, and type C is peaked at negative pressure.

Source: Reprinted with permission from C. Fowler & J. Shanks (2002), Tympanometry, chapter in J. Katz (Ed.) *Handbook of Clinical Audiology* (5th ed.). Philadelphia: Lippincott Williams and Wilkins

A tympanogram that is normal for Y_{tm}, normal for TPP, and normal for TW is considered a completely normal tympanogram or type A (in addition to the type A tympanogram illustrated in Figure 7.6, return to Figures 7.3 and 7.5, which display type A tympanograms that are normal in all respects). Interpretation of a tympanogram classified as type A would indicate a normally functioning middle ear system. It is important to note that this result would obviously be seen in cases of normal hearing but also in cases of any type of sensorineural hearing loss as well, including persons with profound deafness. Therefore, one cannot jump to the conclusion that just because a normal tympanogram exists that the person is hearing normally.

Most significant middle ear pathology—for example, otitis media with effusion—will cause a reduced Y_{tm} with likely wider than normal TW. In cases with wider than normal TW, there often is no discernible peak to the tympanogram, with the results that TPP is incalculable. The tympanogram labeled type B is abnormal for all three designators, Y_{tm}, TPP, and TW, with no obvious peak; as a result, this tympanogram is often also described as "flat."

The lack of a peak is an indication that despite instrumental changes in air pressure in the ear canal, the recorded acoustic admittance is both low and unchanging. This tympanogram is typically seen in stages of otitis media with effusion. Because the fluid effusion in the middle ear space is not compressible, acoustic admittance at the tympanic membrane will not change regardless of the introduction or amount of air pressure into the ear canal. This tympanogram is also seen in cases of occluded ear canals, as debris and occluding foreign objects in the ear canal tend also to not be compressible with changes in air pressure.

A tympanogram with reduced Y_{tm}, despite a normal TPP and normal TW, is suggestive of poor energy flow into a middle ear system. As has already been mentioned, a reduced Y_{tm} may be seen in cases of ossicular fixation, as in otosclerosis. For example, if a middle-aged female demonstrated a 50-dB conductive hearing loss on the pure tone audiometry and the case history resulted in the identification of familial hearing loss, the tympanogram labeled type A_s illustrated in Figure 7.6 would be a likely finding that is consistent with a diagnosis of otosclerosis.

A tympanogram with normal Y_{tm} and TW, but with a negatively valued TPP is depicted as type C in Figure 7.6. The key characteristic of this tympanogram is the presence of a peak with normal Y_{tm}, but shifted into the range of negative middle ear pressure. An illustrative way of describing how this tympanogram occurs is to essentially walk through the development of a case of middle ear effusion. A common cause of developing otitis media might begin with congestion in the nasopharynx and inflammation of the eustachian tube. The inability of the eustachian tube to equalize pressure results in a vacuum created in the middle ear. The resulting vacuum causes a suction effect on the tympanic membrane, pulling it back toward the medial wall of the middle ear cavity. When tympanometry is performed, there is no change in acoustic admittance until the air pressure in the ear canal approximates the vacuum in the middle ear cavity. When negative pressure is introduced into the ear canal, the retracted eardrum is literally pulled back from the middle ear space until it is back in its normal position. The resulting tympanogram shape will show a peak on the tympanogram with normal Y_{tm} and normal TW, but with the TPP in the abnormally negative pressure range (approximately less than -100 daPa). Thus, this tympanogram is typically seen in cases of eustachian tube dysfunction at the beginning of a case of otitis media. As described in Chapter 4, if this abnormality continues, fluid will be pulled from the cellular lining of the middle ear space and fill the cavity, gradually pushing the tympanic membrane back to its normal position. When this occurs, there will be a rounding effect on the shape of the peak of the tympanogram and a gradual decrease in the middle ear pressure. This will cause the tympanogram to develop into a flat-appearing tympanogram. This progression in tympanograms in the process of middle ear effusion development was depicted in Figure 7.4. A tympanogram with excessive Y_{tm}, but with a normal TPP and normal TW, suggests that energy is flowing abnormally easily, that is, without the expected opposition of the structures and their usual tension, into the middle ear system. This tympanogram is clinically important only in the context of some degree of conductive hearing loss, in which case, these findings collectively suggest a break in the ossicular chain somewhere between the tympanic membrane and the stapes footplate. In this case, the tympanogram would retain its normal shape because the tympanic membrane is normal but the tympanogram has excessive Y_{tm}. However, it is important to note that when this tympanogram is seen without significant conductive hearing loss, this probably is evidence of a scarred tympanic membrane that lacks normal tension (that is, it is hyperflaccid). Despite this tympanogram, an individual can have essentially normal hearing sensitivity.

Acoustic Reflex Testing

The measurement of the acoustic reflex is the other test in the acoustic immittance battery. The acoustic reflex is a bilateral contraction of the middle ear muscles, primarily the stapedius muscle, in response to a high-intensity acoustic stimulus (a tone or a band of noise) delivered to one ear. Because the stapedius muscle and its tendon attach to the stapes bone in the middle ear cavity, contraction pulls the ossicular chain posteriorly. The other middle ear muscle and tendon, the tensor tympani, attach to the malleus bone and pull the ossicular chain anteriorly upon contraction but this is usually in response to tactile and nonacoustic stimuli. Therefore, because the stapedius muscle mediates the acoustic reflex, some experts to refer to the acoustic reflex as the stapedial reflex (Wiley & Fowler, 1997).

The principle behind the measurement of the acoustic reflex is that it is a bilateral response to a unilateral stimulus. Technically then, the acoustic reflex could be recorded in either ear, regardless of the ear that was stimulated. With a sufficiently intense acoustic stimulus, the reflexive, simultaneous contraction of the stapedius muscles occurs in each ear, pulling each ear's ossicular chain posteriorly, causing a momentary stiffening of each ear's ossicular chain. The increase in ossicular tension consequently causes an increase in tension of the tympanic membrane. As the tympanic membrane is momentarily tensed, less acoustic energy can flow into it and the acoustic immittance meter used in tympanometry can measure this change in energy flow in the ear canal.

As mentioned above, the acoustic reflex is activated by a high-intensity acoustic stimulus. When a sufficiently intense stimulus is presented, it travels through the outer ear, the middle ear, the cochlea, along the VIIIth cranial nerve, into the brainstem, and into an integrative neuronal center in the lower brainstem called the superior olivary complex. This neural center processes the signal and transmits it to the VIIth cranial nerve (the facial nerve) nuclei on each side, which in turn, transmit a command to contract along the efferent portion of both VIIth cranial nerves to the stapedius muscles, causing them to contract. Therefore, if this test was performed with an activating stimulus presented through the immittance probe tip to a particular ear—for example, the right ear—and then the change in acoustic immittance that signifies a contraction of the stapedius muscle was also measured in that same ear, this would be an ipsilateral acoustic reflex. In contrast, if the probe tip was placed in, for example, the right ear but the activating stimulus was now presented to the left ear, the change in acoustic immittance in response to stapedius contraction could be also measured in the right ear canal, even though the activating stimulus was delivered in the other ear. This is called a contralateral acoustic reflex.

In principle, the acoustic reflex is a simple sensory-reflex initiator-motor effector arc called the acoustic reflex arc. But, because this is a bilateral reflex and because there are two ears, there are actually four measurable acoustic reflex arcs available to measure: right ipsilateral; left ipsilateral; right contralateral; and left contralateral. The conventional practice is that the ear specified (for example, "right") refers to the ear to which the activating stimulus was presented.

The primary clinical application of the acoustic reflex test is the measurement of the acoustic reflex threshold for one or more of the reflex arcs. An acoustic reflex threshold can be obtained consistently across the frequency range with the audiometric octave frequencies 500, 1000, 2000, and 4000 Hz as the typical frequencies tested. The acoustic reflex threshold is defined as the lowest intensity level at which there is a change in acoustic immittance at the tympanic membrane in response to an intense sound. A group of individuals with normal hearing thresholds and normal middle ear function will exhibit a range of acoustic reflex threshold values between 70 and 100 dBHL, with the average occurring at about 85 dBHL (Gelfand, 2002).

Although there is no specified minimum amount of change in acoustic immittance required to identify a presence of an acoustic reflex response, increases in the intensity of the activating stimulus directly lead to greater changes in acoustic immittance; thus, an examiner can quite accurately and easily determine the threshold level of a reflex response. The typical outcome of acoustic reflex testing of a normal individual would be a reflex threshold in the range of 70–100 dBHL. If a reflex is present at intensity levels greater than 100 dBHL, this reflex is said to be present at an elevated level. If a reflex was not elicited at any intensity up to the maximum equipment limits (greater than 110/120 dBHL), the reflex is said to be absent.

As with tympanometry, there are multiple applications and subtests in acoustic reflex threshold testing. In clinical work, measurement of acoustic reflex thresholds is used primarily in the assessment of auditory disorders in corroborating pure tone audiometric and tympanometric findings and to help to determine the location of the auditory disorder. When interpreted very broadly, acoustic reflex thresholds can lead to a gross estimation of peripheral hearing sensitivity.

When the findings of audiometric tests suggest the presence of an auditory disorder, the acoustic reflex threshold findings, especially when all four acoustic reflex arcs are compared, can potentially confirm the abnormal results. The following are several examples of acoustic reflex results and the potential findings that these results likely suggest:

1. *Acoustic Reflexes Within Normal Limits (70–100 dBHL)*   This likely suggests normal hearing sensitivity with no apparent pathology. However, this may be seen in individuals with a mild to moderate sensorineural hearing loss. The reason for normal reflex thresholds in this degree of sensorineural hearing loss is related to the principle of loudness recruitment described earlier. Once the hearing threshold is reached, it takes less intensity relatively speaking to elicit an acoustic reflex.

2. *Elevated Acoustic Reflex Thresholds (100+ dBHL)*   The finding of reflexes present at elevated levels occurs in several conditions and pathologies, specifically, in slight to mild low-frequency conductive hearing loss and additionally, in cases with acoustic neuroma.

3. *Absence of Acoustic Reflex Thresholds*   Absent acoustic reflex thresholds occur in several very different pathologies. Almost any ear with an abnormal tympanogram will also have absent acoustic reflexes when measured in that same ear, regardless of ear in which the activating stimulus was delivered. Ears with significant hearing loss (greater than 70 dBHL) will likely have absent reflexes because the activating stimulus is not sufficiently intense to overcome the hearing loss to elicit the reflex response. Additionally, acoustic reflexes may be absent in cases in which VIIth cranial nerve function is compromised.

Another use of the acoustic reflex threshold measure is the estimation of hearing sensitivity. Several methods have been developed to make these estimations (Popelka, 1981) and all have limited applicability due to the inherent variability in acoustic reflex thresholds in sensorineural hearing loss. In principle, these methods are based on mathematical formulas comparing acoustic reflex thresholds elicited with audiometric pure tones to reflexes elicited with broadband noise. One such method is the Sensitivity Prediction by the Acoustic Reflex (SPAR) test (Jerger et al., 1974). The SPAR test suggests degree of hearing loss/sensitivity within several broad categories, thus assisting in confirming the accuracy of the pure tone thresholds when they come into question. For example, if an individual were to feign a moderately severe or greater hearing loss, the resulting acoustic reflex thresholds would be either elevated or absent. If this individual were to exhibit a normal acoustic reflex threshold as low as 70 dBHL, then a moderate to profound hearing loss could be ruled out.

Clinical Correlations

The acoustic immittance measures of tympanometry and acoustic reflex testing provide objective information regarding the function and status of the hearing mechanism. As with audiologic tests in general, no single test result, especially if abnormal, is adequate to lead to a definitive interpretation unless clarified in the context of other conditions and tests. As with audiologic tests in general, results of acoustic immittance measures should lead to and support a single and unambiguous clinical conclusion. With these caveats in mind, some general, expected clinical correlations can be discussed.

In medically significant middle ear pathology, abnormal tympanometry is usually associated with absent acoustic reflexes in the same ear (that is, on ipsilateral acoustic reflex testing). In addition, abnormal tympanometry usually suggests the likelihood of some degree of conductive hearing loss. The more severe the degree of conductive hearing loss in an ear, the more likely acoustic reflexes will be abnormal (that is, present at elevated levels or absent) when attempting to activate a reflex from this ear (that is, on a contralateral acoustic reflex). In bilateral middle ear pathology, such as bilateral otitis media with effusion, there will likely be abnormal tympanometry in each ear with all acoustic reflexes in all arcs absent and some degree of conductive hearing loss.

However, because some abnormal-appearing tympanograms may be obtained in ears without medically significant ear pathology or any conductive hearing loss, the presence of other causative conditions needs to be determined—for example, tympanosclerotic plaques on the tympanic membrane or the presence of a surgically placed pressure equalizing tube in the tympanic membrane. Conversely, normal tympanometry can be observed in cases with a finding of conductive hearing loss, as is often observed in cases of otosclerosis, or in cases with the test artifact of a collapsing ear canal under supra-aural audiometric earphones.

Normal tympanometry combined with acoustic reflex abnormalities suggest abnormalities in the cochlea or along the VIIth or VIIIth cranial nerve pathways. Certain abnormalities across acoustic reflex arcs (for example, ipsilateral arc present but contralateral arcs absent) are suggestive of retrocochlear pathology.

OTOACOUSTIC EMISSIONS

The otoacoustic emission (OAE) is a measurable by-product of auditory system activity—specifically, the outer hair cells in the cochlea—in response to acoustic stimulation. Because it represents physiologic activity in the cochlea that can be correlated to the presence of normal hearing or, conversely, of the presence of hearing loss, the OAE is a powerful new assessment tool. One of its primary applications is the assessment of the auditory systems of neonates in newborn hearing screening programs.

As one of the five senses, hearing has classically been characterized as a passive, afferent (that is, purely sensory) system that receives stimuli from the environment and, in a series of stages, converts stimuli into neural information to be processed in the brain stem and auditory cortex. An acoustic signal passing through the outer ear strikes the tympanic membrane creating a mechanical vibration that is then transmitted through the ossicular chain and into the cochlea via the oval window. In the cochlea, the mechanical vibration is converted to a fluid-borne traveling wave that courses over the hair cells located in the organ of Corti, causing a conversion to an electrical signal that is transmitted along the nerve pathway to the brain stem and brain. This classic view of the hearing mechanism as a purely passive afferent system was hypothesized by the twentieth-century engineer/scientist, Georg von Békésy, based on a body of work that spanned nearly 50 years and for which he received the Nobel Prize in science. Although Békésy's work was largely confined to observations of cadaver cochleae, his theories remained unchallenged for many decades.

Curiously though, living human and animal subjects performed much better on a variety of hearing tests than the physical capabilities Békésy described would seem to predict. Subsequent researchers explained this gap by hypothesizing the existence of an unknown "cochlear amplifier" or "second filter" (Evans & Wilson, 1973; Evans, 1974). Toward the end of the twentieth century, several investigators provided conclusive evidence of active processing in cochlear structures, thereby revolutionizing the classic view of hearing as a purely passive system. Brownell et al. (1985) reported that the outer hair cells (OHCs) were electromotile, that is, they have the capacity to move when stimulated. Because the OHCs have attachments to the tectorial membrane, OHC movements can cause consequential movement of the tectorial membrane, which in turn creates additional stimulation to the inner hair cells (IHCs), thus providing evidence to support the existence of the hypothetical cochlear amplifier.

Although the exact mechanism of the cochlear amplifier is unknown at this time, it has long been known that there are efferent connections from the auditory brain stem primarily to the OHCs. Thus, the active processing of the outer hair cells and the existence of an efferent nervous system (from the brain stem down to the OHCs) makes the hearing mechanism more that just a passive and afferent receiver of stimulation as had been classically hypothesized.

Interestingly, a reliable measurement of what would later be linked to OHC electromotility had been described by Kemp (1978) as a "cochlear echo" and later termed an otoacoustic emission. Using computer techniques such as signal averaging and sensitive microphone technology, Kemp measured an acoustic signal in the external ear canal that occurred following acoustic stimulation. This acoustic signal, the OAE, is thought to be a by-product of OHC movement. As the stimulus enters the cochlea, the OHCs are activated, by a means not yet known, and pull on the tectorial membrane. It is likely that these consequent motions of the tectorial membrane then create a small, traveling fluid wave that reaches and vibrates structures in the middle ear (possible candidates: the round window; the ossicles via the oval window), in turn creating an acoustic signal in the air of the middle ear, which then could be picked up by a microphone in the ear canal. Whatever the exact origin of the OAE turns out to be, the presence of OAEs is clearly linked to healthy, normally functioning OHCs (Prieve & Fitzgerald, 2002).

Over the last 20 years, numerous studies have been conducted to determine aspects and clinical applications of OAEs. Approximately 50% of normal hearing children and adults have been shown to have a **spontaneous otoacoustic emission (SOAE)** that is measurable in the external ear canal; these are thought to be generated by the cochlea. Because of the small amplitude of the SOAE (approximately ± 10 dBSPL), it is generally inaudible to the person in which it is being measured as well as to any individual listening at the ear. There has not been a significant clinical application of the SOAE, although there is evidence that a very small number (less than 3%) of persons with tinnitus also have an SOAE (Penner, 1990).

However, there is another class of OAE that can consistently be measured in normal ears following the presentation of an auditory stimulus. This type of OAE has been

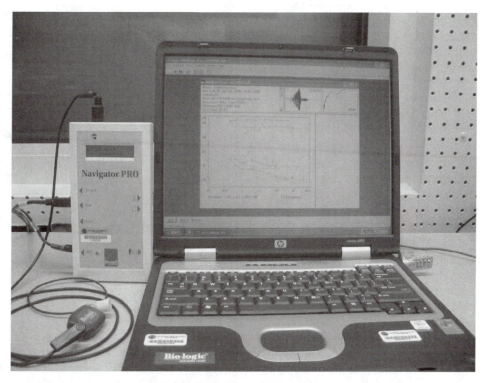

Figure 7.7   Equipment (computer and test box) used to acquire distortion product otoacoustic emissions

Source: Courtesy of Natus Medical, Inc. Navigator® Pro is a registerd trademark of Bio-Logic Systems Corp., A Natus Company

termed an **evoked otoacoustic emission (EOAE)**. A display of the EOAE instrumentation is shown in Figure 7.7. The reliability and clinical correlation studies that have been done with EOAEs have led to a rapid commercial development of the necessary equipment and its widespread clinical use. Because the EOAE technology is housed in computers, much of the test process is automatized; in many cases, the main task of the examiner is the simple placement of probe tip snugly into the ear canal. By using signal averaging techniques, EOAEs can be measured rapidly, often in less than a minute for each ear. Thus, it can be seen that because of this easy measurement of the presence versus the absence of the emission and its relationship to normal hearing function and also the simplicity at which the procedure can be administered simply with a probe tip inserted in the ear, this procedure has a natural application to hearing screening programs. For these reasons, EOAEs have become the procedure of choice in many newborn hearing screening programs. There are two distinct types of EOAEs that are in common clinical use today.

The first type of EOAE is called the **transient evoked otoacoustic emission (TEOAE)**. Historically, the TEOAE was the first EOAE recorded and reported on by Kemp (1978). Technically, the TEOAE is evoked following the presentation of a very brief acoustic signal known as a click. Using a computerized analysis, frequency specific information can be derived from the TEOAE for several bands of mid to high frequencies.

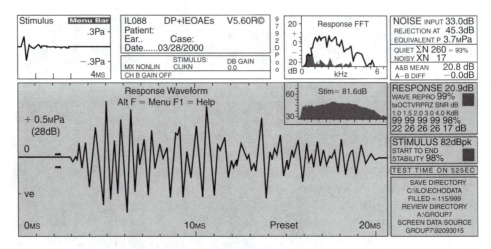

Figure 7.8   Example of a normal TEOAE response from an adult

Source: Reprinted with permission from T. Glattke & M. Robinette (2002), Transient evoked otoacoustic emissions, chapter in T. Glattke & M. Robinette (Eds.) *Otoacoustic Emissions Clinical Applications* (2nd ed.), New York: Thieme

The fundamental value of the TEOAE is that it is essentially present in every auditory system that has normal outer hair cell and cochlear function but generally absent in ears with sensorineural hearing loss of greater than 30 dBHL (Bonfils et al., 1988). A sample display of a TEOAE result is shown in Figure 7.8.

The second type of EOAE that is used in clinical applications is called the **distortion product otoacoustic emission (DPOAE)**. The DPOAE is distinct from the click-evoked TEOAE in that the DPOAE utilizes two tones with frequencies that are mathematically determined to create a difference tone (that is, the distortion product) in the cochlea. The frequencies of the pairs of tones are automatically changed in the DPOAE test sequence and provide quick, direct, and frequency-specific data, which in turn provide additional information to more accurately diagnose a variety of disorders. Figure 7.9 shows a typical DPOAE result.

The powerful application of DPOAE test results in diagnosis can be seen in the following case. Figure 7.10 presents the results of a 35-year-old male complaining of an injury-related hearing loss in the right ear. Although there was no measurable behavioral response for pure tone audiometric testing in the right ear, the DPOAE results revealed the presence of emissions within normal limits for both ears, suggesting a probable case of pseudohypacusis.

One complicating factor to the measurement of otoacoustic emissions is the necessity of a normally functioning middle ear space. Because the signal is traveling from the cochlea through the middle ear cavity and is measured in the external ear canal, the presence of any conductive pathology, such as middle ear fluid, will essentially eliminate the ability to record the otoacoustic emission. Therefore, this factor makes it difficult to determine whether an absent emission is the result of a cochlear or conductive pathology, although either would constitute the need for referral in a hearing screening program.

Patient: Kiddinme, Aryu
Birthdate: 02-02-1986
ID: 605181   Ear: Left
Comment

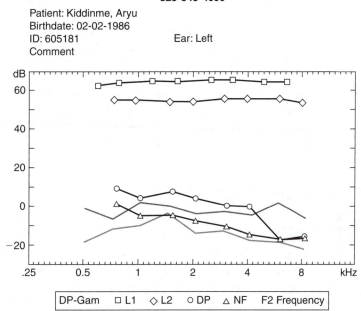

Figure 7.9 Example of distortion product otoacoustic emissions for young adult (left ear only displayed) judged as present through 4000 Hz. DPs are plotted against a normative template (here, Boys Town 65–55, 95th–5th Percentile Reference Set).

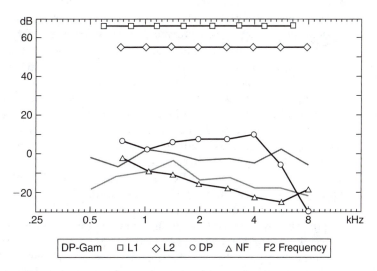

Figure 7.10 DPOAE data from the right ear (o-o) of a 35-year-old adult male complaining of work-related hearing loss who did not respond to pure tone audiometric testing. The finding of a normal DPOAE response in this right ear provides objective data that the pure tone audiometric findings were indicative of feigned hearing loss.

Interpretation of otoacoustic emissions is very straightforward. The presence of an EOAE suggests that there is little or no conductive hearing loss and that the cochlea is likely normal or no worse than a mild sensorineural hearing loss. Interpretation of absent otoacoustic emissions depends on the status of the conductive mechanism. As noted above, if there is conductive hearing loss or abnormality on tympanometric testing, then it is very likely that otoacoustic emissions will be absent and additional comment regarding cochlear function cannot be made based solely on the otoacoustic emissions test. However, if there is no conductive hearing loss and tympanometry is normal, absent otoacoustic emissions suggest the presence of a mild or greater degree of hearing loss, with likely etiology in the cochlea.

EVOKED POTENTIAL AUDIOMETRY

Underlying Principles

The purpose of the normal auditory system is to convert acoustic stimuli from the environment into electrical signals, that is, into voltages (*Note:* another word for voltages is *potentials*) so that structures in the brain stem and the brain can analyze and react to this information. Measurement of the electrical activity in the auditory system provides considerable information regarding both status of hearing as well as the integrity of the structures carrying those electrical signals. Not surprisingly then, the measurement of electrical activity in the auditory system has become critically useful in the practice of audiology, in part because it is physiologic in nature—that is, not requiring a behavioral response from the person being tested—and like tympanometry and otoacoustic emissions, it provides unique data.

In **evoked potential audiometry**, the examiner uses a sensory stimulus (for example, an acoustic stimulus) in an attempt to create an electrical signal in the patient's nervous system in response to that sensory stimulus. In this context, the response was evoked by the use of a stimulus. In contrast, electrical activity recorded in the absence of a stimulus is termed spontaneous activity. The basic measurement technology which underlies evoked potential measures is the recording of electrical brain wave activity from recording electrodes typically placed in different locations on the head in a procedure widely known as **electroencephalography (EEG)**. The EEG recording itself is complex because it contains simultaneous, multiple contributions from many neural generators. The relatively small electrical impulses that are evoked as a consequence of an acoustic stimulus would be lost in this complex electrical activity if it were not for signal averaging and other processing techniques, which minimize the unimportant, ongoing electrical activity and maximize the visibility of the electrical signal associated with the acoustic stimulus. In this way, these voltages are made more prominent for measurement and analysis. The ability to record the hearing-related voltages despite the presence of significant background activity only became possible with the advent and commercial distribution of computer technology, chiefly, the process of computer-assisted signal averaging.

Evoked potentials can be acquired for sensory systems other than auditory (for example, visual or **somatosensory**) so, in general, a test of evoked potentials refers to a type of measurement and not specifically to any one sensory system. **Auditory evoked**

potentials (AEPs) refer to an evoked potential measurement of the auditory nervous system, but not specifically to any one location in the auditory nervous system. The electrical signal initiated in the cochlea of the inner ear travels sequentially from the cochlea along the acoustic nerve (also known as the VIIIth cranial nerve), into and through the brain stem, along the neural connections to the brain, and finally, in the brain itself. Although any one of these general locations could be of interest to an examiner, clinical audiologists tend to focus on the contributions of the cochlea, the VIIIth cranial nerve, and the brain stem.

The data collected in AEP measurement are graphed as a waveform, that is, voltages are plotted across time. For AEPs, the units of time are typically given in milliseconds (msec). Intuitively, the recording of a voltage at different points in time is analogous to distance traveled (it takes time to get from one point in the system to another point), thereby yielding an approximation to location within the auditory nervous system. The technical term for the amount of time that has elapsed between any two points is **latency**. Interestingly, it is the measure of various latencies of the AEP waveform that is critically analyzed, not the amplitude of the voltage of the waveform. Based on the time latency (relative to the initiation of the stimulus) in which AEPs are observed, four categories of AEPs have been recognized that grossly approximate the anatomy of the auditory nervous system. These categories are only broadly defined and each category overlaps the next one.

The first AEP category is a response measured within the first 2 msec following stimulus presentation and this response is called electrocochleography (ECochG). It reflects activity measured from the cochlea and the portion of the VIIIth cranial nerve closest to the cochlea.

The second AEP category is the electrical activity measured within the first 10 msec following stimulus presentation and this response has several names, perhaps most commonly called the auditory brain stem response (ABR), but also known as the brain stem auditory evoked potential (BAEP), the brain stem auditory evoked response (BAER), or the brain stem evoked response (BSER). Technically, the first part of the ABR overlaps with the ECochG. The ABR reflects activity from the VIIIth cranial nerve through the upper brain stem and lower midbrain.

The third category of AEPs is the **middle-latency auditory evoked potentials (MLAEPs)** and these are recorded generally in the range of 15 to 70 msec following the stimulus. The MLAEPs reflect activity from the midbrain and along the neural connections to the auditory cortex.

The final AEP category includes two classes of responses that are generally recorded 50 msec following the stimulus and later. One class of response is the sensory auditory potential recorded from the auditory cortex (brain), which has been called the **late latency response (LLR)**, sometimes also referred to as the "slow" response. The other class of response includes several other responses with the broad name of **processing contingent potentials (PCPs)** (see Stapells, 2002 for a review of all these responses). In general, these cortical-level responses measure the activity in the brain following different types of acoustic stimulation, including speech. Because PCPs represent electrophysiological measures of cortical-level processing, many disciplines other than audiology have an interest in them (as examples, cognitive neuroscience and psychology).

Of all four categories of AEPs, the ABR is the category that seems to be most useful to clinical audiologists as an objective means of assessing the auditory system. Specifically, the ABR is a powerful tool in estimating the hearing of difficult-to-test patients, particularly infants and small children. Just as importantly, the ABR is a sensitive and efficient tool in the differentiation of several auditory system pathologies, particularly for pathologies along the VIIIth cranial nerve, in the skull base, and in the brain stem. While the ABR has some limitations, it is an important and widely used test, and so, the remainder of this section will focus on the procedures and applications associated with the ABR.

Procedures

ABR procedures are straightforward and easily performed. Contemporary ABR systems are housed in commercially available computers that permit control of all stimulus, acquisition, and analysis parameters. There are three procedural stages in ABR testing: patient preparation and electrode placement; response acquisition; and response analysis.

In the first stage, patient preparation and electrode placement, the patient and the family are counseled regarding the procedures, and then surface electrodes are placed on the head at key positions that allow for a noninvasive, far-field recording of the electrical activity inside the skull. Efficient ABR recording is best accomplished with a quiet and comfortable patient. One important characteristic of the ABR, but not all AEPs, is that the response can be recorded not only with patients who are awake but also with patients who are sleeping or have been sedated. This characteristic makes the ABR a feasible test with neonates and young children who may be in a state of natural sleep through the procedure, or possibly have been sedated to induce a sleeping state. After testing for acceptable electrical conductivity through the electrodes, the ABR test can begin.

The next stage, response acquisition, involves two critical technical components: stimulus delivery and response recording. The examiner can control the intensity level of the stimulus, the presentation rate of the stimulus (that is, number of stimuli delivered per second), the total number of stimuli presented, the ear stimulated, as well as other technical parameters (for example, stimulus polarity). Insert earphones or headphones deliver the acoustic stimulus. Two very different types of stimuli are commonly used in ABR testing. One stimulus type is known as a **click**. The click stimulus is well suited for applications that attempt to assess the integrity of neural function because the click activates a greater number of auditory neurons than does any other acoustic stimulus, thus optimizing the response recorded in the ABR. In theory, a click has energy across all frequencies, but not at discrete frequencies as in pure tone audiometry, so a click-evoked ABR is, in theory, ear-specific and intensity-specific but not frequency-specific, as is pure tone audiometry. Therefore, in applications that attempt to estimate hearing sensitivity, stimuli that are more frequency-specific than the click need to be utilized. In ABR testing, a commonly used frequency-specific stimulus is a **tone burst**.

In response recording, several engineering techniques are employed to better view the small voltages coming from the auditory system. The first technique is the use of time-locking (synchronizing) the recording of electrical activity to a specific click stimulus. In other words, the recording system captures only the electrical activity for a set window of time following an individual click stimulus. Other electrical activity not in

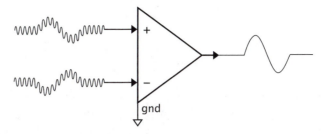

Figure 7.11 Schematic rendition of common mode rejection as employed by a differential amplifier. The high-frequency signal common to both inputs (+, −) is rejected but the low-frequency signal input at "−" is inverted and added to the input at "+"
Source: Reprinted with permission from ASHA (1987), The short latency auditory evoked potential, Rockville: American Speech-Language-Hearing Association

this window is not recorded. Time-locked recording captures the electrical activity most likely evoked by the click and ignores other electrical activity.

The next recording technique is the use of differential amplification and a process termed **common mode rejection** (see the schematic form in Figure 7.11).

Electrodes on the head pick up electrical signals and send those signals to a differential amplifier. In the simplest ABR recording scheme, there are three electrodes: a ground electrode; an electrode connected to the noninverting input; and an electrode connected to the inverting input. The differential amplifier employs an inverting process that transforms the signal at the electrode connected to the inverting input so that it is 180 degrees out of phase with the signal coming from the electrode connected to the noninverting input. In this circumstance, the resulting addition of these two signals, each now 180 degrees out of phase relative to the other, adds to zero, which cancels out what is assumed to be electrical activity unrelated to the test (referred to as "noise"). In this case, signals that are in common to the two electrodes are rejected and not retained for additional processing—hence the term common mode rejection.

However, when different electrical signals are picked up at each of these electrodes, as would be expected in a normal ABR test, the inverting process has minimal effect on the resulting residual voltage, because these signals represent true evoked electrical activity. Signals not in common are not rejected, but rather these residual voltages are then passed on to the next stage of processing. The use of common mode rejection serves to retain the best-quality evoked electrical signals while eliminating activity that is noise. This is also referred to as enhancing the "signal-to-noise ratio."

The final recording technique is the use of **signal averaging**, in which many individual electrical responses are serially added together to form a composite electrical response. In a typical ABR test, more than 1000 stimulus presentations and signal captures are summed to yield one composite waveform for analysis. As each of these responses are averaged, a waveform grows out of the noisy background and creates a definable series of waves that are measurable and repeatable as a response from the auditory system. The use of multiple presentations and signal captures, in the context of time-locking and differential amplification (common mode rejection), permits the visualization of the small voltage evoked response against what would otherwise be an obscuring background of noise.

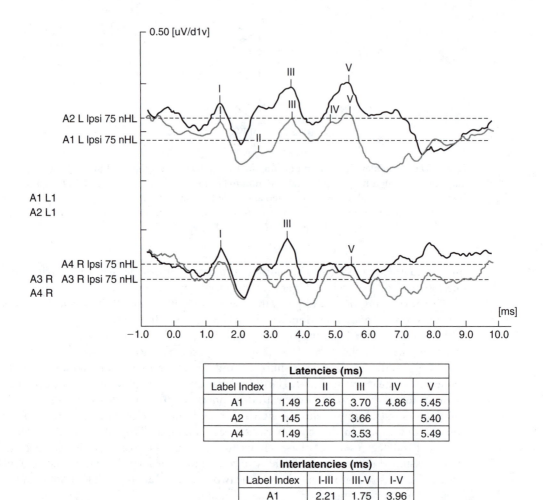

Figure 7.12 Example of ABR waveforms from an adult female. These waveforms were judged as within normal limits for each ear for all latencies and interlatencies. *Note:* interpretation of ABR waveforms is dependent on knowledge of stimulus, acquisition, and other relevant parameters.

Once a waveform is acquired, response analysis can occur. The auditory brainstem response is typically found in the first 10 msec following the stimulus presentation. The signal-averaging process results in a waveform with five identifiable waves. The normal click-evoked ABR waveform for an adult is displayed in Figure 7.12. It has been determined that each of these waves occurs from one or more neural generators as the signal travels up the auditory pathway.

These neural generators are as follows (Møller, 1994):

Wave I   The distal end of the VIIIth nerve

Wave II   The proximal end of the VIIIth nerve as it enters the brain stem

Wave III   The cochlear nucleus (lower brain stem)

Wave IV   Superior olivary complex (lower brain stem)

Wave V   Nuclei of the lateral leminiscus in addition to contribution from other neural generators (mid to upper brain stem)

A basic analysis of a click-evoked ABR waveform includes the determination of three individual wave latencies (**absolute latency**), as well as the determination of three interpeak or **interwave latencies**. Specifically, this analysis includes: the absolute latencies of waves I, III, and V; and the interwave latencies that exist between waves I–III, I–V, and III–V. These latency values are then used to make diagnostic conclusions.

Once these six values have been obtained, they can then be compared to normative data that is matched for age of patient and for similar technical parameters (stimulus, acquisition, and recording). Depending on the clinical application, additional ABR waveforms can be acquired for other intensity levels. Finally, similar measurements are completed for the other ear, thus permitting interaural comparisons for both absolute latencies and interwave latencies.

Clinical Applications

As stated earlier, the ABR can be used for two general purposes: to make estimates of hearing; and to assess the integrity of the physical structures responsible for conducting electrical information through the auditory nervous system. Within these general purposes, there are four specific clinical applications: (1) neonatal hearing screening; (2) estimation of the threshold of hearing sensitivity; (3) differential diagnosis of cochlear versus retrocochlear dysfunction; and (4) intraoperative monitoring during various surgeries.

The first application is the use of the ABR test in neonatal hearing screening. The goal of a hearing screening procedure is to differentiate infants who are normal from those who potentially have a significant hearing loss. A typical screening strategy is to present a stimulus at a fixed intensity level (approximately 30 or 35 dBnHL) to determine whether a response can be recorded. If an ABR waveform is present, it is assumed that the child likely has normal or near normal hearing sensitivity and thus receives a passing result. If no reliable ABR waveform is present, it is concluded that the child is potentially at risk for significant hearing loss. Often in these cases, another test will be conducted at a higher intensity level (for example, 60 dBnHL) to determine whether there is a response at this higher intensity level. The purpose for this is to identify potential severity of the absent ABR and whether it is an indicator of a mild to moderate loss as opposed to something more severe. If time allows, additional testing can be performed at 10-dB increments to try to better estimate the response threshold.

A second application of ABR testing is to estimate hearing sensitivity, that is, to provide an electrophysiologic estimate of the behavioral audiogram when dealing with difficult-to-test populations such as infants or young children, or older individuals who are possibly feigning some degree of hearing loss, all of whom cannot or will not provide a reliable and valid behavioral audiogram (If they could or would, generally that's all we need!). The lack of frequency specificity is a critical limitation of a click-evoked ABR. In contemporary practice recommendations, the use of tone bursts, not clicks, is recommended for threshold estimation in children because tone bursts have greater frequency specificity (American Speech-Language-Hearing Association, 2004). Additionally, a currently evolving methodology, the auditory steady-state response (ASSR), is stated to be an even better means of improving frequency specificity (Sininger & Cone-Wesson, 2002). The ABR employing frequency-specific stimuli (such as tone bursts) and the ASSR are the primary recommended procedures for hearing sensitivity estimation applications in young children (American Speech-Language-Hearing Association, 2004).

The ABR remains intensity-specific, so the process of determining the level of hearing sensitivity is rather simple in that the lowest intensity level at which a reliable ABR waveform can be identified will indicate an estimate of the threshold of hearing sensitivity (or alternately, the degree of hearing loss). In this application, a series of ABR waveforms is acquired at progressively lesser intensity levels. As the intensity of the auditory stimulus (click or tone burst) is reduced and approximates threshold, the amplitude of the key waveforms will be reduced correspondingly to the point that several will disappear and often, only wave V remains. In addition, as the intensity is reduced the latency of all waves will be delayed (that is, they appear at a later time than normal). This is consistent with the fact that fewer neurons fire at lower intensity levels and thus require a slightly longer time for the stimulus to travel through the auditory pathway. A plot of change in waveform as a function of change in stimulus intensity is known as a **latency-intensity function** and is represented in Figure 7.13. In this example, it can be seen that the threshold is likely near or better than 20 dBHL in view of the still present wave V at that intensity level.

The third clinical application of ABR testing is its use in differentiating different types of a hearing loss—chiefly, cochlear versus retrocochlear. This type of interpretation involves multiple interaural comparisons of the absolute and interwave latencies.

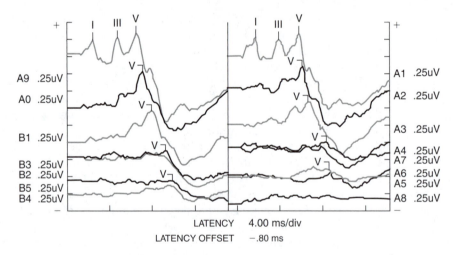

Figure 7.13 ABR latency-intensity function obtained on a normally hearing 3-year-old-male. Left side tracings were obtained following stimulation of left ear and right side tracings were obtained following stimulation of right ear. Presentation levels (intensities) were as follows: A1 and A9 @ 75 dBnHL; A2 and A0 @ 60 dBnHL; A3 and B1 @ 45 dBnHL; A4/A7 and B2/B3 @ 25 dBnHL; A5/A6 and B4/B5 @ 20 dBnHL; A8 was a silent control—presentation level set to 0 dBnHL. Note the rightward movement of the peak labeled "V" as intensity level decreased.

In the case of a unilateral retrocochlear lesion such as an VIIIth cranial nerve tumor, one typical outcome is an asymmetric delay of the absolute latencies of waves III and V, but with wave I grossly unaffected. Consequentially, there will be abnormally prolonged I–III and I–V interwave latencies on the side of the tumor. These asymmetric abnormalities are significant evidence of the possibility of retrocochlear pathology signaling the need for medical intervention. Thus, the ABR test procedure has become very valuable as a measure prior to other more involved and more expensive radiological procedures that are performed to confirm the presence or absence of a retrocochlear lesion.

A fourth clinical application of the ABR test is in the monitoring of the response during neuro-otologic surgery. Similar to the monitoring of heart rate during operative procedures, surgeons operating on the brain stem and skull base often require reports of neurological activity during the extremely delicate surgeries involving these structures. This need has created another viable use of the ABR test.

SUMMARY

A Glimpse into the Profession Revisited

In Jonas' case, all the physiologic tests described in this chapter can be employed to answer his parents' and physicians' questions regarding the status of his hearing in each ear. The immediate assessment of his normally formed left ear using otoacoustic emissions revealed the presence of OAEs, a finding that is indicative of hearing within normal limits in this ear. Tympanometry was within normal limits, indicating normal outer and middle ear systems. This is an important finding because speech and language development typically proceeds within normal limits when hearing is within normal limits in at least one ear. Tympanometry was abnormal in the right ear and otoacoustic emissions were absent in the right ear. Subsequent ABR testing was within normal limits in the left ear (confirming otoacoustic results). On the ABR for the right ear, there was no response to air-conducted stimuli, but there was a response for bone-conducted stimuli, suggesting a probable moderate to severe conductive hearing loss. Subsequent imaging by CT scan revealed an abnormally formed ossicular chain. An otolaryngologist conferred with Jonas' parents and provided a timetable for cosmetic repair of the right external ear, later in Jonas' childhood. Discussion of possible surgical modification of his narrow ear canal and of his malformed ossicular chain will be deferred until Jonas is in his teenage years.

CHAPTER REVIEW

❑ The progressive inclusion of new technologies and a greater understanding of the function of the auditory mechanism have led to the development of new instrumentation and measurement techniques that facilitate the measurement of hearing and the identification and diagnosis of problems in the auditory system.

❑ Acoustic immittance testing has become a routine part of the audiological test battery, as it is a specific measurement of the function of the middle ear and of the tympanic membrane.

❑ Because of its ease in measurement, acoustic immittance testing can easily be applied to a hearing conversation program in the schools to identify children that are either currently suffering from or are at risk of developing some form of otitis media.

❑ It also further confirms pure tone audiometry and assists in the differentiation of various causes of hearing loss.

❑ In addition, the acoustic reflex test in the acoustic immittance battery presents some indication of the integrity of the auditory pathway.

❑ Evoked otoacoustic emissions have become a simple yet valuable procedure to determine the presence or absence of normal outer hair cell function. This clearly has direct application to the hearing screening program for infants and preschoolers as well as other difficult-to-test populations.

❑ Auditory evoked potentials are a precise and accurate way of predicting hearing sensitivity without the need of a behavioral response from the patient. With the use of computer-enhanced electroencephalography and the noninvasive placement of electrodes, a measurement can be obtained from the cochlea, auditory nerve, and auditory brain stem in response to acoustic stimuli.

❑ The resulting waveform can then be used to interpret the presence or absence of hearing loss and to what degree, can differentiate a cochlear from a retrocochlear lesion, and can be used for the purposes of newborn hearing screening as well as in monitoring intraoperatively the status of neurologic function.

❑ The addition of these physiologic measures into audiologic testing has further refined the ability to effectively and accurately obtain information about the status of the hearing mechanism. This information can then be used to supplement the information obtained through the normal behavioral measurement process.

ACTIVITIES FOR DISCUSSION

1. Why is there a place for physiological testing in audiology?

2. Who are likely candidates for physiological testing?

3. Can physiological tests be wrong, inaccurate, or misleading?

4. What are the latest developments in physiological testing?

REFERENCES

American Academy of Audiology. (1997). Audiologic guidelines for the diagnosis and treatment of otitis media in children. *Audiology Today, 4* (4).

American National Standards Institute. (1987). Specifications for instruments to measure aural acoustic impedance and admittance (aural acoustic immittance). ANSI S3.39-1987. New York: American National Standards Institute.

American Speech-Language-Hearing Association. (2004). Guidelines for the audiologic assessment of children from birth to 5 years of age. Rockville: ASHA.

American Speech-Language-Hearing Association. (1997). Guidelines for audiologic screening. Rockville: ASHA.

Bonfils, P., Piron, J., Uziel, A., & Pujol, R. (1988). A correlative study of evoked otoacoustic emission properties and audiometric thresholds. *Archives Otolaryngology, 245*, 53–56.

Brownell, W., Bader, C., Betrand, D., & de Ribaupierre, Y. (1985). Evoked mechanical responses of isolated cochlear outer hair cells. *Science, 227,* 194–196.

Evans, E. (1974). The effects of hypoxia on the tuning of single cochlear nerve fibers. *Journal of Physiology, 238* (1), 65p–67p.

Evans, E., & Wilson, J. (1973). The frequency selectivity of the cochlea. In A. Moller (Ed.), *Basic Mechanisms in Hearing*. New York: Academic Press.

Fowler, C., & Shanks, J. (2002). Tympanometry. In J. Katz (Ed.), *Handbook of clinical audiology* (5th ed., pp. 175–204). Baltimore: Lippincott Williams and Wilkins.

Gelfand, S. (2002). The acoustic reflex. In J. Katz (Ed.), *Handbook of clinical audiology* (5th ed., pp. 205–232). Baltimore: Lippincott Williams and Wilkins.

Jerger, J., Burney, P., Mauldin, L., & Crump., B. (1974). Predicting hearing loss from the acoustic reflex. *Journal of Speech and Hearing Disorders, 39,* 11–22.

Kemp, D. (1978). Stimulated acoustic emissions from within the human auditory system. *Journal of the Acoustical Society of America 64,* 1386–1391.

Liden, G., Peterson, J., & Bjorkman, G. (1970). Tympanometry. *Archives Otolaryngology, 92,* 248–257.

Møller, A. (1994). Neural generators of auditory evoked potentials. In J. Jacobson (Ed.), *Principles and applications in auditory evoked Potentials.* Needham Heights, MA: Allyn and Bacon.

Penner, M. (1990). An estimate of the prevalence of tinnitus caused by spontaneous otoacoustic emissions. *Archives of Otolaryngology, 116,* 418–423.

Popelka, G. (1981). *Hearing assessment with the acoustic reflex.* New York: Grune and Stratton.

Prieve, B., & Fitzgerald, T. (2002). Otoacoustic emissions. In J. Katz (Ed.), *Handbook of clinical audiology* (5th ed., pp. 440–466). Baltimore: Lippincott Williams and Wilkins.

Roup, C., Wiley, T., Safady, S., & Stoppenbach, D. (1998). Tympanometric screening norms for adults. *American Journal of Audiology, 7,* 55–60.

Shanks, J., Stelmachowicz, P., Beauchaine, K., & Shulte, L. (1992). Equivalent ear canal volumes in children pre- and post-tympanostomy tube insertion. *Journal of Speech and Hearing Research, 35,* 936–9 941.

Sininger, Y. & Cone-Wesson, B. (2002). Threshold prediction using auditory brainstem response and steady-state evoked potentials with infants and small children. In J. Katz (Ed.),: *Handbook of clinical audiology,* 5th ed. Baltimore: Lippincott Williams and Wilkins; 298–322.

Stapells, D. (2002). Cortical event-related potentials to auditory stimuli. In J. Katz, (Ed.): *Handbook of clinical audiology,* 5th ed. Baltimore: Lippincott Williams and Wilkins; 378–406.

Wiley, T. & Fowler, C. (1997). *Acoustic immittance measures in clinical audiology: A primer.* San Diego: Singular.

Wiley, T. & Stoppenbach, D. (2002). Basic principles of acoustic immittance measures. In J. Katz, (Ed.): *Handbook of clinical audiology,* 5th ed. Baltimore: Lippincott Williams and Wilkins; pp. 159–174.

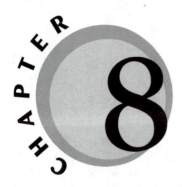

CHAPTER 8

Pediatric Audiology: Screening and Evaluation

Key Terms

CASE STUDY

A Glimpse into the Profession

Brandon is a new member of a kindergarten class. His teacher has noticed, however, that he is not always attentive and does not seem to listen and hear consistently. She was concerned that he might have a hearing problem and was pleased to receive notification that the annual hearing screening was about to take place. The questions that she hopes will be answered by screening are, "Does a hearing problem exist, or is there another reason for Brandon's inattentiveness?" "If he does not pass the screening, what is his hearing sensitivity?" Finally, "Based on the hearing test and immittance screening results, what type of referral should be made for further assessment and treatment?"

OVERVIEW OF THE SCREENING PROCESS

The purpose of any **screening** program, whether it is for hearing, speech, or vision, etc., is to separate those persons who exhibit problems from those who have no apparent problems in an efficient and effective manner. The goal of speech/language and hearing professionals is to identify communication disorders as early as possible so that intervention can begin to ameliorate or minimize the problems. To accomplish this goal, audiometric screening is an important component of the scope of practice for audiologists, speech-language pathologists (ASHA, 1996b), and other health professionals.

Setting Screening Levels—Sensitivity versus Specificity

Hearing screening has been an established practice in educational settings and presumably all who have attended the public schools should have experienced a screening procedure at one time or another. With this high volume of testing, the criteria for screening need to effectively identify those persons with potential problems but in a way that screening can be accomplished expeditiously. If time and staffing were not factors, actual hearing threshold testing could be performed on every single person to accurately identify hearing loss. In contrast, if the goal of screening is just to fulfill a legal mandate as quickly as possible, then many individuals with problems could be missed for the sake of efficiency. There needs to be a balance between the thoroughness in effectively referring those persons with a possible disorder and the efficiency in which screening programs are administered with the time and resources that are available. Parameters used to describe this balance are **sensitivity** and **specificity**, as explained by Johnson (2002):

> Sensitivity—The ability of the screening procedure to identify the target population accurately (hit rate or number of individuals who actually have hearing loss).
>
> Specificity—The ability of the procedure to not identify (e.g., to pass) those who truly do not have the disorder the screening program is designed to identify.

Table 8.1 A 2 × 2 table showing the ideal outcome of a screening procedure

	Optimal Screening Results	
	Diagnostic Results	
	+	**−**
Screening Results **+**	10	0
−	0	90

Screening criteria should be set so that the highest level of sensitivity and specificity can be realized. Unfortunately, in the real world, there clearly will be cases in which individuals with hearing loss will be missed and those with normal hearing will be incorrectly identified.

Table 8.1 displays a 2 × 2 table that can be used to determine the efficiency and accuracy of a hearing screening protocol. The abscissa across the top of the table indicates the diagnostic results indicating the actual hearing levels compared to the screening results obtained along the ordinate of the table. The numbers that are displayed show an example of optimal screening results for 100 children being screened. In the upper left quadrant, the 10 children that in fact have hearing problems were identified as such. In the bottom right quadrant the 90 children with normal hearing sensitivity showed that they passed the screening test. In this case, no children that actually had a hearing loss were missed in the screening, and conversely, no children with normal hearing failed the hearing screening measure. The prevalence of hearing loss in this example is 10 out of 100 or 10%.

Table 8.2 displays screening results that might occur with very strict criteria in terms of the intensity level and frequency used in the screening procedure. This is an indication of very high sensitivity in that it accurately identifies everyone with hearing loss. But the upper right quadrant indicates 25 children who were tested positive for hearing loss through

Table 8.2 This table displays a highly sensitive screening protocol, but resulting in a large number of false positive (FP) results

	High Sensitivity/Low Specificity	
	Diagnostic Results	
	+	**−**
Screening Results **+**	10	25 FP
−	0	65

Table 8.3 A highly specific screening protocol, but resulting in a large number of false negative (FN) results

Low Sensitivity/High Specificity

		Diagnostic Results	
		+	−
Screening Results	+	6	0
	−	4 FN	90

the screening procedure but in fact had no hearing problems. Thus, the high sensitivity in this example is realized at the expense of many **false positive** (FP) results, which reduces the efficiency of the screening program because of the need to retest these individuals.

Table 8.3 displays screening results using criteria that is set at a level that allows for easier passing of the screening procedure. This is an indication of low sensitivity but high specificity in the result. The lower left quadrant shows four individuals who in fact had a hearing loss but passed the screening. Although this procedure is highly efficient in conducting a screening program, the accuracy is diminished because of the 40 percent of individuals with hearing loss who were **false negative** (FN) results and were missed because this screening protocol was used.

Unfortunately, no screening criteria can possibly show ideal results with the absence of false positive or false negative responses. Clearly the greatest concern is the number of false negatives that may occur with criteria that allows for missed cases of persons with hearing problems. However, reality dictates that the efficiency of the program is influenced by the cost of time and money in its fulfillment.

EARLY IDENTIFICATION OF HEARING IMPAIRMENT

The value and importance of early identification of infants with hearing impairment is well documented (Yoshinaga-Itano, Sedey, Coulter, & Mehl, 1998; Yoshinaga-Itano, 1995; Kenworthy, 1993; Elssmann, Matkin, & Sabo, 1987). The obvious benefits relate to early intervention and habilitation of the impairment. In addition, recognizing the presence of a hearing loss at an early age can facilitate the early treatment of speech and language deficits as well as minimize the possible delays that could occur in academic performance and social development (Kenworthy, 1993). Because of the variety of characteristics associated with hearing loss and the fact that speech and language are just developing, hearing loss will often go undetected during the first two years of life. Until recently, the average age of identification in the United States had been 30 months of age (Harrison & Roush, 1996), and some children with mild to moderate impairment are often not identified until school age (Elssmann, Matkin, & Sabo, 1987). The Center for Disease Control and Prevention report that approximately 12,000 infants are born in the

United States each year with some form of hearing loss, making it the number one birth defect in America. It is not surprising then that optimal guidelines and criteria for infant hearing screening has been of particular interest for many years.

Universal Newborn Hearing Screening

In 1970, The **Joint Committee on Infant Hearing (JCIH)** was formed to address the important issue of **universal newborn hearing screening**. The committee is presently comprised of representatives from the American Academy of Audiology; the American Academy of Otolaryngology-Head and Neck Surgery; the American Academy of Pediatrics; the American Speech-Language-Hearing Association; the Council on Education of the Deaf, whose members include representatives from six deaf advocacy and deaf education organizations; and the Directors of Speech and Hearing Programs in State Health and Welfare Agencies.

The initial and subsequent JCIH recommendations (JCIH, 1972; JCIH, 1982; JCIH, 1991) did not advocate universal newborn hearing screening but rather a **high-risk register** to determine referral for an evaluation. A register utilizes specific indicators to determine the potential risk for hearing loss. These indicators include low birth weight, congenital infections, the general health of a baby at birth, craniofacial anomalies, and whether or not there are any hereditary issues with deafness in the family. However, only about 50 to 70% of infants with sensorineural hearing loss exhibit at-risk indicators associated with a high-risk register (Diefendorf, 2002; Kileny & Lesperance, 2001). Because of this low identification rate and high average age of identification, The National Institute on Deafness and Other Communication Disorders (NIDCD) released a statement recommending that "all infants admitted to a neonatal intensive care unit be screened for hearing loss before hospital discharge and that universal screening should be implemented for all infants within the first three months of life" (NIDCD, 1993). Soon after, the JCIH endorsed this recommendation for universal newborn hearing screening (UNHS) (JCIH, 1994). The implementation of UNHS programs and subsequent studies have confirmed the effectiveness of early detection of hearing impaired infants through universal screening (Prieve & Stevens, 2000; Spivak et al., 2000; Vohr et al., 1998; Vohr & Maxon, 1996).

The most recent recommendations made by JCIH is the Year 2000 Position Statement: Principles and Guidelines for Early Hearing Detection and Intervention Programs (JCIH, 2000). Eight principles outline this statement, most notable being the recommendation for the use of electrophysiologic measures as part of routine hospital care after birth and before one month of age. Specifically, otoacoustic emissions (OAEs) and auditory brain stem response (ABR) technology have been implemented successfully in UNHS programs (Finitzo, Albright, & O'Neal, 1998; Mason & Hermann, 1998; Doyle et al., 1997). Another important principle is the recommendation for follow-up of appropriate audiologic and medical evaluations before 3 months of age and intervention of permanent hearing loss before 6 months of age (JCIH, 2000). A coalition of numerous organizations and the United States Public Health Service along with state health departments created the **Healthy People 2010** initiative (a follow-up to the 2000 initiative). Their recommendations related to hearing are exactly aligned and concur with the principles stated by JCIH. The most recent data from the National Center on

Hearing Assessment and Management (NCHAM) indicate that over 92% of the 4 million-plus infant births reported by UNHS programs from all 50 states in 2005 were screened for hearing before one month of age. This figure is up from 22% in 1998.

Unfortunately, the actual diagnostic evaluations performed on those children who were referred before three months of age is still reportedly less than 60%. For this reason, a quality UNHS program is more than just a screening procedure. It requires a series of steps from initiating the program to follow-up with data collection to be truly effective.

A Model Screening Program

The following is a model newborn hearing screening program established in 2001 by the California Department of Health Services. It is comprised of four major components:

Outreach and Awareness Campaign

Independent audiologists, hearing clinics, and other contractors who provide hearing screening services will conduct an outreach and awareness public media campaign in order to educate the general public regarding the screening program. This will include the development of materials for pregnant women, families with newborn hearing infants, primary care physicians serving them with information about the value of hearing testing and the test results that are obtained.

Screening

Ideally all the children born in each state would be screened for hearing. The Department of Health Services assures the quality of the screening by certifying each hospital's hearing screening program. This certification is designed to assure that appropriately trained individuals actually are performing the tests with properly calibrated equipment and are using the appropriate policies and procedures set forth by the program.

Geographically Based Newborn Hearing Coordination Centers

Despite the implementation of the hearing screening procedures, as often as 50% of the time, infants who fail the screening do not receive the necessary services to determine the significance of the hearing loss and to confirm its presence. A solution to this problem is the use of coordination centers following the screening services. These centers provide the necessary follow-up to the screening services to ensure that the infants who do not pass, receive prompt evaluation and appropriate intervention as needed. Without this particular component, the benefit of an early screening program is greatly diminished.

Data System

A comprehensive data management system should be used by each of the hospital programs and coordination centers and a tracking system will consolidate the data into a statewide database at the Department of Health Services. This is an essential tool for monitoring activities, recording test results, tracking follow-up appointments, and providing case management for children needing assistance.

Clearly, UNHS programs have become the new standard for early identification of hearing loss in infants and children. They are an effective screening procedure for the early detection of hearing and have the potential of making a significant shift in the average age in which intervention can begin for hearing-impaired children.

ASHA Guidelines—Birth to Age Five

The American Speech and Language Hearing Associations (ASHA) has published several sets of guidelines for audiologic screening. The most recent guidelines were developed in 1996 and the recommendations for infants and preschoolers are summarized in the following outline. In consideration of the earlier discussion regarding minimizing false positive and false negative responses in a hearing screening program, the ASHA guidelines are suggestive of an ideal set of criteria that is not only accurate in its administration but also an efficient way of conducting a hearing screening program (ASHA, 1997). Each state, however, has developed its own set of guidelines that are some variation to those suggested by ASHA, which indicate that instead of a certification requirement, audiologists' credentials are defined by degree and licensure.

The screening protocols are separated into categories based on chronological and developmental disabilities. The first three set of guidelines listed below are for screening hearing impairment, and the fourth section is specific to screening outer and middle ear disorders of all children and youth.

Screening for Hearing Impairment—Birth to 6 Months of Age

1. The personnel performing this screening should be limited to licensed and certified audiologists (ASHA, 1996a) or support personnel under the supervision of an audiologist (ASHA, 1981), ideally as part of a UNHS program.

2. The recommended screening is with the use of one or two physiologic measures—auditory brainstem response (ABR) or evoked otoacoustic emissions (EOAE) with the infant in a quiet or sleeping state.

3. The screening should include an educational component designed to inform parents about the process of hearing screening, the results, and follow-up procedures.

4. Referral criteria is based on the absence of a reliable response in either ear with a follow-up confirmation of auditory status within 1 month, but no later than 3 months after the initial screening.

Screening for Hearing Impairment—7 Months to 2 Years of Age

1. The personnel performing this screening should be limited to licensed and certified audiologists, who are the only professionals who have the knowledge and skill to screen this age group (AHSA, 1997).

2. Children of this age should be screened if they were not tested at birth as part of a UNHS program, if they exhibit any of the high-risk indicators, are at-risk for fluctuating or progressive hearing loss, or as requested by a parent or other professional.

3. For those children who can condition to visual reinforcement audiometry (VRA), screen with earphones (supra-aural or insert) using 1000-, 2000-, and 4000-Hz tones at 30 dBHL.

4. For those children who can condition to play audiometry (CPA), screen with earphones using 1000-, 2000-, and 4000-Hz tones at 20 dBHL.

5. Sound field testing can be substituted for earphone screening, recognizing the limitation of not obtaining ear-specific results.

6. EOAE or ABR screening is suggested as an alternative procedure when behavioral methods are ineffective.

7. As with other age groups, the screening should include an educational component to inform parents.

8. Screenings failed at any frequency in either ear should be referred for an audiologic evaluation of hearing status within 1 month, but no later than 3 months after the initial screening.

Screening for Hearing Impairment—3 to 5 Years of Age

1. The personnel performing this screening should be limited to licensed and certified audiologists (ASHA, 1996a), licensed and certified speech-language pathologists (1996b), or support personnel under the supervision of an audiologist (ASHA, 1981).

2. Preschool children should be screened who exhibit any of the high-risk indicators, are at-risk for fluctuating or progressive hearing loss, or as requested by a parent or other professional.

3. Condition the child to the desired motor response (raising the hand, verbal response, play activity) with at least two trials at a presumed suprathreshold level.

4. If the child can reliably participate in conditioned play audiometry (CPA) or conventional audiometry, screen with earphones using 1000, 2000, and 4000 Hz at 20 dBHL.

5. Modifications to these procedures include screening in sound field for those who do not accept earphone placement, recognizing the limitations; and using visual reinforcement audiometry (VRA) for preschool children who cannot be conditioned for play audiometry.

6. A pass result is determined if the child's responses are judged to be clinically reliable at least 2 out of 3 times at each frequency in each ear.

7. The child should be referred for an audiologic assessment within 1 month, but no later than 3 months after the initial screening, if there is not a reliable response at least 2 out of 3 times at any frequency in either ear or if the child cannot be conditioned to the task.

Screening for Outer and Middle Ear Disorders, Birth Through 18 Years

1. The personnel performing this screening should be limited to licensed and certified audiologists (ASHA, 1996a), licensed and certified speech-language pathologists (1996b), or support personnel under the supervision of an audiologist (ASHA, 1981). Screening for infants should be conducted by primary care practitioners as part of a well-baby examination (Lim, 1989).

2. Screen all infants and children, 7 months to 6 years of age. If this is not possible, screen children with the following characteristics (Bluestone & Klein, 1996):

- A first episode of acute otitis media prior to 6 months of age
- Infants who have been bottle-fed
- Children with craniofacial anomalies stigmata, or other findings associated with syndromes known to affect the outer and middle ear
- Ethnic populations with documented increased incidence of outer and middle ear disease (e.g., Native American and Eskimo populations)
- A family history of chronic or recurrent OME
- Those in group day care settings and/or crowded living conditions
- Those exposed to excessive cigarette smoke
- Children diagnosed with sensorineural hearing loss (Pappas, 1985), learning disabilities, behavior disorders, or developmental delays and disorders

3. Visually inspect the ears to identify risk factors for outer and middle ear disease, and to ensure that no contraindications exist for performing tympanometry (e.g., drainage, foreign bodies, tympanostomy tubes). Using an otoscope, examine the external ear canal and tympanic membrane for obvious obstructions or structural defects, and then using properly calibrated equipment, perform tympanometry in each ear.

4. The criteria for referral is based on tympanometric results that reveal reduced peak admittance or compliance of <0.2 mmho for infants, and <0.3 mmho for children 1 year to school age. Referral is also recommended if the tympanometric width is >235 daPa for infants or >200 daPa for children older than 1 year.

5. Also, referral for a medical examination is appropriate if a previously unidentified structural defect is present, or ear drainage, obstructions, impacted cerumen or foreign objects, blood or other secretions, stenosis or atresia, otitis externa, and perforations or other abnormalities of the tympanic membrane are apparent.

For a detailed review of screening criteria, refer to the ASHA Guidelines for Audiologic Screening (ASHA, 1997).

HEARING CONSERVATION IN THE SCHOOLS

Hearing conservation in elementary and secondary education is a vital program because of the significant and dramatic impact hearing loss can have on all aspects of a child's life. Numerous investigations have documented the effects of hearing loss on speech and language development and academic performance (Bess, Dodd-Murphy, & Parker, 1998; Carney & Moeller, 1998; Davis et al., 1986; Blair, Peterson, & Viehweg, 1985; Bess & McConnell, 1981). Several studies have also suggested that at any given time, 5 to 12% of school-age children have hearing loss that can impact them educationally (Bess et al., 1998; Niskar et al., 1998; and Montgomery & Fujikawa, 1992). The public schools have the responsibility to identify all children with hearing loss, to refer such children for diagnosis and treatment, and to determine if program modification or special placement is needed. A comprehensive hearing conservation program in the schools should, therefore, "identify all children with hearing impairment, whether temporary or permanent; help families secure remediation; identify and prevent conditions which may contribute to loss of hearing; interpret test results and recommendations of hearing specialists to teachers, parents and child and provide classroom and program adaptation to meet the special educational needs of children with impaired hearing" (State of California Health and Welfare Agency, Department of Health Services, Children's Medical Services, Branch, 2001).

The Test Environment

One of the most difficult aspects of performing hearing testing in the schools is to identify a location with the least amount of interference from noise and other loud sounds. To appreciate the necessity of a quiet environment, examiners need only test their own hearing in an average classroom to experience the difficulty in listening for pure tone stimuli when competing with background noise. Typical criteria used to specify SPL levels that noise should not exceed are derived from the American National Standards Institute maximum permissible noise levels for threshold testing (ANSI, 1991) and adjusted for screening at 20 dBHL (ASHA, 1997). These acceptable levels are: 41.5 dBSPL at 500 Hz, 49.5 dBSPL at 1000 Hz, 54.5 dBSPL at 2000 Hz, and 62 dBSPL at 4000 Hz. Practically speaking, a sound level meter needed to take these measures is typically not accessible by a professional administering screening in a school setting. An alternative to precise SPL measurements to determine the acceptability of a particular room for testing is to perform a "biologic calibration." This procedure is accomplished simply by examiners recording their own hearing thresholds in a quiet environment and comparing those thresholds with results obtained in the environment about to be used for testing. A 10-dB or greater shift in any of the hearing thresholds indicates that the environment is inappropriate for hearing screening.

Who to Test

A common result of screening children is the identification of hearing loss caused by different forms of otitis media. The incidence of this particular disorder occurs more frequently in younger children such as preschoolers and kindergarten children. Therefore, it is appropriate to start a hearing screening program by testing kindergarten and preschool classes when applicable. This would be followed up by a second screening at the first and/or second grade level, then again with two- to three-year intervals throughout each child's educational experience. A suggested sequence of grades to be screened could be the first three or four years of schooling as recommended by the ASHA guidelines, fifth grade, seventh or eighth grade, and tenth or eleventh grade. Thus, the children are tested three or more times in their elementary years and then once each in middle school and again in high school.

In addition to the standard grades just mentioned, other specific groups of children should also be included in the annual screening. Because some children may have missed the hearing screening at a particular school and then relocated, it is essential that all new children to the school be screened regardless of the grade. Children who are diagnosed with other disabling conditions and may be predisposed to hearing loss should be screened as well. Finally, if a teacher or parent has a concern about a particular child, it is important to recognize this request and include them in the screening process.

The Screening Protocol

The process for screening children in schools can be carried out in two basic steps. The first step is to screen the designated groups of children in an efficient manner by using the sweep screening approach. The goal, as indicated earlier, is to separate those children suspected of hearing loss from the children who have no hearing problems. The screening criteria should be selected in order to separate these two groups with the highest level of sensitivity and specificity. The second step will vary based on the recommended guidelines. In some states, a second screening is conducted on the same day as recommended by ASHA (1997). Other guidelines recommend a threshold test on the same day, while others suggest a second screening or threshold test within two to three weeks of the initial screening.

When conducting sweep screening, specific frequencies need to be selected and the intensity level predetermined that will most accurately distinguish the two groups. The most common frequencies selected are 500, 1000, 2000, and 4000 Hz. In some programs and as recommended by the ASHA guidelines, the screening sequence is limited to only three frequencies, not including 500 Hz. The purpose for this alteration is due to the potentially high fail rate from the presence of background noise at that frequency, causing an increase in false positives. Eliminating 500 Hz, however, has the potential of increasing the false negative rate for those children that might be at the beginning stages of otitis media with effusion accompanied by a low-frequency hearing loss. Although many states include 500 Hz, particularly if tympanometry is not part of the hearing screening, the use of three frequencies is often a compromise to increase the efficiency of screening large numbers of students.

The intensity level is also determined by the effect of background noise during the screening procedure. Although ideal circumstances would dictate a screening program using four frequencies at the upper limit of the normal hearing range (15 dBHL), most hearing conservation programs use an intensity level of 20 to 25 dB, recognizing that the testing environment in the schools is not equivalent to a sound-treated room. The ASHA recommended frequencies and intensity level include 1000, 2000, and 4000 Hz at a level of 20 dBHL (ASHA, 1997).

Screening Procedures

The task of performing a hearing screening on 300-plus students on a given day in a typical elementary school can be rather arduous because of its repetitious nature. Therefore, it is recommended that consistent procedures be established in order to minimize potential errors that may occur (incorrect earphone placement or testing the same ear twice). When instructions are given to an entire classroom of children or to a smaller group of children rather than individually, the apprehensive child recognizes the simplicity of the task and is not intimidated by the procedure as easily as they might be during individual instruction. To do this, the audiometer can be set at 2000 Hz or 4000 Hz at a high-intensity level so that the tone can be heard from a distance. The tone can then be presented to the group and all the children can raise their hands as a practice for the actual test. As each child is tested individually, they also can be reinstructed.

Following class instruction, the children can be brought to the testing room individually or in small groups (4–5 for each examiner) for screening. The benefit of bringing in several children at one time is to allow each of them to observe one another participate in the screening, which reduces the anxiety of the younger age groups. It also dramatically increases the speed and efficiency of the screening process. A drawback of this technique is the noise the children generate as they await their turn. Each child should be positioned ideally at a right angle in a way that they are unable to see the operation of the audiometer but the profile of the child can be seen by the examiner. The accuracy of the response is not only determined by hand raising, but also by other subtle responses such as the child's facial expressions and the promptness with which they respond to each tone. Switching to the other ear without informing the child will often cause them to switch to their other hand, verifying the accuracy of the result. For difficult-to-test children, reinstruction or verbal reinforcement throughout the procedure may be necessary to complete the screening.

A suggested sequence of presentation is to begin with a 1000-Hz tone at 40 dB to familiarize the child with the stimulus. The intensity level is then reduced to 20 or 25 dB at 1000 Hz (depending upon the particular protocol) to begin the screening. The sequence would then continue with a stimulus presented at 2000 Hz and 4000 Hz followed by the appropriate response. Without changing the frequency, the examiner switches the stimulus presentation to the other ear and the three frequencies would be presented in reverse order.

Threshold Testing

With some guidelines, a rescreening during the same session or later in the day following reinstruction is recommended. However, the protocol in many hearing conservation programs replaces the second screening with a threshold test performed on the same day. The procedure used for this threshold testing is the conventional modified Hughson-Westlake technique, measuring thresholds at the screening test frequencies of 1000 Hz, 2000 Hz, and 4000 Hz. Some guidelines also suggest the addition of 500 Hz as part of the threshold testing. The reason for the immediacy of the testing is to minimize the false positive rate by separating those children who may not have understood the screening task or may have been reluctant to participate during the initial screening. After providing additional instruction and assistance, many of these children will pass the threshold test. This second test also accurately confirms the results for those children who in fact failed the initial screening.

In many cases, a child will fail an initial screening and the rescreening or threshold test because of a temporary shift in hearing from negative middle ear pressure or serous fluid in the middle ear secondary to a cold or illness on the day of screening. Some lines recommend rescreening or a second threshold test at least two weeks following the initial screening to separate those children who have had a temporary shift in hearing from children who have chronic or permanent hearing disorders.

Referral Criteria

Following the second screening, the criterion used for referral is failure to respond to any one of the test frequencies for either ear at the screening level of 20 or 25 dBHL. Applying the same criterion for threshold testing would result in a referral if a threshold was measured at an intensity greater than the screening level for any of the test frequencies. However, some programs have established less strict criteria so that the number of false positive responses are reduced and consequently overreferring is minimized. For example, a referral is indicated if a test results in hearing threshold levels of 30 dBHL or greater for two or more frequencies in an ear or a hearing threshold level of 40 decibels or greater for one of the frequencies tested. When this type of criteria is used, a careful review of the results should be made prior to recording a passing score because of the potential for passing a child with an educationally significant hearing loss. For example, if testing were performed and the results indicated thresholds of 25 dB at 1000 Hz, 35 dB at 2000 Hz, and 25 dB at 4000 Hz, this referral criteria would result in a pass and not require a referral. However, studies have shown that hearing thresholds at these levels cause learning difficulties in an educational setting (Bess, Dodd-Murphy, & Parker, 1998; Davis et al., 1986; Blair, Peterson, & Viehweg, 1985). Therefore, careful scrutiny of the results should be conducted prior to passing borderline cases using less strict criteria. The simple principle, "when in doubt, refer," should be applied whenever conducting hearing screening.

Guidelines for Hearing Screening

The ASHA guidelines for hearing-impairment screening for school-age children, 5 through 18 years of age are summarized as follows:

1. The personnel should be limited to licensed and certified audiologists (ASHA, 1996a), licensed and certified speech-language pathologists (ASHA, 1996b), support personnel under the supervision of an audiologist (ASHA, 1981), or audiometrists/audiometric technicians in states that certfication and licensure laws permit.

2. Screen on initial entry to school, entrance to special education, grade repetition, or new to the school, and annually in kindergarten through third grade and in seventh and eleventh grades. Other years should be screened if: parent/care provider, health care provider, teacher, or other school personnel have concerns regarding hearing, speech, language, or learning abilities; a family history of hereditary hearing loss; recurrent or persistent otitis media; craniofacial anomalies; findings associated with a syndrome known to include sensorineural and/or conductive hearing loss; head trauma with loss of consciousness; or reported exposure to potentially damaging noise levels or ototoxic drugs.

3. Screen via conventional audiometry or conditioned play audiometry with supraaural or insert earphones using 1000, 2000, and 4000 Hz at 20 dBHL.

4. Reinstruct and rescreen within the same screening session in which a child fails.

5. Refer all who fail the rescreen or fail to condition to the screening task, at any frequency in either ear for audiologic confirmation of hearing status within one month but no later than three months after initial screening.

Tympanometry in Hearing Screening Programs

An important purpose for hearing screening is to identify those children with hearing loss caused by otitis media. Because of this fundamental purpose, it seems logical that a measurement technique designed specifically for the identification of tympanic membrane compliance and middle ear function would be a more appropriate technique to be used in hearing screening. Many programs throughout the country, therefore, are recommending that tympanometry be added to the testing protocol in their hearing conservation programs. Unfortunately, the implementation of this recommended procedure is still rare.

Ideally, tympanometric screening should be performed on all young school-aged children in preschool and kindergarten through the third-grade level. A simple screening tympanometer can perform this test on both ears in less than one minute with consistently accurate results, and it can be conducted on the same day as the pure tone hearing screening. If this routine use of tympanometry is not feasible, the tympanometric procedures should be included as part of the rescreening or threshold testing for those children who failed the initial screening.

The inclusion of tympanometry helps confirm the presence of middle ear fluid that is consistent with a measured hearing loss. It also will assist in the appropriate direction for referral. For example, if a child fails the hearing screening and the tympanometric test results show the presence of fluid with a reduction in the tympanic membrane compliance, the appropriate referral would be to a physician for medical treatment of the middle ear disorder. A follow-up screening or audiologic assessment would then be conducted to confirm a recovery of hearing sensitivity following treatment. Conversely, if a hearing loss is identified but tympanometry reveals normal tympanic membrane compliance, the combination of these results would be suggestive of a possible sensorineural hearing loss. In this case, a more appropriate referral would be directly to an audiologist for an audiologic evaluation. Incorporating tympanometry into a hearing screening program increases the ability to verify a potential ear disorder and make a more expeditious referral to the proper health professional for diagnosis and treatment.

Organizational Planning and Reporting

The following are suggested guidelines designed to assist in the initiation and management of a hearing conservation program and may need to be modified to fit unique situations (State of California Health and Welfare Agency, Department of Health Services, Children's Medical Services Branch, 2001):

Contact with Administration

1. Meet with appropriate administrators early in the school year and explain the purpose of the program followed by a written plan.
2. The plan should include the number and age groups of students as well as the number of days needed to complete the screening.

3. Outline and explain the need for a quiet, convenient testing room for screening and threshold testing. If necessary, inspect proposed testing sites—what is quiet and convenient to a school administrator may not be quiet and convenient enough to meet testing needs. Also ensure that power outlets are within close proximity to the testing locations.

Scheduling

1. Discuss and agree upon a schedule for screening and threshold testing at each school in order to minimize the disruption to regular school activities.
2. Announce the screening dates to the staff and confirm the test locations within the schools and the number of students to be tested on each scheduled day.

Testing

1. Ensure that the audiometers are calibrated and operating correctly.
2. Verify that the examiners are properly trained and licensed or certified when necessary.
3. Review the schedule of classes and instruct the support staff on the retrieval of children from the classroom in a timely manner to maintain a good flow during the testing.

Test Forms and Reporting

1. Forms for each child should be provided prior to the test date to have them filled out and ready to record the test data. Some programs record certain groups or a classroom of children on a single form.
2. Upon completion of the screening procedures, all forms are to be collected to insure proper referral for threshold testing.
3. Record the names of children to be referred and provide a form for the audiologist/physician to complete following their evaluation in order to ensure the testing is performed and recommendations are made.
4. An annual report that summarizes the results for each school provides a means to track the screening program from year to year.
5. Report yearly program results to the state department of health services.

Follow-up Procedures

1. Outline referral criteria and procedures for the teachers and administrators.
2. Provide notification to parents and the school principal of those children who fail the threshold evaluation.
3. Know what medical/audiological, educational and rehabilitation resources are available locally for proper referral.

4. Obtain the medical and/or audiological reports for each child referred and provide this information to the appropriate person or persons for the purpose of closing a case or providing additional services such as special education or hearing aid evaluations.

PEDIATRIC EVALUATION

The goals in evaluating an infant or a small child are to identify the presence of a hearing disorder and then determine its characteristics such as the degree of the impairment as well as the cause of the disorder. Obviously, these goals are similar to evaluating an adult or school-age child but special test procedures need to be employed to overcome certain obstacles with which you are faced when testing an infant or child's hearing. The first and most obvious obstacle is the limited cognitive capabilities of this group in responding behaviorally to an auditory stimulus. In place of a simple hand raise or the repeating of words presented, other forms of behavioral responses need to be used to determine whether or not the auditory signal is heard. These types of responses may come in the form of a head turn, eye movement, a pointing gesture, or a reflexive action. Second, the short attention span of this pediatric group limits the time available to perform a thorough evaluation. The standardized testing protocols must be modified to obtain the most important information as soon as possible before that precious time is gone and the responses are either unreliable or are no longer obtainable. A third obstacle involves the use of conventional pure tone test signals. Hearing testing using pure tones presented at low intensity levels is not a very exciting experience even for adults and requires a certain degree of concentration by the listener. So it is not surprising that pure tones generally hold very little interest and may not by very effective stimuli to a small child or infant (Moore, Wilson, & Thompson, 1977). They may respond initially to this unique sounding auditory signal, but in most cases, their desire to respond to it diminishes rapidly. A modification to pure tones such as pulsing or warbling may extend the number of responses while maintaining the frequency specificity of the test stimulus.

Speech measures are usually more reliable and carry greater interest for this population resulting in more accurate auditory thresholds (Northern & Downs, 1991). Using familiar names and words, naming head and facial body parts, or pointing to color pictures are ways to modify the testing process and thereby increase the number as well as the reliability of the responses. Finally, the willingness of a pediatric patient to participate in the testing procedure can easily make or break the evaluation and its validity. A reluctant child, a crying child, an undisciplined child, or one that is "bouncing off the walls" will cause the testing results to be extremely difficult if not impossible to obtain. Familiarity with the environment and the examiner on a second or third visit, and practicing the testing tasks or "games" at home when appropriate, can significantly improve the chances of having a child agreeable to participate in the testing.

Interestingly, a large number of infants and children seen by an audiologist have normal hearing. A referral for an evaluation is often for the purpose of ruling out a hearing loss rather than identifying or confirming the presence of a hearing loss. Many children are referred to determine whether or not a diagnosed speech or language disorder has resulted from a decrease in hearing sensitivity. Other children are seen to monitor the temporary effect of otitis media on hearing ability. Therefore, an abbreviated evaluation or screening procedure may be sufficient to accurately diagnose normal hearing. The advent of electro-physiologic testing, which was discussed in Chapter 7, has particular value in this type of assessment as well as part of the more complete evaluation process. Immittance testing that reveals a normal tympanogram and measurable acoustic reflexes can confirm an open ear canal, normal middle ear function, and recognition of the reflex signal through the auditory pathway. The presence of otoacoustic emissions when screened at normal levels is a strong indicator of normal hearing function. Combining the immittance and otoacoustic emission test results obtained from a willing patient with behavioral testing using special techniques can culminate in a reliable conclusion regarding a child's hearing sensitivity.

Special Pediatric Test Protocols

There are a series of behavioral tests that have been developed and categorized sequentially based on the mental and chronological ages of infants and children. Although these test techniques are primarily utilized for children, they can also be applied to the other difficult to test populations as discussed in Chapter 9.

Behavioral Observation Audiometry

The actual observation of behavior should be the beginning of any special test used to measure the hearing of an infant or young child. It is important to note various factors of the child's relationship with adults and other children such as their general alertness, appropriate behaviors, motor function, and methods of communication. With this information in hand, more controlled test procedures can then be applied. A logical starting point might be the use of gross measures discussed previously such as the clapping of hands or calling the name of the child and then observing any response or change in behavior. Another technique is the use of a set of noisemakers such as rattles, bells, squeak toys, etc. Special toy noisemaker kits have been designed in an attempt to provide a representation of sounds across the frequency spectrum. Introducing a variety of stimuli to a patient, presumably an infant, and then monitoring the responses is a test procedure called **behavioral observation audiometry (BOA)**. The BOA technique is a measurement of an unconditioned response to sound and should be used along with other electrophysiologic measures to test infants from birth to about 5 months of age.

There are several types of responses to auditory stimuli that can be presented by a child. The most obvious is localization to sound. For example, if an infant is sitting on her or his mother's lap, the presentation of noisemaker stimuli from behind may elicit a head-turning response. It is important to note that with infants younger than 3 or 4 months, the ability to localize a signal has not yet developed sufficiently to provide a distinct measurable response. Another behavior observed as a response to louder auditory signals are reflexes such as the *auropalpebral reflex,* eye blink or tightening of the eyelids, or the *Moro reflex,* a startle response characterized by a sudden jerking motion. If a child is moving during the presentation of a signal, a response may be a quieting or cessation of activity or movement of the infant as she or he is trying to identify a change in acoustic signals or in search of the location of the signal. In addition to noisemakers, speech signals can also be used when performing BOA. However, frequency-specific stimuli are no longer recommended as part of a BOA procedure (Diefendorf, 2002). It needs to be understood that this observation procedure is a fairly gross measure of hearing sensitivity and that children do not respond

Table 8.4   Minimal response levels to noisemakers, warble tones and speech in sound field for infants, 0 to 24 months

Age	Noisemakers	Warble Tones	Speech
0–8 weeks	58–70 dB	78	40–60
5 wks–4 mos.	50–60	70	47
4–7 mos.	40–50	51	21
7–8 mos.	30–40	45	15
8–13 mos.	25–35	38	8
13–15 mos.	25–30	32	5
15–21 mos.	25	25	5
21–24 mos.	25	20	3

Source: Adapted from N. Matkin 1977. Assessment of hearing sensitivity during the preschool years. In F. H. Bess (Ed.). *Childhood Deafness.* New York: Grune & Stratton.

to sound at threshold levels. Generally, these hearing results are more often the level at which the stimulus has caught the attention of an infant or child and they were willing to respond rather than an absolute measure of hearing sensitivity (Diefendorf and Gravel, 1996). This measurement is called a **minimal response level (MRL)** (Matkin, 1977). Typical MRLs and the gradual shift to threshold as infants age is displayed in Table 8.4.

Visual Reinforcement Audiometry

As infants reach 5 to 6 months, the ability to condition them to respond to a specific stimulus improves. An effective method to test these small children up through the age of 2 using a conditioned response is called **visual reinforcement audiometry (VRA)**. The developmental age of the infant being tested will influence the accuracy of the results. However, studies have shown that infants ages 6 to 12 months exhibit a high success rate of testability even if the child is high-risk or has special needs (Widen, 1990; Wilson, Folsom, & Widen, 1983; Thompson, Wilson, and Moore, 1979). The fundamental premise behind VRA is the use of the operant conditioning paradigm of stimulus-response-reinforcement to elicit a response from the patient. The auditory stimulus will cause a child to respond, which results in a visual reinforcement that is of interest to the child. This type of procedure requires a sound booth with the use of speakers or earphones and hidden visual reinforcement that is within close proximity to the acoustic stimulus. It also typically necessitates two examiners to effectively perform the procedure.

The process by which VRA is performed is as follows:

1. The child being tested is placed on his or her parent's lap or in a high chair facing an audiologist or an assistant in the sound booth (Figure 8.1). Speakers are placed at an angle of 45 to 90 degrees from the child sufficient to require a distinct head turn to the auditory stimulus. The examiner is outside the sound booth or in the control room of a sound suite operating the clinical audiometer.

2. The visual reinforcers are then located near the sound source. These reinforcers are usually animated animals such as a drum-playing monkey or a rocking parrot housed

Figure 8.1 An example of a testing arrangement in a sound-treated test booth for visual reinforcement audiometry (VRA)

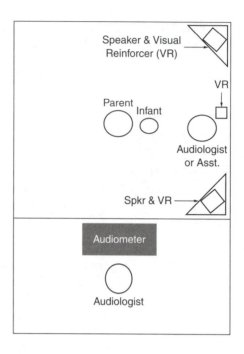

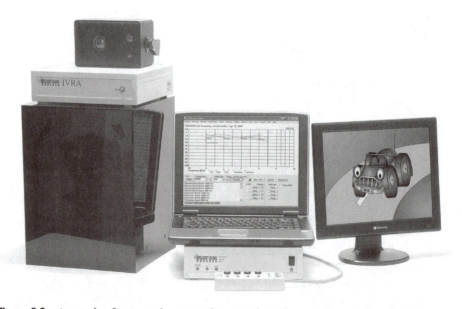

Figure 8.2   A sample of animated toys used in visual reinforcement audiometry (VRA).
Source: Courtesy of Intelligent Hearing Systems

in a smoke glass casing so that the child does not initially notice them. In addition, a third animated toy such as a barking dog is often placed directly in front of the child; it can be used to redirect a child's attention back to a midline position in readiness for the next stimulus presentation. Recently, advanced equipment has been developed which displays computer-generated images on a monitor as shown in Figure 8.2. This design further enhances the interest of the child in responding to the reinforcer.

3. The first step in the procedure requires a pairing of the acoustic stimulus to the visual reinforcement. This is accomplished by presenting either the examiner's voice, a loud warble tone, or a narrow band noise while simultaneously lighting up the smoke glass container with the animated toy. This procedure is designed to condition the child to make a connection between stimulus and reinforcement. The pairing may need to be performed two or three times for the child to realize the relationship between the two. Once the visual reinforcement has been presented the first time, the child will obviously show great interest in seeing it again. The assistant will need to bring the child's attention back to midline either with the use of a hand puppet or a toy (Figure 8.3).

4. Following the conditioning, testing begins with the presentation of the stimulus at a test level that presumably will be audible to the child and elicit a head-turn response (Figure 8.3). The initial response confirms that, in fact, the child is conditioned to look for a visual reinforcement in response to an auditory stimulus. The intensity of the signal can then be decreased and an ascending technique is used in an attempt to identify hearing thresholds.

It is important to note that despite the reliability and effectiveness of the VRA procedure, the end result may still not be a hearing threshold but rather an MRL. As in BOA measures, a speech detection threshold is often the first test that is performed with VRA due to its higher level of accuracy as compared to pure tone stimuli. However, a child's attention span is relatively short and will only allow a certain number of reliable responses. Therefore, the frequencies of 500 Hz and 2000 or 3000 Hz are used initially for testing in order to yield information from both the low frequency and high frequency ranges.

Pure tones are not used in a sound field environment because of the occurrence of dead spots in the sound booth that occur from the reflection of a pure tone waveform, which causes a cancellation of that signal. By slightly altering or modulating the frequency of the signal with a warble tone, the effect of pure tone cancellation is eliminated. Narrow band noise has also been considered as a stimulus to obtain hearing information from a child. However, narrow band noise provides less frequency-specific information because of the presence of potential acoustic energy across a much greater frequency spectrum.

The VRA procedure is most commonly performed using sound field speakers with the pairing of stimulus to reinforcement. However, this type of testing will yield responses only from the better ear. If the child being tested will tolerate the use of earphones, an attempt should be made to perform the procedure in this manner in order to obtain ear-specific information.

An alternative form of operant conditioning audiometry is to substitute the visually reinforcing signal with something that is tangible or edible. Tangible reinforcement operant conditioning audiometry (TROCA), described by Lloyd, Spradlin, and Reid (1968), employs the use of a tangible reinforcer such as a piece of candy, cereal,

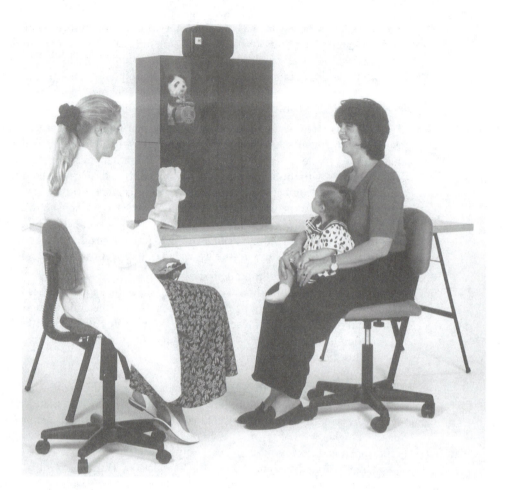

Figure 8.3 Infant's head-turn response during visual reinforcement audiometry (VRA) to see an animated reinforcer following signal presentation. Photograph also shows the second audiologist or assistant ready to return the infant's attention to midline position with the use of a hand puppet.
Source: Courtesy of Intelligent Hearing Systems

or some token to maintain the interest of more difficult to test children. The procedure used is similar to VRA in that the child is again conditioned to respond to a tone, but rather than a head-turning response, the child is conditioned to flip a switch or push a button in order to receive a tangible reward. Unfortunately, this test procedure requires special equipment as well as more time and patience for it to be effective. It will often take many trials of conditioning for the child to understand the task. For these reasons, TROCA is not commonly used in most clinics. When performed properly, however, it can ultimately produce some very reliable and accurate test results.

Conditioned Play Audiometry

The testing of three- and four-year-old preschool children will also require the use of operant conditioning in obtaining behavioral responses. As children age, the type of response and form of reinforcement used in the testing process need to change to coincide with changes in their behavior. An effective test designed to measure hearing of this age group is called conditioned play audiometry (CPA). This protocol is accepted among audiologists and is effective for children as young as 30 months of age (Diefendorf, 2002; Thompson, Thompson, & Vethivelu, 1989; Thompson & Weber, 1974). CPA is a simple procedure that can be employed in a regular audiology clinic setting or by using a portable audiometer in a school setting. The essence of this procedure is to make the hearing test an enjoyable game that would entice the child to participate. The procedures are as follows:

1. The child is seated in front of a table with an assistant positioned next to him or her and the examiner facing the child through the sound booth window. A modification of this arrangement would be for the examiner to be seated next to the child with a portable audiometer and then the examiner performs the testing as well as provides assistance. The child is asked to participate in a fun game listening to different sounds.

2. A game in the form of pegs and a pegboard; blocks or small plastic animals and a bucket; or a series of plastic rings for stacking are placed on the table in front of the child. The basic concept of this procedure is for the child to place a peg in a pegboard, drop blocks or plastic toys into a bucket, or stack rings each time a signal is heard (see Figure 8.4). Children are conditioned with assistance to respond to tones by placing the toy object in their hand and holding it up to their ear to begin "playing the game." Once the child is conditioned to the task, accurate hearing thresholds can be obtained.

3. Again, valuable information in the low and high frequencies in each ear should be measured first before the interest of the child declines. If the child still shows interest in the game after initial thresholds are measured, additional frequencies can be tested to complete the audiogram. It is also important to vary the rhythm of stimulus presentation so that the child is not just responding as part of the game and ignoring the actual acoustic signal. If the child does respond without a stimulus presentation, it is vital that the peg or block is placed back in the child's hand to listen again for an accurate signal before responding. Ensuring that the child must respond to the acoustic signal to play the game increases the accuracy of the test results. A large supply of toys or tokens to play the game is suggested, since many children assume the game will be over once they have completed placing all pegs or dropping all the blocks. The ability of the examiner to provide verbal or social praise is a critical element to the CPA protocol. Although the play activity helps maintain the interest of the child, it is not the reinforcement. The ongoing verbal reinforcement is essential to maximize the response behavior of the child.

As these procedures are attempted, children may be unable or unwilling to perform many tasks because of the newness of the environment and the comparisons

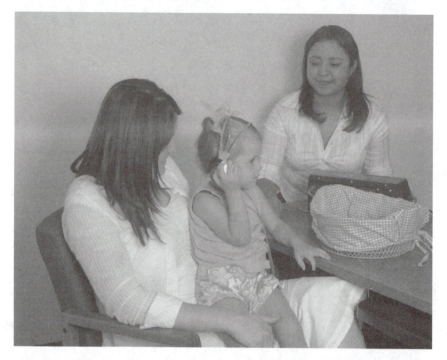

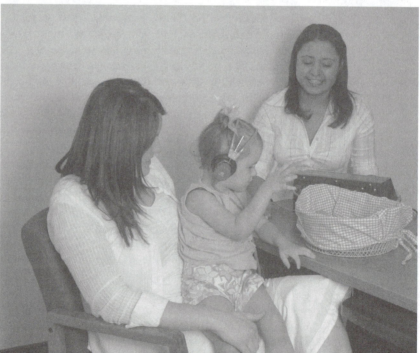

Figure 8.4 Arrangement used in testing with conditioned play audiometry (CPA) procedures. The first photograph shows the child listening for the signal with a toy placed next to the headphones. The second photograph shows her response to the stimulus by dropping the toy into the basket.

they might make between the clinical environment and a physician's office in which a child recalls experiences of discomfort or pain as part of certain medical procedures. For this reason, it is often appropriate to attempt the procedure on the first visit despite a child's reluctance so that it can be portrayed as an enjoyable and entertaining experience. The follow-up appointment can then yield more accurate test results because of the child's familiarity with the environment, the procedures, and greater willingness to participate and respond appropriately. Participation of the parents in practicing the games at home between appointments can also facilitate the reliability of the test results.

Modifications to Conventional Audiometry

The transition from special test protocols such as operant conditioning to conventional audiometry often requires some slight modifications to standard procedures in order to maintain the interest of a 4-year-old or timid 5-year-old. The familiarization and threshold search stimulus presentations of conventional testing may need to be reduced because of the short attention span of the children being tested. In addition, the frequency sequence could be altered as indicated before so that information in the low and high frequencies is obtained for both ears and then additional frequencies can be tested if time and the child's attentiveness will permit. Responses to stimuli may also need to be altered to accommodate the circumstances of the patient. For example, children may be reluctant or inconsistent when raising a hand in response to each tonal stimulus. The inability to consistently respond may necessitate a reinstruction by asking them to see how quickly they can raise their hand or how high they can raise their hand when they hear the tone. An alternative to this typical response would be for the child to respond verbally by saying "yes" or "I hear it" to each tone. Regular verbal reinforcement also is essential for a child to maintain interest throughout the test procedure. These types of modifications to the conventional procedures will increase effectiveness in your testing as well as improve the accuracy.

Speech Testing with Children

As indicated earlier, an infant or preschooler will respond to speech with greater reliability. A measurement of the speech detection threshold (SDT) for children younger than 2 years old is the first test of choice, using their name or nonsense sounds as stimuli. At the age of 2 or 3, more precise results using speech audiometry may be obtained by using simple questions such as "Where is your mommy?" Another alternative is to condition them to point to various body parts such as "Point to your nose, point to your mouth, point your eye" and so forth. This can usually be accomplished with the help of their parent in physically taking the child's hand in assisting them to point until they understand the concept and can do it on their own. The end result can yield a fairly accurate threshold for speech.

Speech recognition thresholds can also be obtained using standard spondees in the form of pictures or objects, which creates a game quite enjoyable for children as they are asked to point to different pictures; resulting in precise threshold levels without requiring the child to verbally respond. Although these different forms of speech audiometric testing do not provide frequency specific information, at a minimum it will allow for a reasonable indication of hearing thresholds for speech and can rule out severe levels of hearing loss.

SUMMARY

A Glimpse into the Profession Revisited

The initial screening outcome for Brandon required a rescreening with the same results: a failed response at all frequencies for both ears at 20 dBHL. Tympanometry was then performed, revealing normal tympanic membrane compliance for both ears. Because the failed screening indicated the need for a referral, but the normal tympanometric results were not consistent with a middle ear disorder, a medical referral was contraindicated. Brandon was seen by an audiologist for a complete audiologic evaluation. A mild, flat sensorineural hearing loss was diagnosed. Following a visit to his pediatrician for medical clearance, Brandon was seen again by the audiologist to begin audiologic rehabilitation with amplification.

CHAPTER REVIEW

❑ The screening and evaluation of the pediatric population is a fundamental part of the practice of audiology and audiometry.

❑ Hearing screening is an essential process used in detecting hearing impairment in infants and children. The criteria designed to accurately separate persons with hearing problems from the general population needs to incorporate a high level of sensitivity and specificity in order to fulfill the goals of the screening program.

❑ When establishing a screening program, it is important to maximize the effectiveness of the screening procedure in order to appropriately separate those children with normal hearing from those with potential hearing problems, while minimizing the number of false positive or false negative results.

❑ Early identification is a critical component of audiologic practice and necessitates the implementation of early hearing detection, evaluation, and intervention programs in order to quickly ameliorate or minimize the potential impact a hearing loss can have on a child's life.

❑ The JCIH Year 2000 Position Statement and the Healthy People 2010 initiative have established principles and guidelines to facilitate universal newborn hearing screening across the country. Recent studies have confirmed the value of these programs in the early detection of hearing-impaired infants.

❑ A hearing conservation program is an essential component of any health service in elementary or secondary education. The implication of hearing loss is significant and far-reaching, particularly in preschool and young school-aged children.

❑ Once a screening program has been conducted and the children with failed responses have been identified, rescreening or threshold tests and tympanometry should be performed to confirm the hearing loss and to make a proper referral.

❑ Throughout this testing process it is important to have an organized plan to interface with administrators and teachers to make the process as efficient as possible while minimizing the effect it has on the children's daily academic activities.

❑ The selection of the testing site is also critical to minimize the impact that background noise will have on the accuracy of the testing.

❑ When conducted properly, hearing conservation programs can be an effective means to help in the identification of significant hearing impairment in children.

❑ The evaluation of infants and young children requires the use of special test procedures to obtain a reasonable measure of hearing sensitivity. The inclusion of visual reinforcers, toys or game-type activities, and ongoing verbal encouragement are particularly effective in eliciting responses from small children.

ACTIVITIES FOR DISCUSSION

1. In the Case Study, why wasn't Brandon's hearing loss diagnosed at an earlier age?

2. How can more universal newborn hearing screening programs be implemented to increase the number of infants screened and improve the effectiveness of follow-up procedures?

3. Who should be responsible for hearing conservation programs in the schools; for administering the program and performing the hearing screening procedures?

4. Why is visual reinforcement audiometry more effective than behavioral observation, and why are younger children (12–18 months) quite often easier to test than older children (2–3 years old)?

REFERENCES

American National Standards Institute. (1991). *Maximum permissible ambient noise levels for audiometric test rooms* (ANSI S3.1-1991). New York: Acoustical Society of America.

American Speech-Language-Hearing Association Audiologic Assessment Panel 1996. (1997). *Guidelines for audiologic screening.* Rockville, MD: Author.

American Speech-Language-Hearing Association. (1996a). Scope of practice in audiology. *ASHA, 38*(Suppl.16), 12–15

American Speech-Language-Hearing Association. (1996b). Scope of practice in speech-language pathology. *ASHA, 38*(Suppl. 16), 1–4.

American Speech-Language-Hearing Association. (1981). Employment and utilization of supportive personnel in audiology and speech-language pathology. *ASHA, 23,* 165–169.

Bess, F. H., Dodd-Murphy, J., & Parker, R. (1998). Children with minimal sensorineural hearing loss; prevalence, educational performance, and functional status. *Ear and Hearing, 19,* 339–354.

Bess, F. H., & McConnell, F. E. (1981). *Audiology education and the hearing impaired child.* St. Louis: C. V. Mosby Company.

Blair, J. C., Peterson, M. E., & Viehweg, S. H. (1985). The effects of mild sensorineural hearing loss on academic performance of young school-age children. *The Volta Review, 87*(2), 87–93.

Bluestone, C. D., & Klein, J. O. (1996). Otitis media, atelectasis, and eustachian tube disfunction. In C. D. Bluestone, S. E. Stool, & M. A. Kenna (Eds.), *Pediatric Otolaryngology* (3d ed., vol. I, pp. 388–582). Philadelphia: Saunders.

California Department of Health Services. (2001). *Manual for the school audiometrist.* Health and Welfare Agency, Children's Medical Services Branch.

Carney, A., & Moeller, M. P. (1998). Treatment efficacy: Hearing loss in children. *Journal of Speech and Hearing Research, 41,* 61–84.

Davis, J., Elfenbein, J., Schum, D., & Bentler. (1986). Effects of mild and moderate hearing impairment on language, educational and psychosocial behavior of children. *Journal of Speech and Hearing Disorders, 51,* 53–62.

Diefendorf, A. O. (2002). Detection and assessment of hearing loss in infants and children. In J. Katz (Ed.), *Handbook of clinical audiology* (5th ed.). Baltimore: Lippincott, Williams & Wilkins.

Diefendorf, A. O., & Gravel, J. S. (1996). Visual reinforcement and behavioral observation audiometry. In S. E. Gerber (Ed.), *Handbook of pediatric audiology* (pp. 55–83).Washington, DC: Gallaudet University Press.

Doyle, K., Burggraaff, B., Fujikawa, S., Kim, J., & MacArthur, C. (1997). Neonatal hearing screening with otoscopy, auditory brainstem response, and otoacoustic emissions. *Otolaryngology-Head and Neck Surgery, 116,* 597–603.

Elssmann, S. A., Matkin, N. D., & Sabo, M. P. (1987). Early identification of congenital sensorineural hearing impairment. *The Hearing Journal, 40,* 13–17.

Finitzo, T., Albright, K. & O'Neal, J. (1998). The newborn with hearing loss: Detection in the nursery. *Pediatrics, 102,* 1452–1460.

Harrison, M., & Roush, J. (1996). Age of suspicion, identification and intervention for infants and young children with hearing loss: A national study. *Ear and Hearing, 17,* 55–62.

Johnson, C. D. (2002). Hearing and immittance screening. In J. Katz (Ed.), *Handbook of clinical audiology,* (5th ed.). Baltimore: Lippincott, Williams & Wilkins.

Joint Committee on Infant Hearing. (2000). Year 2000 position statement: Principles and guidelines for early hearing detection and intervention programs, *Audiology Today,* Special Issue.

Joint Committee on Infant Hearing. (1994). 1994 position statement. *Audiology Today, 6,* 6–9.

Joint Committee on Infant Hearing. (1991). 1990 position statement. *ASHA, 33,* 3–6.

Joint Committee on Infant Hearing. (1982). 1982 position statement. *ASHA, 24,* 1017–1018

Joint Committee on Infant Hearing. (1972). Supplementary statement on infant hearing screening. *ASHA, 16,* 160.

Kenworthy, O. T. (1993). Early identification: principles and practices. In J. G. Alpiner & P. A. MacCarthy, *Rehabilitative audiology: Children and adults* (pp. 53–71). Baltimore: Lippincott, Williams & Wilkins.

Kileny, P., & Lesperance, M. (2001). Evidence in support of a different model of universal newborn hearing loss identification. *American Journal of Audiology, 10,* 65–67.

Lim, D. J. (Ed.). (1989). Recent advances in otitis media: Report of the Fourth Research Conference. *Annals of Otology, Rhinology, and Laryngology, 98* (Suppl. 139), 4, 2.

Lloyd, L. L., Spradlin, J. E., & Reid, M. J. (1968). An operant audiometric procedure for difficult-to-test patients. *Journal of Speech and Hearing Disorders, 33,* 236–245.

Mason, J., & Hermann, K. R. (1998). Universal infant hearing screening by automated auditory brainstem response measurement. *Pediatrics, 101,* 221–228.

Matkin, N. (1977). Assessment of hearing sensitivity during the preschool years. In F. H. Bess (Ed.), *Childhood deafness.* New York: Grune and Stratton.

Montgomery, J., & Fujikawa, S. (1992). Hearing thresholds of students in the second, eighth, and twelfth grades. *Language Speech and Hearing Services in the Schools, 23,* 61–63.

Moore, J. M., Wilson, W. R., & Thompson, G. (1977). Visual reinforcement of head-turn responses in infant under 12 months of age. *Journal of Speech and Hearing Disorders, 42,* 328–334.

National Center on Hearing Assessment and Management (NCHAM) (2005). Utah State University, InfantHearing.org

National Institute on Deafness and Other Communication Disorders (NIDCD) (1993). National Institutes of Health Consensus statement: Early identification of hearing impairment in infants and young children. Bethesda, MD: Author.

Niskar, A. S., Kieszak, S., Holmes, A., Esteban, E., Rubin, D., & Brody, D. J. (1998). Prevalence of hearing loss among children 6 to 19 years of age: *The Third National Health and Nutrition Examination Survey. JAMA, 279,* 1071–1075. et al., 1998.

Northern, J. L., & Downs, M. P. (1991). *Hearing in Children* (4th ed.). Baltimore: Williams & Wilkins.

Pappas, D. G. (1985). *Diagnosis and treatment of hearing impairment in children.* San Diego: College-Hill Press.

Prieve, B., & Stevens, F. (2000). The New York State universal newborn hearing screening demonstration project: Introduction and overview. *Ear and Hearing , 21,* 85–91.

Spivak, L., Dalzell, L., Berg, A., Bradley, M., Cacace, A., Campbell, D., DiCristofaro, J., Gravel, J., Greenberg, E., Gross, S., Orlando, M., Pinheiro, J., Regan, J., Stevens, F., & Prieve, B., (2000). The New York state universal newborn hearing screening demonstration project: inpatient outcome measures. *Ear and Hearing, 21,* 92–103.

Thompson, M. D., Thompson, G., & Vethivelu, S. (1989). A comparison of audiometric test thresholds for two-year-old children. *Journal of Speech and Hearing Disorders, 54,* 174–179.

Thompson, G., & Weber, B. A. (1974). Responses of infants and young children to behavioral observation audiometry (BOA). *Journal of Speech and Hearing Disorders, 44,* 80–90.

Thompson, G., Wilson, W. R., & Moore, J.M. (1979). Application of visual reinforcement audiometry (VRA) to low-functioning children. *Journal of Speech and Hearing Disorders, 54,* 174–179.

Vohr, B. R., Carty, L., Moore, P., & Letourneau, K. (1998). The Rhode Island Hearing Assessment Program: Experience with statewide hearing screening (1993-1996). *Journal of Pediatrics, 133,* 353–357.

Vohr, B. R., & Maxon, A. (1996). Screening infants for hearing impairment. *Journal of Pediatrics, 128,* 710–714.

Widen, J. E. (1990). Behavioral screening of high-risk infants using visual reinforcement audiometry. *Seminars in Hearing, 11,* 342–356.

Wilson, W. R., Folsom, R.C., & Widen, J. E. (1983). Hearing impairment in Down's syndrome children. In G. Mencher & S. Gerber (Eds.), *The multiply handicapped hearing impaired child.* New York: Grune & Stratton.

Yoshinaga-Itano, C., Sedey, A., Coulter, D. K., & Mehl, A. L. (1998). Language of early and later identified children with hearing loss. *Pediatrics, 102,* 1161–1171.

Yoshinaga-Itano, C. (1995). Efficacy of early identification and intervention. *Seminars in Hearing, 16,* 115–120.

Assessing Special Populations

Key Terms

CASE STUDY

A Glimpse into the Profession

Sally is a fifth-grader who recently failed the hearing screening performed at her elementary school. The retest showed the same results, so a pure tone threshold test was conducted, which indicated a moderate to severe hearing loss in both ears. These results seemed unusual because of Sally's ability to respond appropriately to speech at normal conversational levels. She was referred for a complete audiologic evaluation. A case history revealed a negative history of hearing loss in the family and a medical history that was unremarkable. Sally's mother reported that she has not noticed any difficulty in communicating with Sally and was unaware of any hearing difficulty. The results of the testing identified a moderate hearing loss, which was somewhat better than the thresholds obtained at school. Speech audiometric results were also inconsistent with the pure tone findings, indicating significantly better speech reception thresholds. Immittance testing revealed normal type A tympanograms and normal acoustic reflexes. With these conflicting results, it was determined that additional special testing procedures needed to be implemented in an attempt to more accurately identify Sally's hearing sensitivity.

OVERVIEW OF SPECIAL ASSESSMENT

Behavioral audiometric procedures used to assess hearing function, as described in Chapter 6, can be reliably used for most individuals from children to the elderly. However, there are certain groups of individuals that require significant modification of testing procedures in order to obtain a more meaningful measure of auditory function. These populations include developmentally disabled adults, elderly patients diagnosed with a form of dementia, deaf individuals with minimal residual hearing, and those individuals who, for whatever reason, attempt to **feign** or exaggerate a hearing loss.

When clients cannot fully cooperate with the hearing professional, the success of the examination will largely depend on the ability of the professional to establish a relationship with the patient, assess the unique challenges that the patient brings to the conventional testing process, and adapt the more rigorous science of audiologic testing to achieve a meaningful diagnosis. With each of these unique groups, a variety of special techniques and modifications to standard protocols needs to be utilized in the evaluative process. This chapter addresses this special assessment and includes those tests requiring special audiological equipment as well as simple techniques that can be performed in a remote setting using a portable audiometer.

EVALUATING ADULTS WITH SPECIAL NEEDS

Assessing the Cognitively Disabled

Conventional audiometry incorporates the process of soliciting a behavioral response in order to obtain accurate hearing measures. If a patient's cognitive ability is compromised, that person's ability to fully cooperate with the audiologist is likewise compromised and the potential accuracy of standard testing methods with any cognitively impaired patient is questionable. In the latter part of the twentieth century, two trends have emerged that have had a dramatic impact on this need for special testing techniques to assess clients who are cognitively disabled. First, there has been a migration of individuals with cognitive or developmental disabilities, from segregated institutional settings into more mainstream community and family-related settings (Ray, 2002). This transition has been brought on by the passing of numerous public laws for the benefit of disabled individuals such as the Individuals with Disabilities Education Act (IDEA) and the Americans with Disabilities Act (ADA) as discussed in Chapter 1. Today, a majority of individuals classified with cognitive or developmental disabilities live either on their own or with their families rather than in a public care system (Amado, Lakin, & Menke, 1990). This societal integration has resulted in a greater demand on the audiology professional to develop successful strategies in the hearing assessment of this challenging patient population.

A second factor involves the demographic shift in the aging of North Americans. The recent U.S. census has indicated that individuals over the age of 65 are the fastest growing segment of the U.S. population. It is estimated that by the year 2020, these senior citizens will represent almost 17% of the total population (Weinstein, 2002). As indicated in Chapter 1, this is also the most common age group to develop hearing impairment; this will create an obvious increase in the need for hearing assessment and rehabilitation. However, chronological age, which refers to actual age, and physiological age, which indicates how the body functions, do not necessarily coincide. The impact of physiological age makes the elderly population indeed one of the most heterogeneous groups of individuals, which requires a significant amount of creative adaptability when approaching hearing assessment. Although the vast majority of elderly patients can be evaluated using conventional test procedures, there is an unfortunate and growing number of this group that begin to experience a progressive deterioration in cognitive function. This type of disorder affecting the central nervous system is called **dementia**. The most well known form of dementia is **Alzheimer's disease**, which has devastating effects on an individual's memory and ability to communicate.

When evaluating a patient who is cognitively or developmentally disabled, or an elderly victim of dementia, the normal testing protocols need to be modified by the audiologist to accommodate the unique presentation of each patient. In our growing elderly population, for example, there is a high likelihood that hearing loss exists, accompanied by increased difficulty processing speech. Special consideration must then be made to ensure that the professional and the patient are able to adequately communicate while gathering information to build a case history, give and receive instructions during testing procedures, explain the results, and provide patient counseling. A simple solution to effectively dealing with the hearing impairment is for the examiner to enunciate more clearly and at a slower rate of speech, or communicate with the patient through earphones so that the amplitude of the examiner's voice can be increased to an effective level. Additionally, regular reinstruction using different wording may be used to facilitate the patient's ability to understand the task.

Another challenge exhibited by clients with reduced cognitive function is the inability to focus on any task for extended periods of time. This lack of attention to a diagnostic examination may necessitate a critical streamlining of procedures in order to obtain key information in a time frame far more limiting than in routine testing. Other factors affecting a disabled patient's ability to respond cooperatively may include visual impairment, which will limit the ability to respond to an examiner's visual reinforcers or speech testing performed by the use of pictures. Also, patients with restricted motor function (such as clients confined to a wheelchair or those having limited mobility in their hands and arms) may require modification of traditional response methods.

While inattention, visual impairment, and limitations in motor function pose significant challenges to testing for hearing impairment, a greater challenge can be the patient's unwillingness to participate in the test process at all. Cognitively impaired clients may not understand what is taking place and may either passively ignore the examiner entirely, or conversely, become physically or verbally abusive to the audiology professional or family members assisting in the procedures. Because of this broad range of challenges common to the cognitively impaired, the examiner is faced with no small difficulty in achieving a meaningful compromise between optimal testing procedures and the often considerable limitations of each client. The art of adapting testing methodology to the needs of the cognitively disabled requires patience, creativity, resourcefulness, and a commitment to achieve a meaningful diagnostic outcome on the part of the examiner. The purposeful adaptation of testing to meet the needs of the cognitively impaired generally falls into three broad categories: variations in the testing stimuli, the test environment, and the assessment of patient response.

Variations in Testing Stimuli

Pure tones are the common stimuli used in standardized testing, but these often hold no intrinsic interest for individuals with reduced cognitive function. Stimulus changes, such as using warble tone stimuli or pulse tones, may present a sufficient variation to produce a reliable response from the patient. Other signals presented through the audiometer such as narrow band noise may also facilitate a reasonably reliable response. A common test signal used for this group, although not highly calibrated, is signal noisemakers, mentioned in the previous chapter. A simple toy such as a rattle, a bell, a squeak toy, or a drum may be a sufficient change in the auditory stimuli to elicit an appropriate response. Caution should be exercised, however, in interpreting these results, recognizing the gross nature of the testing procedure. This type of testing essentially confirms hearing ability at higher-intensity levels and will allow the examiner to rule out a severe to profound hearing loss. But any further interpretation of these results is not reliable due to the inaccuracy of the stimulus used. Speech stimuli can be a valuable source of obtaining a more accurate indication of hearing sensitivity and is at a higher interest level for many patients with cognitive disabilities. Rather than using a standard word list, simple commands such as requesting that the patient sit down, stand up, or turn their head to your voice may provide some reliable information. Often a simple conversation about daily activities, such as what patients ate for breakfast or if they'd like to go have lunch may be simple enough for them to understand and, in turn, provide a reliable response to speech stimuli.

Variations in Test Environment and Procedures

Some disabled patients may feel uncomfortable entering an enclosed sound booth and have an adverse reaction to this type of environment. This situation necessitates using a basic exam room with a portable audiometer and normal conversational speech or noisemakers to perform behavioral testing. In addition to changing the environment, the sequence of the normal testing process may need to be significantly altered. For example, testing may begin by obtaining a response to speech initially because of its higher interest level followed by attempts to acquire a response to other stimuli such as pure tones. The presentation of pure tones may involve a simple minimal response level in the low-frequency range such as 500 Hz, quickly followed by a 2000- or 3,000-Hz stimulus to obtain some measure of hearing ability in both the low and high frequencies. Ear-specific data is preferred with the use of supra-aural earphones or insert phones but may be rejected by the patient, requiring speakers to obtain data from the better ear. Constant communication with the patient with regular reinforcement is also a necessity to maintain attention to the procedures.

Variations in Patient Response

The use of hand raising or a response switch may be beyond the capabilities of many disabled patients. Specific head turns to certain stimuli or imitative behavior may be the only measurable response from the patient. Often, when developmentally disabled individuals hear pure tones, they will attempt to imitate that pure tone, which provides a very reliable response to the stimulus. Another type of observed response may be the actual discontinuation of activity. If a patient is particularly active exhibiting repetitive behaviors and movements, the sudden cessation of the activity or change in behavior is often a way to observe attention to the new stimulus.

By applying some of these simple techniques and modifications to the standard protocol of a hearing assessment and by observing unique response behaviors, fairly reliable information regarding hearing sensitivity can be obtained from patients with cognitive or developmental disabilities.

Measuring Hearing in the Deaf Population

An adult or teenager who has been diagnosed with deafness generally has measured hearing thresholds in the profound hearing loss range greater than 90 dBHL. Despite the minimal hearing ability that remains, deaf individuals routinely have their hearing evaluated for several reasons. First and foremost is the need to monitor the stability of the remaining residual hearing. In addition, hearing measures are often obtained to determine cochlear implant candidacy as well as verifying hearing aid benefit. The process by which a deaf individual is evaluated follows the same pattern and protocol that is used for conventional audiometry, but with some variations. With many patients, the only measurable hearing thresholds are in the low-frequency range (corner audiogram), and so a threshold at 125 Hz is often added to the test protocol to determine the extent of low-frequency residual hearing.

Another important aspect of evaluating patients diagnosed with deafness is to reconfirm the reliability of the test results. Because of the severity of hearing loss and the minimal amount of hearing that remains, the quality of the signal may not be as distinct and clear for these patients as compared to a hearing-impaired patient with a greater amount of residual hearing. In addition, the numerous hearing tests they have had throughout their life, increases the familiarity with the testing protocol and so they tend to anticipate the presentation of the test stimulus. It is important, therefore, to verify each threshold due to the potential of having an increased number of false positive responses.

Deafness typically causes a severe limitation in speech recognition ability. A speech awareness or detection threshold measure may need to take the place of speech recognition threshold testing to obtain a viable measure of response to speech. Instead of a word recognition test, a speechreading test or word list combining auditory and visual modes can be used as part of assessment. This modified procedure is important to show the patient's ability to integrate auditory and visual information for functional communication.

When pure tone thresholds are measured in the severe to profound range, the ability to make comparisons between air conduction and bone conduction test results is compromised due to the equipment limitation in bone conduction testing, with the maximum intensity levels occurring between 60 and 80 dBHL. Although the hearing loss is predominantly sensorineural in nature, the presence or absence of an air bone gap or conductive component cannot always be verified with the pure tone audiometric results. Tympanometric results can assist in characterizing a hearing loss and some assumptions can be made with regard to whether the loss is sensorineural or mixed, but it can be difficult to make a definitive diagnosis of type in some profound hearing loss cases.

PSEUDOHYPACUSIS

On occasion, audiologists will be faced with testing individuals who are not cooperative and who willfully attempt to falsify their test results. The classic term used to describe this type of case is **pseudohypacusis**, which literally means "false hearing loss." **Functional, exaggerated,** or **nonorganic hearing loss** are other terms used to describe someone who has attempted to fabricate or exaggerate a hearing loss with no apparent organic disorder in evidence. This type of patient is particularly challenging for the audiologist—first to identify the possible presence of pseudohypacusis and then to obtain true hearing thresholds without cooperation from the patient. As indicated in Chapter 4, pseudohypacusis can fall into two categories. If an individual willfully attempts to exaggerate or falsify the hearing test results, it is often called **malingering** or feigning a hearing loss. However, if the patient is suffering from a severe emotional disorder in which the underlying cause of the problem is at a subconscious level, the disorder is often termed **psychogenic, conversion,** or **hysterical deafness.**

There are a number of factors that underlie the reasons for feigning a hearing loss. Children may use this as a mechanism to gain attention or as an excuse for poor academic performance. Adults may attempt to exaggerate or completely feign hearing loss for the purposes of obtaining some form of compensation. These results can often be seen in medical-legal cases—the determination of fault in an auto accident, or an industrial worker's compensation claim after working in a noisy environment. Some studies have suggested that the most frequent occurrence of pseudohypacusis in adults is directly related to the amount of monetary compensation that could be received (Rintelmann & Schwan, 1999). For children, pseudohypacusic cases can be as simple as two children who have decided to play a game during the annual hearing screening, or it could be a more serious case of a child apparently hungering for attention from her or his peers or family.

Signs of Potential Functional Hearing Loss

One of the first signs that a functional hearing loss might exist is the underlying reason for the evaluation—a referral for testing as part of some form of legal action or a determination of financial compensation. Although the majority of patients are honest in their responses during testing, the possibility that someone coming in for one of these reasons and might supply inaccurate information must be taken into consideration.

When a person comes to the clinic with the express purpose of exaggerating or feigning a hearing loss, they exhibit behaviors that are not typical of average patients. Instead of being alert and naturally compensating with visual cues as seen in patients with true hearing loss, these patients may overly exaggerate their inability to hear. This unnatural behavior may begin as soon as they enter the clinic and continue throughout the whole testing process. A hearing-impaired individual's difficulties are consistent, both in conversation and in response to questions and test procedures. Pseudohypacusic cases will often exaggerate their inability to hear, straining to hear the examiner's voice, raising the level of their own voice, or in some cases actually pretending that they have difficulties speaking, thinking that speech always has a direct correlation to hearing loss.

When performing the actual audiological evaluation, an obvious result of pseudohypacusis is the inconsistency in responses from test to test (Chaiklin & Ventry, 1965). It is difficult for these individuals to retain the exact same level of loudness perception to provide similar thresholds. The average person receiving a hearing test may show minor fluctuations from test to test of 5 or 10 dB. However, when changing frequencies and performing tests on pseudohypacusic cases, these thresholds can fluctuate quite drastically by as much as 20 to 30 dB. In addition to this variability, the perception of a speech signal is unlike the perception of a pure tone signal. This difference in loudness causes the speech recognition thresholds to be significantly better than the pure tone average by as much as 15 dB or more. As the speech testing is administered, the response of only half of a spondee or the substitution of rhyming words during word recognition testing may also occur.

Bone conduction thresholds that have been measured at a significantly poorer level than air conduction thresholds causing a negative air-bone gap is another indicator of pseudohypacusis. In cases of a unilateral hearing loss, a **shadow curve** appears that represents hearing thresholds measured from the normal ear. If the loss is functional, the patient may choose to wait to respond until the stimuli have reached high-intensity levels, thus negating the crossover effect and confirming the functional nature of the loss.

Simple Techniques

When audiologists or audiometrists suspect possible functional hearing loss during hearing screening and/or threshold testing conducted in the schools, a series of simple techniques can be performed to eliminate the majority of cases needing referral.

1. *Reinstruction*—Many cases of pseudohypacusis in children can be resolved simply by providing some form of reinstruction to the child. This can be done in a very nonaccusatory fashion in order to protect the examiner from falsely accusing a child with a true hearing loss or placing the child in a defensive situation. One effective reinstruction procedure is as follows: "There seems to be a problem with the test results. I am not sure that these results are correct and so I would like to try to do the test again. Please listen carefully to these instructions. Raise your hand as soon as you hear the tone even if it is very soft. Don't wait until the tone gets loud before you raise you hand." If children are feigning a hearing loss, this is a very neutral way of telling them exactly what they are already doing and that you recognize that fact. They are waiting until the tone gets loud before they respond in order to exaggerate or fabricate a hearing loss. By telling them not to do exactly what they have been doing, they may realize that you have discovered their inappropriate behavior. In this way, you will not put them on the defensive, but rather give them an "out" as if they did not understand the instructions in the beginning. In most cases, a miracle will occur and suddenly the child will have normal hearing sensitivity.

2. *Ascending-descending variations*—When an individual attempts to feign a hearing loss, they create certain loudness perception references in order to be consistent in their responses to louder signals. An examiner can disrupt this loudness perception reference by altering the traditional "down 10 dB, up 5 dB" sequence and varying the intensity level to try to focus in on the threshold. Another variation is to use 2-dB interval steps instead of 5-dB interval steps beginning at zero without any reference to louder signals. By slowly increasing the intensity and presenting a signal in 2-dB increments, the patient will eventually tire of hearing so many signals and finally respond at a lower level than their previous result.

3. *The yes or no answer test*—This third procedure is an effective way of improving hearing thresholds particularly with children who persist in continuing with the feigning behavior. The test needs to be performed rapidly before the child realizes the essence of the procedure. The child is given the following instructions, "Please say yes when you hear the tone and say no when you don't." By immediately presenting a tone at a high-intensity level that elicits a "yes" response and then lowering the stimulus level, hopefully you will receive a "no" response from the child, indicating that they actually heard the tone at that intensity level. Continue this technique until a true threshold is reached or until they realize their error in responding "no" and signifying that they did indeed hear the tone. A variation to this procedure is to have the patient "count the tones" that are presented in groups of two or three tones at one intensity level. The child will begin to make intentional errors when counting, but will still respond at low levels.

Special Clinical Tests

If the attempts to perform a hearing test using these simple techniques still result in questionable or inconsistent results, there are several special tests available to acquire more accurate thresholds. A specific description of these tests is beyond the scope of this textbook, but a brief explanation is appropriate. The reader who is interested in their background and detailed description should refer to chapters by Martin (2002) and Rintelmann and Schwan (1999). The most obvious tests employed to determine true sensitivity are electrophysiologic in nature, requiring no behavioral response from the patient. Otoacoustic emissions testing or the use of acoustic reflexes to predict hearing sensitivity are two simple procedures that can be done fairly quickly to rule out nonorganic hearing loss. If necessary, a more exhaustive measure using auditory brain stem response procedures can verify true thresholds. In addition, some behavioral tests still being used are worth mentioning.

One of the first and most effective tests to identify malingering in cases of a supposed unilateral hearing loss is the **Stenger test** (Stenger, 1907). This is based on the Stenger principle that indicates when a tone is introduced simultaneously into both ears but at different intensity levels, only the louder tone will be perceived. If the louder tone is presented at a level just below the admitted hearing threshold of the so-called "poorer" ear, the malingering patient will not respond, thinking that the tone is the only one being presented. If it were a true hearing loss in that ear, the patient would still respond to the softer tone heard in the normal or better ear. The results of this test can easily detect pseudohypacusis behavior. In fact, it has been recommended by some that it should be performed as a standard test on anyone with a unilateral hearing loss, because of its ease of administration. Recently, the **varying intensity story test (VIST)** was developed by Martin, Chaplin, and Marchbanks (1998). The patient listens to a story in one ear. The intensity level of the story varies rapidly and is difficult for patients to remember which parts of the story are above their supposed threshold level and which are below that level. The patient is then asked several questions about the story and a threshold can be estimated based on their correct answers to questions about sections of the story that were presented below their admitted threshold.

Some older tests were developed to identify cases of malingering and have some historical significance but are not commonly used today. The **Doerfler-Stewart test** (Doerfler & Stewart, 1946) and the **sensorineural acuity level (SAL) test** (Jerger & Tillman, 1960; Rintelmann & Harford, 1963) cause a patient to lose their loudness reference by introducing noise during the testing. The **Lombard test** utilizes the natural phenomenon of raising our vocal intensity when talking in the presence of loud background noise. When noise is presented to an ear with a hearing loss, no change in vocal level should occur unless the hearing sensitivity is much better than what is admitted. **Delayed auditory feedback (DAF)** applies the auditory-vocal feedback loop in a slightly different manner. People rely on simultaneous feedback of their own voice to maintain good continuity in speech. If the vocal feedback is mechanically delayed, significant dysfluency occurs. The application as a test of pseudohypacusis is realized when the intensity of the vocal feedback is presented below the presumed hearing thresholds. If the hearing thresholds are accurate, no dysfluency will be present. But if the admitted thresholds are not a true level of hearing sensitivity, the delayed feedback will cause the patient to slow their speech rate or elicit stuttering or other errors in fluency.

A first impression of the behavioral tests just described might be that they are highly effective and valid techniques in confirming the presence of a false or exaggerated hearing loss. Although the results may provide some qualitative information and verify that the patient is uncooperative or malingering, an estimate of the true hearing thresholds is not always obtained. This reason combined with the advent of new electrophysiologic techniques has caused these tests to have limited use today.

SUMMARY

A Glimpse into the Profession Revisited

The case study introduced at the beginning of the chapter portrayed a fifth-grade girl named Sally. Recall that the school screening and initial threshold testing suggested a significant moderate to severe hearing loss. But her responsiveness in normal conversation was not consistent with the loss. A complete hearing evaluation resulted in several inconsistent results. As one might have guessed, Sally is exhibiting behavioral findings that suggest malingering. The first signs were the variation in thresholds from test to test. In particular, the speech reception thresholds measured at levels substantially lower than the pure tone results is a strong indicator of an exaggerated or feigned hearing loss. A word recognition score of 84% at the same intensity level as the supposed hearing thresholds also suggests that the pure tone findings are questionable. Because simple reinstruction was ineffective, changes in ascending and descending tone presentation and the administration of the Modified Stenger test elicited threshold levels near the normal range of hearing (see Figure 9.1). Otoacoustic emission testing confirmed this suspicion with normal findings at all frequencies in both ears. Further investigation into Sally's motivation behind this malingering behavior revealed a popular fellow classmate who received considerable attention because of her severe hearing impairment. Upon parental consent, Sally was referred for a psychological evaluation.

Figure 9.1 Case study results for Sally depicting normal hearing in the left ear and a moderate hearing loss in the right ear for the first test. The speech recognition threshold was significantly better (35 dBHL) than the pure tone average (53 dBHL) for the right ear. Following reinstruction and the use of special test techniques, pure tone thresholds and speech recognition threshold were measured within normal limits.

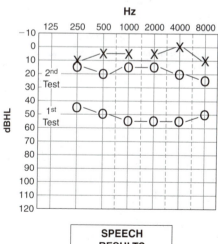

	SPEECH RESULTS	
	R	L
SRT	35	5
2nd SRT	15	
WRS	84%	100%
LVL	55	45

CHAPTER REVIEW

- There are certain patients who require an alteration in the routine audiological test battery in order to obtain more accurate information regarding their hearing ability.

- In particular, developmentally disabled adults and elderly patients can be effectively tested when applying procedures that are consistent with their capabilities. These procedures come in the form of basic observation or the addition of special reinforcers to facilitate responses.

- Profoundly hearing-impaired individuals often require variations in test procedures as well. Because of their limited capacity to process speech and the frequent difficulty in discerning the presence of a stimulus,

care must be taken to verify the accuracy of the test results.

- Another special population that requires unique techniques to obtain accurate results are those uncooperative individuals with apparent pseudohypacusis or nonorganic hearing loss. Patients exhibiting these types of problems feign or exaggerate a hearing loss for many reasons such as the need for attention or for financial gain. There are several simple techniques that can be applied to improve the test results or completely eliminate the apparent functional hearing loss. In addition, a variety of special clinical tests can be implemented for those difficult to test patients.

ACTIVITIES FOR DISCUSSION

1. In the Case Study, is it possible for someone like Sally to convince an audiologist or other professional that a hearing loss does exist?

2. There is some disagreement between professionals, insurance companies, and administrators in skilled nursing facilities as to the amount of audiological services that

is warranted for elderly patients with limited cognitive ability. Why?

3. How far along the sequence of services—identification, evaluation, diagnosis, and treatment—could someone feigning a hearing loss proceed before the true hearing ability is discovered?

REFERENCES

Amado, A. N., Lakin, K. C., & Menke, J. M. (1990). Chartbook on services for people with developmental disabilities. Minneapolis, University of Minnesota, Center for Residential and Community Services.

Chaiklin, J. B., & Ventry, I. M. (1965). Patient errors during spondee and pure tone threshold measurement. *Journal of Auditory Research, 5,* 219–230.

Doerfler, L. G., & Stewart, K. (1946). Malingering and psychogenic deafness. *Journal of Speech Disorders, 11,* 181–186.

Jerger, J., & Tillman, T. A. (1960). A new method for the clinical determination of sensorineural acuity level (SAL). *Archives of Otolaryngology, 71,* 948–955.

Martin, F. N. (2002). Pseudohypacusis. In J. Katz (Ed.), *Handbook of clinical audiology* (5th ed.), Baltimore: Lippincott, Williams & Wilkins.

Martin, F. N., Champlain, C. A., & Marchbanks, T. P. (1998). A varying intensity story test for simulated hearing loss. *American Journal of Audiology, 7,* 39–44.

Ray, Carri (2002). Mental retardation and/or developmental disabilities. In J. Katz (Ed.), *Handbook of clinical audiology* (5th ed.), Baltimore: Lippincott, Williams & Wilkins.

Rintelmann, W. F., & Harford, E. (1963). The detection and assessment of pseudohypacusis among school-age children. *Journal of Speech and Hearing Disorders, 28,* 141–152.

Rintelmann, W. F., & Schwan, S. A. (1999). Pseudohypacusis. In F. E. Musiek & W. F. Rintelmann (Eds.), *Contemporary perspectives in hearing assessment.* Boston: Allyn & Bacon.

Stenger, P. (1907). Simulation and dissimulation of ear diseases and their identification. *Deutsche Medizinsche Wochenschrift, 33,* 970–973.

Weinstein, B. E. (2002). Hearing loss in the elderly: A new look at an old problem. In J. Katz (Ed.), *Handbook of clinical audiology* (5th ed.). Baltimore: Lippincott, Williams & Wilkins.

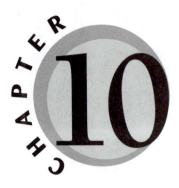
Hearing Rehabilitation: Helping Individuals with Hearing Loss

Nancy E. McCoy

Key Terms

CASE STUDY

A Glimpse into the Profession

Mr. Barnes is a 75-year-old man who comes to the office at the urging of his wife, who complains that she must repeat herself frequently, that she misses out on many family functions because he cannot hear what's going on, and that he turns the TV up louder than is comfortable for her. Mr. Barnes reports that he feels his hearing is not too bad and that he would be fine if she would just stop mumbling to him. He does admit that he sometimes misunderstands his grandchildren with their little voices, and that he turns the TV louder than his wife does. Mrs. Barnes further reports that they have regularly been traveling in their RV since retirement, but that conversations in the cab of their vehicle are often strained because Mr. Barnes cannot hear over the engine and road noise. She adds that they frequently enjoy taking tours of resort areas or wilderness trails, but that she worries he is only understanding a fraction of the interesting lectures. Testing reveals that Mr. Barnes has a bilateral sensorineural hearing loss, which is mild in the low frequencies and severe in the high frequencies. He has been medically cleared for amplification by his otolaryngologist.

REHABILITATION STRATEGIES

The purpose of this chapter is to acquaint the reader with the various types of rehabilitation strategies that may be used to help individuals with hearing loss, as well as their families and significant others. Once a hearing loss has been identified, where medical or surgical solutions are not possible or not desired, the question then arises, "What next?" This chapter discusses the issues that come to play in answering that question. It is not intended as a comprehensive review of all areas of aural rehabilitation. For that, the reader is referred to excellent texts such as those listed in Appendix A. Rather, this chapter provides an overview or survey of the most pertinent issues involved in aural rehabilitation. Audiology and speech pathology students will go on to study this field in greater depth.

SCOPE AND DEFINITIONS

Aural Habilitation versus Rehabilitation

Hearing rehabilitation, also called *aural rehabilitation* or *auditory rehabilitation,* involves the various processes, techniques, and devices used to help an individual with a hearing loss regain skills and abilities that were present before the onset of the loss. In other words, these are methods to help that individual overcome the handicap as much as possible and improve communication function at home, at work, and in social situations. For a child who is born with hearing loss, or who loses hearing prior to developing verbal communication, the term *aural habilitation* is more appropriate. The child is not relearning skills that he once had. Instead, he must be taught many of the skills that come naturally without instruction to the child with normal hearing. Because of this, the challenges in aural habilitation are often greater than in aural rehabilitation, although many of the same strategies and devices can be utilized.

Scope of Practice

Before the development of electric hearing aids, aural rehabilitation consisted primarily of two approaches: (1) maximizing the use of residual hearing through auditory training and (2) maximizing the use of visual cues in communication through speechreading or lipreading training. However, since the 1950s, when electric hearing aids were developed that could be worn on the body, amplification devices have taken a primary role in the rehabilitative process. For many patients, appropriately fit hearing aids—along with orientation counseling and follow-up care—address most of the communication problems, so that no further rehabilitation is required. For a smaller group of patients, appropriately fit hearing aids do not solve enough of the communication problems, and other types of services must be employed to complete the rehabilitation process. These include auditory training, speechreading training, compensatory strategies to improve communication, other kinds of assistive listening devices, and various kinds of counseling. Rehabilitation can be provided in individual or group sessions, as well as by computer or distance programs through the Internet.

Professionals

Hearing habilitation or rehabilitation services are provided by a number of professionals, including audiologists, hearing aid dispensers, speech-language pathologists, teachers, psychologists, and rehabilitation counselors. Anyone involved in helping the hearing-impaired individual or family cope with a hearing handicap and overcome or minimize its effects on communication, education, and employment can be considered a hearing rehabilitation service provider. Likewise, any activity, strategy, or device that aids in this process can be considered a rehabilitative tool.

THE USE OF HEARING AIDS

The single best rehabilitative tool is the hearing aid. Therefore, when an individual has a handicapping hearing loss, the rehabilitative process usually begins here. What follows is a brief overview of the many issues involved in the selection and fitting of hearing aids.

Medical Referral

Prior to the fitting of hearing aids, each patient should be examined by a physician, preferably an otolaryngologist, who will determine that no medical condition exists that would preclude such a fitting. Hearing aid dispensers and dispensing audiologists are required by federal law to advise their patients of the need for a medical evaluation prior to purchasing hearing aids (FDA, 1977). In some states, a medical referral is required when certain conditions exist. An example of some of these conditions is as follows:

- Visible congenital or traumatic deformity of the ear
- History of, or active drainage from the ear within the previous 90 days
- History of sudden or rapidly progressive hearing loss within the previous 90 days
- Acute or chronic dizziness
- Unilateral hearing loss of sudden onset within the previous 90 days
- Significant air-bone gap (determined by pure tone air conduction and bone conduction audiometry (HADEC, 1996)

Adults who do not wish to see a physician prior to purchasing hearing aids may sign a waiver, which releases the dispenser of any liability regarding medical referral. However, for children 16 years of age or younger, a waiver may not be accepted and the otolaryngologist must be seen prior to the hearing aid fitting (FDA, 1977). In addition, in many states an audiologist must provide the audiological testing and hearing aid recommendation for children 16 years or younger, although a hearing aid dispenser may fit the hearing aids. Hereafter in this chapter, the term "dispenser" will be used to refer either to a hearing aid dispenser or dispensing audiologist.

Candidacy

Anyone with a handicapping hearing loss that cannot be corrected with medicine or surgery, or who chooses not to have surgery, may be considered a candidate for hearing aids. That includes infants, children, adults, senior citizens, or individuals with various other handicapping conditions. That is not to say that everyone meeting this criterion will achieve similar success with hearing aids. Most patients with hearing loss in both ears are candidates for binaural amplification (in both ears), although certain aspects of the ear, the audiogram or the patient's abilities and lifestyle may preclude the fitting of two hearing aids. In addition, not everyone who is a candidate for amplification will be motivated to seek help with hearing aids. A dispenser may determine from the audiogram that a patient has a handicapping hearing loss and should benefit from amplification. However, the patient may either be unaware of the problem, in denial of the problem, or not feel that the problem is sufficient to warrant the use of hearing aids.

Hearing Aid Design and Components
Components

There are three main components to a hearing aid: the microphone, the amplifier, and the receiver. The **microphone** is a transducer, which picks up acoustical energy and converts it to electrical energy. The **amplifier** takes the electrical signal and boosts the intensity and shapes the frequency response. The **receiver** is another transducer, which

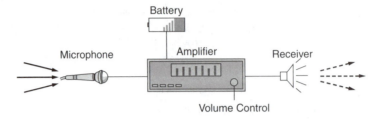

Figure 10.1 Basic components of a hearing aid

acts as a speaker and converts the amplified electrical signal back to acoustical energy for delivery to the ear. All hearing aids will have a **battery** that supplies power to perform these functions. Many hearing aids also have a **volume control** that the user can operate, to adjust the intensity or loudness of the aid for varying speakers or acoustic environments. For some hearing aids, volume is adjusted with the use of a remote control. For others, volume is adjusted automatically by the amplifier, based on the intensity of varying input signals, so that a user-adjusted volume control is not necessary. Figure 10.1 shows a schematic drawing of these basic components.

Some hearing aids come equipped with a **telecoil**, or T-switch, which shuts off the microphone, picks up electromagnetic energy, and converts it to an electrical signal to be amplified and converted to acoustic energy. This hearing aid feature allows the patient to use the telephone without experiencing acoustic feedback from a live microphone, which is heard as a high-pitched whistling. Other uses will be discussed later in this chapter.

Styles

There are four major and two minor styles of air conduction hearing aids in use today. The major styles are shown in Figure 10.2. In the **behind-the-ear** (**BTE**) style, the components of the aid are housed in a small case that fits over and behind the ear, and the amplified sound travels through tubing and a custom-fit earmold placed inside the ear.

Figure 10.2 Examples of the four major types of air conduction hearing aids
Source: Courtesy of Widex, Inc.

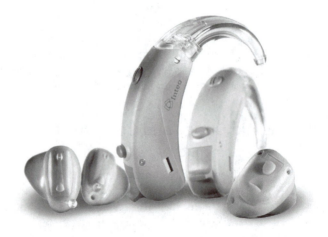

BTE AND EYEGLASS TUBE TYPE

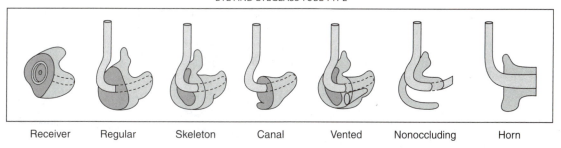

| Receiver | Regular | Skeleton | Canal | Vented | Nonoccluding | Horn |

Figure 10.3 Basic types of earmolds
Source: Courtesy of Westone Labs

This style accounted for 43% of all hearing aids sold in the United States during the first three quarters of 2006 (Kirkwood, 2006). However, most hearing aids sold (57% in the same period) are fit entirely in the ear, with nothing behind the ear. The standard **in-the-ear (ITE)** instrument fills the entire bowl or concha of the ear and can be readily seen. The **in-the-canal** instrument protrudes from the canal of the ear, but does not enter the upper portion of the concha or the helix of the ear. The **completely-in-the-canal** instrument fits deep in the canal and virtually disappears in most ears.

The remaining 3% is comprised of (1) eyeglass instruments, where the components are housed in the temple piece of the eyeglass and the receiver connects to an earmold; (2) body-style instruments, where the components are housed in a case the size of a cigarette pack, and a cord leads from the case on the body to a button receiver placed in the ear; or (3) various kinds of specialty aids. Figure 10.3 illustrates a variety of earmolds used in behind-the-ear, eyeglass, and body-style hearing aids.

Specialty Aids

1. A **bone conduction** instrument is considered when none of the air conduction instruments discussed above is feasible, usually because of a congenitally absent or incomplete ear canal (microtia) or a chronically draining ear. A bone vibrator is placed on the mastoid area and held in place by a tension band, much like the vibrator used in bone conduction audiometry, and a body-style or behind-the-ear instrument is used to amplify sound and drive the vibrator. For this type of instrument to work, the patient must have normal or near-normal cochlear sensitivity, as determined by bone conduction testing.

2. **CROS** and **BICROS** instruments are used for unilateral hearing losses where the poor ear cannot be aided directly (CROS), or for bilateral and asymmetrical losses where only the better ear is an appropriate candidate for direct amplification (BICROS). In these cases the poor ear cannot be aided directly because there is no measurable hearing to stimulate, because speech discrimination is so poor that amplified sound would be distorted and unusable, or because the patient cannot tolerate amplified sound in that ear. In the CROS fitting, a microphone is placed on the bad ear, and the

signal is routed—by a wire or a wireless FM radio signal—to an amplifier and receiver placed in the good ear. The good ear receives the sound, but the patient can hear from the bad side, which is helpful in group situations or noisy environments. In the BICROS fitting, the good ear has some impairment and is a candidate for amplification. A second microphone is placed on that ear and the patient receives amplified sound from both sides, but only in the better ear.

3. All the instruments discussed so far can be removed by the patient for sleeping and bathing, but there are other types of **implantable aids**, which are surgically implanted and are not removed by the patient.

    a. In the bone conduction implant, the vibratory portion of the instrument is implanted in the mastoid bone, and the microphone, amplifier, and driver are housed in a small case that snaps onto the protruding implant post. This eliminates the need for a headband, which is cumbersome and can easily slip out of position. Like the standard bone conduction aid, this device is used only for patients with outer and/or middle ear pathology, who have relatively good cochlear hearing. A picture of this device can be seen in Figure 10.4.

    b. The middle ear implant is a device recently developed for patients with sensorineural hearing loss and normal middle ear function, who have had problems with traditional air conduction hearing aids. These problems range from persistent acoustic feedback, even with a properly fitted earmold, to chronic outer ear infection, to inability to relieve the occlusion effect (hearing one's own voice as if one is in a barrel) when the instrument or earmold is placed in the ear.

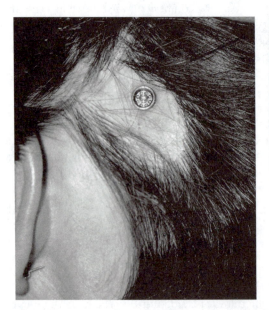 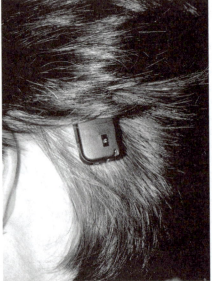

Figure 10.4 Bone-anchored hearing aid (BAHA). Left view shows the external mount and right view shows the electronic portion of the BAHA system attached.

Source: Courtesy of Cochlear

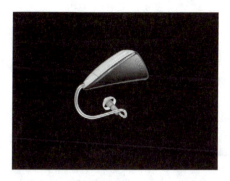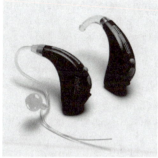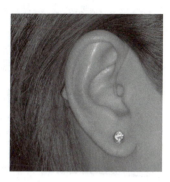

Figure 10.5 Example of mini-BTE open-fit hearing aids (not illustrated to scale)
Source: (a) Courtesy of Oticon, Inc. (b) Courtesy of Unitron Hearing Inc. (c) Courtesy of Widex, Inc.

This fitting contains an external portion—usually consisting of a microphone, amplifier, and transmitter—and an internal portion, which is implanted in the middle ear and affixed to one of the ossicles. The external portion sends a signal to the implant, which vibrates the ossicles and sends the amplified signal to the cochlea, thus bypassing the air conduction system of the outer ear.

c. The **cochlear implant** is a device for patients who have hearing loss so profound (and sometimes severe) that they can derive little benefit from conventional air conduction hearing aids. This device will be discussed in greater detail later in the chapter.

4. In these days of instant gratification and disposable commodities, we now have hearing aids that can be fitted on the spot, because a custom-fit earmold or in-the-ear shell is not used. These modular or one-size-fits-all instruments work for some patients, and have the advantage of providing instant benefit, without having to wait the standard 1–3 weeks for a custom product to be built.

There has been a recent surge of mini-BTE products that utilize various sizes of preshaped thin tubing and fitting domes to couple to the aid and channel sound to the ear. These are primarily used in high-frequency hearing losses where a standard earmold coupling is likely to cause occlusion and an unpleasant sound of the patient's own voice. If the product is successful but the preshaped dome is unacceptable, it can be exchanged for a custom earmold. These products fit in the behind-the-ear category of instruments discussed above. Some examples are illustrated in Figure 10.5.

Technology

After the invention of the transistor in 1948, hearing aids were developed that could be worn on the body, which revolutionized the way that hard-of-hearing people functioned. No longer tethered to bulky tabletop amplifiers, they were free to move out into more workplace opportunities and social situations. Since those early days, the technological advances that have revolutionized every aspect of modern life have gradually been applied to hearing aids, creating more improvements in the lives of patients, and vast changes in the way that hearing aids are manufactured and dispensed. A brief description of the current hearing aid technologies follows. Any of these technologies can be placed in each of the styles of instruments discussed above in "Styles."

Standard Analog

In the year 2006 (January–September), approximately 11% of the almost 1.8 million hearing instruments dispensed in the United States were of analog technology, (Kirkwood, 2006) which is considered standard or basic. The dispenser or manufacturer chooses one of several different amplifiers that best matches the frequency and intensity characteristics of the patient's audiogram. The dispenser can then fine-tune the amplifier to the patient's needs with the use of one or more screw-set potentiometers, much like dimmer switches for lights. The patient has a volume control to regulate the loudness. If the patient's hearing changes such that the chosen amplifier no longer meets his or her needs, the aid must be sent to the factory for a different circuit, or a new aid must be purchased. Analog instruments can include various output-limiting circuits that control the intensity of the loudest signals, so that they do not violate the patient's loudness discomfort level.

Digitally Programmable Analog

Silicon chip technology was applied to hearing instruments in the late 1980s, so that now the frequency and intensity characteristics of the analog instrument are **digitally programmable** by a personal computer or a dedicated programmer supplied by the manufacturer. Cables connect the instrument to the programmer or computer, and the dispenser selects the best program for the user, with the help of the manufacturer's software and fitting strategies. Once the program is burned into the internal chip, the cables are disconnected and the instrument operates as the program dictates. The signal is still analog, but the instructions it uses to amplify have been digitally programmed. This type of technology accounted for approximately 30% of all hearing aids sold in 2000, but by 2005 it was replaced almost entirely by full digital signal processing (Kirkwood, 2005) and by 2006 it had been phased out entirely but the features and benefits of this circuitry type are still used in most hearing aids today. (Kirkwood, 2006). The advantages over standard analog technology are as follows:

1. The computer software and silicon chip allow more precise fit to the contour of the hearing loss, which means that sound will be more accurately reproduced for each patient.

2. Because each amplifier has a wider range of intensity, if the patient's hearing changes, the instrument can be reprogrammed to the new hearing levels at the dispenser's office, so it does not need to be upgraded at the factory or replaced.

3. Many of these instruments divide the frequency range into two or more **independent bands or channels,** so that sound processing can be better tailored to specific frequency regions on the audiogram. This is useful in steeply sloping high-frequency losses, for example, where the patient may have very different levels of comfort and discomfort in the low frequencies versus high frequencies.

4. Many of these instruments also have **multiple memory** chips, meaning they have the capability to store more than one program in memory. This means that different programs can be tuned for best hearing in different listening environments. For example, program 1 can be set for quiet, program 2 for noisy situations, and program 3 for music and TV. It's like having two, three, or more hearing aids in one, and the patient can access these programs with a switch, button, or remote control.

Digital Signal Processing

The latest level of technology, which as of 2006 has taken over 90% of the market share, employs not only digital programming, but full **digital signal processing (DSP)** (Kirkwood, 2006). In these instruments, the analog signal is digitized, or converted to binary computer code, in a step between the microphone and amplifier. The amplified signal is then changed back to acoustic energy by a digital-to-analog converter or the receiver. All the advantages of digitally programmable aids discussed above are present in DSP instruments, as well as several additional benefits:

1. *Digitizing the signal* allows for much greater flexibility in the amplification process. Certain sounds can be eliminated, such as microphone hiss and circuit noise, while other sounds can be enhanced, such as the consonant sounds of speech, which are so critical for understanding. The number of channels can be increased, to allow for independent processing of smaller bands of frequency and a more precise fit to each audiogram. The result is a cleaner, more "transparent" signal presented to the patient, and the processor has greater flexibility for fine-tuning various signals to the individual's perception of sound.

2. Many of the DSP instruments *automatically adjust the gain* or degree of amplification, depending on the intensity of the input signal. The goal is to amplify soft sounds so that they are audible, amplify average sounds so they are comfortable, and manage loud sounds so they are loud but not uncomfortable. Therefore, the user does not need to adjust a volume control manually to increase soft sounds or reduce loud sounds, and many of these instruments eliminate the user-adjust volume control altogether.

3. DSP instruments can employ special **noise reduction** circuits, which attempt to separate speech signals from background noise, so that they may be processed differently. Although these circuits do not eliminate all noise, many users report that they can tolerate noisy environments much better, which results in less fatigue and greater enjoyment in more situations.

4. Many of the DSP instruments include **directional microphone** systems, which change from omnidirectional (picking up signals from all directions) to directional (picking up signals from the front and reducing signals from the sides or behind). The patient uses a button or remote control to access these different microphone modes. Some instruments have adaptive directionality circuits, which continually search for the direction of background noise and automatically reduce amplification from those directions, even as the patient or the noise moves around in the environment.

5. Some DSP instruments have elegant **feedback reduction** circuits, which detect acoustic feedback and quickly move to reduce or eliminate it, without affecting the amplification of important speech cues in the frequency range near the feedback. This allows the patient to use the telephone without fumbling for switches, or to receive a hug from a loved one without the embarrassment of a whistling hearing aid.

The beauty of digital signal processing is that as the hearing aid performs ever more sophisticated operations, the user has less worry about operating several controls. However, those users who prefer to have volume controls, switches, or remote controls still have those features as options.

Selection, Fitting, Verification, and Follow-up Care

While hearing aids have become easier for the patient to use, with each new development in technology, the process of dispensing hearing aids to the patient has become more complex. The number of viable options for devices and features has grown dramatically, such that the process of choosing the best system for each patient is often a challenge for the dispenser. However, this process can be broken down into several discrete steps or phases.

Selection

The dispenser asks a number of questions when choosing the proper amplification for each patient. Information to answer these questions comes from the audiogram and the physical ear, as well as the patient's age, abilities, and lifestyle. The first of these questions is: Should the patient have one hearing aid or two? As mentioned earlier, when a patient has fairly symmetrical hearing loss in both ears, hearing aids are fit to both ears. This is critical with children, where the auditory reception of language must be optimized for communication and learning. The main advantages of binaural hearing aid fittings are as follows:

1. Sounds in the environment can be located or localized when both ears are fit and balanced.
2. Sounds can be heard from both sides, which means less volume is needed in each aid to achieve the same perception of loudness. This also translates to better hearing in group situations like classrooms.
3. With information coming from both ears, the brain has more to work with, in terms of focusing on the signal and tuning out unwanted noise (Schow & Nerbonne, 2002).

There are some circumstances when a monaural fitting is more appropriate, such as when one ear is not a candidate for amplification because of significant asymmetry between the ears or because of chronic drainage. In addition, monaural amplification is chosen for some adults because of the patient's physical or mental limitations, personal preference, or budgetary constraints.

The second question the dispenser asks is: What type or style of instrument is best? Young children are always fitted with behind-the-ear aids, for several reasons. As young ears are still growing, replacing earmolds as they become loose is easier and less expensive than remolding the shells of custom in-the-ear aids. As children play and occasionally get hurt, soft earmolds are less likely to damage ears than are the hard shells of in-the-ear aids. Information about the degree and configuration of a child's hearing loss is often sketchy until their listening and test-taking skills develop, and behind-the-ear models generally have greater flexibility to fit a variety of hearing losses. In addition, anyone with a profound hearing loss, and many with a severe hearing loss, must be fit with behind-the-ear aids, because the in-the-ear styles have insufficient power for the hearing loss.

Adults are more likely to choose one of the in-the-ear styles, if appropriate for the degree of hearing loss, based largely on cosmetic factors. There are some acoustical advantages to the ITE styles, however, which relate mostly to the benefits of microphone placement in the concha or canal, rather than above or behind the ear. In addition, children whose ears reach adult size during the preteen years may eventually switch to in-the-ear fittings, if appropriate for the hearing loss. It should be noted that the behind-the-ear model has seen a resurgence in popularity in the past few years, due largely to the cosmetic and acoustic appeal of the new open-fit mini-BTE products for high-frequency hearing loss.

The third question usually asked is: What technology is needed? The range of choices here is quite large, and the process used to narrow the range to one or two options is not exact. All dispensers have preferences for certain levels of technology, based on their experience, familiarity, and comfort with the hardware and software of the various manufacturers. Most adult patients have preferences, too, based on what they have read about hearing aid technology or heard from other hearing aid users; their own previous experience with hearing aids; or financial issues. And parents will naturally want the very best technology for their hearing-impaired children, although insurance benefits and third-party payment policies may dictate otherwise.

Digital signal processing (DSP) hearing aids are roughly twice the cost of analog hearing aids in the same style, but are they twice as good? Research is being conducted in academic, manufacturing, and clinical settings to answer this and other questions about DSP technology, but meanwhile DSP instruments have garnered over 90% of market share. All hearing aids, if fit appropriately to the frequency and intensity requirements of the hearing loss, will improve hearing in quiet environments. But theoretically, the more sophisticated programmable and DSP hearing aids, as well as directional microphones, should provide greater improvement in groups and background noise. Therefore, many dispensers focus on the lifestyle, to determine what communication demands are placed on patients as they go about their daily life. The choice of technology and features within the technology is matched to these communication needs.

The fourth question to ask is: How much amplification is needed? In order to be certain that the hearing aids will be appropriate, the dispenser needs to match hearing aid performance with the degree, type, and configuration of the hearing loss, as determined in the basic audiogram. The three main performance characteristics to select are gain, maximum output, and frequency response.

1. **Gain** is a measure of how much the hearing aid boosts intensity, and is expressed by the formula: output minus input equals gain. For example, if a 60 dBSPL (sound pressure level) signal is sent into the hearing aid microphone and the amplified signal is measured at 90 dBSPL at the receiver, the gain of the aid is 30 dB. The amount of gain selected is based on the degree of the hearing loss, although the gain is not equal to the degree of hearing loss. Experience has shown that most patients are well fitted and comfortable with an instrument whose gain is somewhere between one-third and one-half of the hearing loss. Dispensers and manufacturers use several different formulas to determine the gain needed for each hearing loss.

2. **Maximum output** is a measure of the loudest sounds that an aid will produce. An input signal of 90 dBSPL will put the instrument into saturation, meaning that additional increases in input will not result in any increase in output. This maximum output level should be compared to the patient's loudness discomfort level (LDL) and adjusted as needed, to be sure that no sounds that the hearing aid produces will violate that level.

3. **Frequency response** is a measure of the range of frequencies amplified by the aid. The output of the aid can be expressed graphically as a function of frequency, as seen in Figure 10.6. The dispenser attempts to match the frequency response to the pure tone configuration of the hearing loss, by choosing the appropriate hearing aid circuit and modifying the response of that circuit with potentiometers or computer programming.

Often, the process of hearing aid selection is one of trial and error. In fact, the patient undergoes a trial period of at least 30 days with the amplification system that is selected, and has the option of returning it for a refund or exchanging it for another choice if he is not satisfied.

Impressions

The dispenser will take impressions of the patient's ear canals so that the earmolds or hearing aid shells can be built to an exact fit by the earmold laboratory or hearing aid manufacturer. This process is much like taking a dental impression. The finished impressions are then mailed to the manufacturer, along with an order form. The advent of laser scanning technology now allows the manufacturer to more accurately reproduce the impression in the final shell, and a few dispensers have the capability of scanning the impressions in the office and then emailing the dimensions of the ear, along with the order form, to the manufacturer.

Fitting

When the instruments are received from the factory, or at the time of the fitting, the dispenser will analyze the gain, output, and frequency response characteristics of each aid in a specially designed test box, such as that seen in Figure 10.7. This is done to make sure that the hearing aid performance meets the needs of the hearing loss, and to have a record of that performance for comparison, should adjustments or

OSPL90 - Output Sound Pressure Level

Input: 90 dB SPL. Technical setting: A0

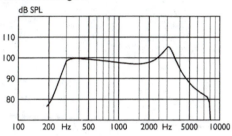

Full-on Gain

Input: 50 dB SPL. Technical setting: A0

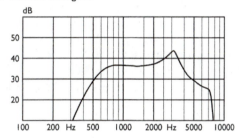

Measurements according to American
National Standard ANSI S 3.22-2003 and S3.7.
Supply voltage: 1.4 Volt
Coupling system: Sound outlet sealed at coupler reference plane

0 dB SPL ref. 20 μPa		**Delta 8000**
Peak OSPL90		105 dB SPL
HF Average OSPL90		98 dB SPL
Peak Full-on Gain		44 dB
HF Average Full-on Gain		38 dB
HF Average Reference Test Gain		21 dB
Frequency Range		370-7600 Hz
Total Harmonic Distortion	500 Hz	.5 %
Total Harmonic Distortion	800 Hz	.5 %
Total Harmonic Distortion	1600 Hz	.5 %
Battery Current		1.2 mA
Equivalent Input Noise Level		17 dB
Attack Time		20 ms
Release Time		25 ms

Figure 10.6 Typical hearing aid specifications and response curves showing gain, maximum output, and frequency response.

Figure 10.7   Example of equipment to analyze hearing aids

Source: Courtesy of Frye Electronics, Inc.

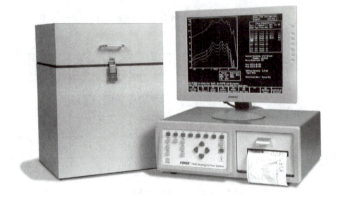

repairs be needed in the future. In addition, the dispensers will make sure that the physical fit of the instrument is good, and make shell or earmold modifications as needed. They will also orient patients or their parents or other caregivers on how to insert and remove the instruments, as well as change batteries and perform daily or periodic maintenance.

Verification

The dispensers will use one or more of several methods that can provide verification that the fitting is appropriate for the hearing loss. They can measure aided hearing for tones and speech in the sound field, and compare these results to the unaided audiogram, in order to derive aided benefit or **functional gain.** They can measure the real-ear *aided* response of the aid, using a probe microphone placed in the ear canal, and compare this to the real-ear *unaided* response, or to a target curve to show aided benefit or **real-ear gain** (or output.) A view of the real-ear testing process is shown in Figure 10.8. For adult patients, dispensers can ask patients through informal interview how well they are hearing, and if they are satisfied with the fitting. Or, they can administer any one of several hearing **handicap scales** or questionnaires, before and after the fitting, to more formally evaluate how well patients feel the hearing aids have reduced their hearing handicap (Alpiner et al., 1974; Newman et al., 1991; Schow & Nerbonne, 1982; Schow & Nerbonne, 1977; Ventry & Weinstein, 1982; and Ventry & Weinstein, 1983).

All these outcome measures give the dispenser confidence in the fitting, and they can demonstrate the aided benefit to the patient or family. In addition, insurance carriers and other third-party payers are sometimes requiring outcome measures, to justify the fitting of hearing aids that employ more sophisticated, and thus more expensive, technology.

Follow-up Care

Once the fitting is complete, the patient returns to the dispenser's office for periodic follow-up care. During these visits, the programming or potentiometers can be adjusted

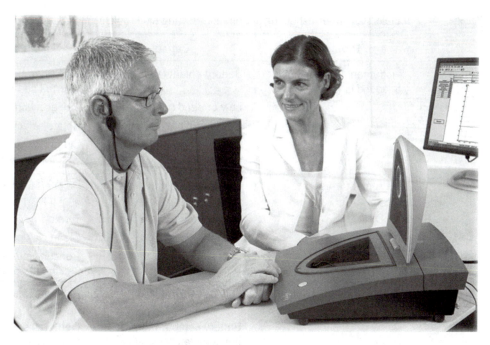

Figure 10.8   Real-ear measurement of hearing aid benefit using probe microphone
Source: Courtesy of Interacoustics

and fine-tuned, based on patients' experience using the instruments in their daily life, or based on the observations of parents, teachers, and other school professionals. As these adjustments are made, additional verification measurements can be repeated, as needed. During these visits, the dispenser also helps the patient and family members make a psychological adjustment to amplification, and reinforce the instructions on manipulation and maintenance of the instruments. The number of visits needed varies with each patient, but should be provided as needed, until both the dispenser and the patient or parents are satisfied with the fitting. Once that milestone has been reached, the patient returns for routine hearing aid checks, cleaning, and hearing reevaluation on a semiannual, annual, or as-needed basis. Young children are usually seen more frequently until a complete picture of unaided and aided hearing levels is obtained, and then yearly as long as hearing levels are stable.

Troubleshooting Hearing Aid Problems

All hearing aids will break down from time to time, such that repairs will be required, either in the dispenser's office or in the factory. Adult patients, as well as speech pathologists, teachers, school nurses, and aides who work with hearing-impaired children may encounter problems as they make regular hearing aid inspections and listening checks. Some of the more common problems they will encounter, as well as possible solutions, are shown in Table 10.1. For problems that cannot be solved with these strategies, the

Table 10.1 Troubleshooting of Common Hearing Aid Problem's

Problem	Cause	Possible Solution
Instrument has no sound or sound is weak	Battery polarity reversed	Make sure battery is inserted correctly
	Low or dead battery	Replace with fresh battery
	Instrument not turned on	Rotate volume control
	Clogged wax guard	Clean wax guard
	Volume turned down	Turn up volume control
Instrument whistles	Improper seating in ear	Reinsert the instrument until It fits securely
	Volume control too high	Turn down volume control
	Clogged wax guard	Clean wax guard
	Excessive wax in the ears	Consult your hearing health care professional
Sound is distorted or intermittent	Low battery	Replace battery
	Battery compartment is not completely closed	Gently close the battery compartment
Buzzing sound	Low battery	Replace battery
Swelling or discharge in ear		Check with your physician

Source: Adopted from Schow & Nerbonne, 2002

patient or family should be referred back to the dispenser. Schools with large programs for hearing-impaired children will usually employ or contract with an audiologist to provide these services.

COCHLEAR IMPLANTS

Although hearing aids have helped millions of people and have improved with each decade, there are many individuals with profound hearing loss who derive little to no benefit from them. However, beginning in 1972—and particularly in the last 20 years—new devices called cochlear implants have been developed that enable these people to hear and appreciate the world of sound around them (Holmes, 2002).

Instrumentation and Function

The cochlear implant consists of an external portion, which is worn on the head and body, and an internal portion, which is surgically implanted in the mastoid bone and cochlea. Therefore, this device bypasses the peripheral hearing mechanism that is damaged (outer ear, middle ear, and sensory cells of the cochlea), and stimulates the auditory nerve directly.

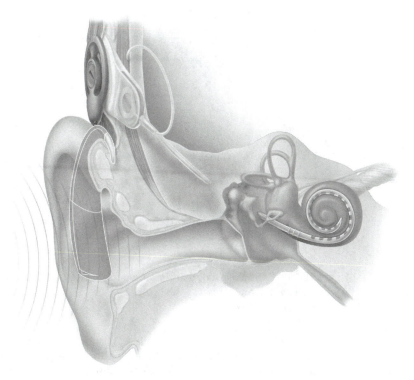

Figure 10.9 Illustration of cochlear implant, with external microphone, ear-level processor, magnetic connection to internal receiver, and electrode implanted into cochlea
Source: Courtesy of Cochlear Americas

Figure 10.9 shows the external portion as it is worn on the head, as well as the implanted internal portion. A microphone at the ear picks up sound and converts it to an electrical signal. The signal then travels through a cord to a **speech processor**, where it is encoded and processed, based on a variety of manufacturer strategies. This processor is housed in a small case worn on the body, or it may be housed with the microphone in a case that looks like a behind-the-ear hearing aid. From the speech processor, the signal travels back up to the **external transmitter coil**, which is held in place behind the ear by a magnet embedded in the implanted internal receiver. The processed signal is sent from the external transmitter through the skin to the internal receiver by FM radio waves. The internal receiver then sends the signal to the implanted **electrode**, which passes through the mastoid bone and middle ear and enters the cochlea through the round window. This electrode array is inserted in the cochlea up to a depth of 30 mm, and stimulates the auditory nerve fibers, which are sensitive to a range of different frequencies. The neural signal travels to the brain and is perceived as sound. All this occurs with almost no time delay. Figure 10.10 shows an example of the implantable electrode and an external ear-level processor.

Surgery for the implant is performed under general anesthesia, sometimes on an outpatient basis, and then the patient waits 4–6 weeks for healing to occur before the external device is connected and programmed. The patient will then undergo many

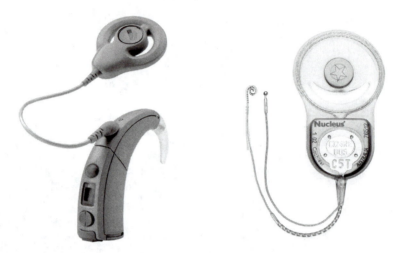

Figure 10.10   Example of external sound processor (left) and internal receiver and electrode (right) of a cochlear implant
Source: Courtesy of Cochlear

rehabilitation sessions to program and adjust the device, a process called mapping, and to train patients to make the best use of the sounds they receive. Sound from the cochlear implant is rather crude relative to that produced by modern hearing aids. In fact, adults often report that speech initially sounds like cartoon characters or a 1960s transistor radio. But with time and training, many patients begin to make more sense of what they hear, and they report a more natural sound.

Candidacy and Historical Perspectives

The first cochlear implant device was implanted in an adult in 1972, and it consisted of a single electrode implanted in the basal or high-frequency end of the cochlea. Patients could hear sounds across the frequency spectrum at fairly soft intensities, but they could not discriminate between different frequencies above about 1000 Hz. This means that they could detect the presence of environmental sounds and hear some of the rhythm and pitch features of speech, but few could understand speech through audition alone. However, many patients appreciated an improvement in their speechreading skills, as well as greater ability to monitor their own speech. Initially, the cochlear implant was approved only for late-deafened adults, but in 1980 the Food and Drug Administration (FDA) approved the single-channel device for children over the age of 2 (Wilson, 2000).

In the 1980s several multielectrode cochlear implants were developed for adults, and these were FDA-approved for children over the age of 2 in 1990. These devices have the advantage of stimulating many auditory nerve fibers along a much wider frequency range, so that the patient can distinguish one frequency from another. In addition, the speech processors have become more sophisticated, such that many patients are now demonstrating the ability to understand speech without speechreading, and some are able to communicate over the telephone. Cochlear implant users are now as young as 12–18 months and as old as patients in their eighties.

The benefits that individuals receive from the cochlear implant can vary widely, depending on many factors, including their age at the onset of deafness and the length of time between onset and implantation. Late-deafened adults who have oral communication skills and a recent memory for sound, as well as young children whose brains are very malleable, are the best candidates and generally derive the greatest benefit. Until recently, only those patients with profound hearing loss in both ears, who received little benefit from hearing aids, were considered candidates. However, some patients with severe hearing loss are beginning to be implanted, as well as adults with congenital or early-onset deafness.

All patients or families investigating the cochlear implant must undergo an extensive candidacy evaluation. They must meet the unaided hearing criteria and they must demonstrate little benefit with conventional hearing aids after a 3- to 6-month trial period. They must have no medical contraindications, such as middle ear infections or absence of auditory nerve fibers. And they must meet the psychological criteria, in terms of motivation, mental health, and appropriate expectations. These evaluations, as well as postimplant hookup and rehabilitation, are performed by a cochlear implant team, consisting of the surgeon, audiologist, speech pathologist, psychologist, teachers, the patient, and family members.

The cochlear implant is not for everyone who is deaf. Adults who were born deaf or were deafened prior to developing oral language cannot expect to understand speech, even if they can hear many of the components of speech with the device. They have passed the critical time period for developing auditory skills, so the benefits are limited—even with extensive training. Some who have been implanted appreciate the awareness of speech and environmental sounds, and others are bothered by an assault of sound and reject the device.

Many adults in the Deaf Community, who identify themselves as part of a rich culture with a unique and beautiful language, American Sign Language, are opposed to the use of cochlear implants—particularly with children. They feel that the implant turns deaf children into "hearing robots" and robs them of the opportunity to find the culture in which they belong—deaf culture. However, 90% of deaf children are born to hearing parents, who naturally want their children to be part of the hearing world, or perhaps part of both worlds (Scheetz, 1993). The controversy over cochlear implants for children rages on. But meanwhile, children are being implanted in greater numbers each year.

AUDITORY ASSISTANCE IN THE CLASSROOM

Hearing-impaired children have unique challenges in school, as they are developing communication skills and learning academic subjects through an impaired auditory system. Even if that auditory system is optimized with appropriate hearing aids or a cochlear implant, the hearing-impaired child does not function like a normal hearing child. In addition, noisy and reverberant classrooms put hearing-impaired students at a much greater disadvantage than their normal hearing classmates.

Classroom Acoustics

A 1980 study of noise levels in classrooms found a range of 42–66 dB SPL in occupied classrooms—even in those classrooms specifically sound treated for hearing-impaired students—with a median level of 56 dBSPL (Sinclair, 1980). This noise level is distributed fairly evenly throughout the classroom. The same study found that the average level of the teacher's voice is 65 dBSPL at a distance of 3 feet. A **signal-to-noise ratio** can be calculated by subtracting the average noise level from the average speech level. This means that the child who sits 3 feet from the teacher hears his or her voice at an S:N ratio of +9 dB, meaning that the speech is 9 dB louder than the background noise. But speech, unlike classroom noise, decreases in intensity as the distance from the speaker increases. In fact, each doubling of the distance from the speech source reduces the intensity of that speech by 6 dB. So a child 6 feet from the same teacher hears his or her voice at an S:N ratio of +3 dB (59–56 dB). A child sitting 12 feet from the teacher loses more volume still, and hears the voice at an S:N ratio of −3 dB (53–56 dB), which means that the noise is now louder than the speech!

Other studies have shown that hearing-impaired children need an S:N ratio of at least +10 dB, and preferably +20 dB, to function effectively. Yet even for the child sitting just 3 feet from the teacher, this criterion is not met, and those at greater distances from the teacher are at a considerably greater disadvantage (Gengel, 1971; Olsen, 1988).

Reverberation, or the echo caused by sound reflecting off walls and other hard surfaces, adds another dimension to the problem. When the reflected sound overlaps with the direct signal from the teacher, the student wearing hearing aids has greater difficulty sorting out the primary signal from the echo. Add this reverberation to the ongoing background noise, and you have a listening environment that is severely compromised for learning. Classrooms that are sound-treated with acoustical ceiling tiles, carpet, soft wall textures, and the like can cut down on reverberation, and many of the digital hearing aids can reduce the level of the background noise. However, only special classroom amplification systems can address the problem of distance from the teacher.

FM Technology

Various kinds of group amplification systems have been used in classrooms for the hearing impaired for several decades, but the majority of systems in use today, called **FM systems,** employ FM radio signals. The frequency band of 72–76 MHz (megahertz), which is below the FM (frequency modulated) dial on commercial radios, has been designated for use in educational settings. Due to an expanded need, the FCC recently designated the band of 216–217 MHz for use with hearing assistance technology. The teacher wears a microphone and FM radio transmitter, which sends the signal out into the classroom. The student wears a receiver tuned to the same frequency as the teacher's transmitter. This receiver picks up the signal and delivers it to his ears, either by a button receiver in a custom earmold, or by direct audio input to his personal hearing aids or cochlear implant. Both the transmitter and receiver are housed in small cases that can be clipped to a belt or worn in a pocket. With this system, the hearing-impaired student hears the teacher's voice as if his ear is just a few inches from her mouth, and this is true whether or not she faces him. Adjacent classrooms can utilize FM systems by tuning the devices to different frequencies in the designated range. And because these systems are battery operated, they can be taken out of the classroom for field trips.

Sound Field Reinforcement Systems

Many students with minimal hearing loss, unilateral hearing loss, or fluctuating hearing levels due to chronic otitis media do not use personal hearing aids. Yet they suffer from the same deleterious effects of noise, reverberation, and distance from the teacher, which places them at a disadvantage for learning. Another type of FM system can be used to amplify the entire classroom using speakers similar to a public address (PA) system (see Figure 10.11). The teacher still wears a microphone and FM transmitter, and the signal is sent to an FM receiver and amplifier. However, the amplified signal is sent to one or

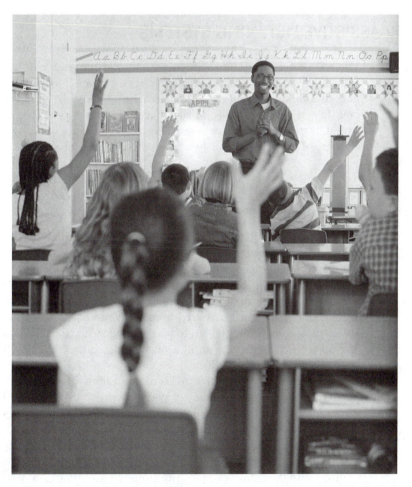

Figure 10.11 Example of FM sound field classroom system.
Source: Courtesy of FrontRow for Active Learning

more speakers placed around the room, so the student does not wear a receiver. This allows all students in the classroom to hear at an improved S:N ratio, not just those with hearing impairment or those with hearing aids, and the teacher is free to move about the room. These systems have also been found to be effective for other special needs students, such as those learning English as a second language, those with language disorders, or those with other developmental disabilities.

Fortunately, a new national standard (ANSI/ASA S12.60-2002) for maximum background noise (35 dB) and reverberation time (0.6–0.7 seconds) in unoccupied classrooms was published in 2002. To the extent that it can be implemented in classrooms for hearing-impaired children, this educational issue may be resolved somewhat through architectural engineering. However, classroom FM systems will still play an important role in learning for the hearing-impaired student.

OTHER ASSISTIVE LISTENING SYSTEMS

There are other situations or listening environments where hearing-impaired children and adults experience communication difficulty, even if they use appropriate amplification. In addition, some individuals have a hearing loss that is not severe enough to warrant the use of hearing aids, or they have chosen not to use hearing aids, yet they still have difficulty hearing or understanding in specific communicative situations. There are a variety of devices available to address these specific needs.

Devices for Telephone

Hearing aid users often have a problem using the telephone, because the close proximity of the handset to the hearing aid microphone causes acoustic feedback. Many hearing aids come equipped with telecoil circuits that bypass the hearing aid microphone, as described earlier in the "Hearing Aid Design and Components" section. Instruments with multiple memories can incorporate a telecoil as one of the memories, or one of the acoustic programs can be tailored to minimize feedback with the telephone. Some instruments automatically convert to telecoil mode when the telephone is placed at the ear, and other instruments remain in acoustic mode but eliminate feedback with a special feedback cancellation circuit.

Cell phones have revolutionized communication for the world, but hearing-impaired persons have encountered many obstacles trying to use them. Historically, cell phones were exempt from the FCC ruling, which required that all phones be compatible with telecoil circuits used in hearing aids by 1991 (Ahlman, 2006). Therefore, success was hit-and-miss as hearing aid wearers searched for cell phones they could use without getting feedback. Additionally, digital hearing aid wearers using digital cell phones had to contend with the radio frequency (RF) interference coming from the cellular signal, and this occurred even in cells phones made to be compatible with the hearing aid telecoil. However, a 2003 FCC ruling required a phase-in period for the wireless industry to become compatible with hearing aids, so now there are cell phone models that are rated for their compatibility with hearing aids—both in the microphone mode and the telecoil mode (Ahlman, 2006).

For those individuals who do not use hearing aids, or who are unable to use their aids on the telephone, a variety of telephone amplifiers are available. They are built into the handsets or can be attached to the base of standard desk phones, or they come in portable units that can be coupled to the listening portion of any handset. The local telephone companies make these available at no cost for hearing-impaired customers who submit an application signed by their doctor, audiologist, or hearing instrument specialist. These devices have volume controls, so that other members of the household with normal hearing can also use them. In addition, for customers who have difficulty hearing their telephone ring, the local telephone company will supply a special ring amplifier.

Individuals with severe or profound hearing loss who cannot understand amplified speech use special **telecommunication devices for the deaf (TDD)**. These devices attach to the telephone and use a keyboard to send typed messages electronically over the phone lines to other TDD users. Rather than speak and listen, these individuals type and read. Some TDDs are portable, some have answering machines built in, and the local telephone company makes basic devices available at no cost with a signed application. When an individual with a TDD wants to call someone who does not have the device, he may call a relay service. This service employs hearing operators with TDDs, who relay spoken messages by typing them and typed messages by speaking them. Persons without TDDs can call TDD users in the same way.

Many of the newer cell phones incorporate text messaging capability, such that friends and family members, hearing or deaf, can call each other anywhere, without using relay operators. And, of course, those with personal computers can join the Internet revolution, by researching information, surfing the net, joining chat rooms, or emailing. Because so many of the Internet activities do not require hearing, this revolution has broadened the social and employment horizon and leveled the playing field for many deaf individuals.

Devices for Television

Couples and families often have conflicts over the television volume when one or more members is hearing-impaired, and even hard-of-hearing people who live alone may play their television so loud that neighbors complain. A variety of devices can be used to resolve these conflicts. Remote speakers can be plugged into the television and placed near the hard-of-hearing person, or the person may use earphones that plug into a jack on the front of the TV set, provided this does not cut out the standard speakers for other family members.

A **personal FM system**, similar to those described earlier for classrooms, can be used to reduce the distance from the TV, amplify the signal, and improve the S:N ratio.

Infrared systems work like FM systems, but they use an invisible infrared light beam to carry the audio portion of the television signal. A transmitter placed on top of the set picks up the signal from a jack into the TV, or a microphone placed nearby, and sends

Figure 10.12   Example of personal infrared system receives
Source: Courtesy of TV Ears, Inc.

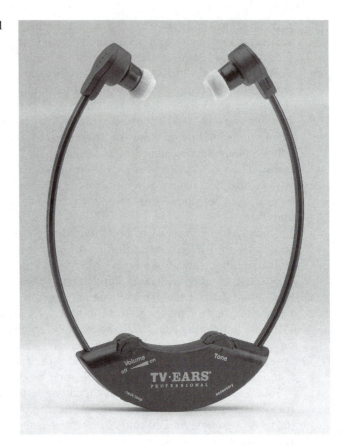

the infrared signal to a receiver worn by the listener. The receiver converts the infrared signal back to acoustic energy and the user can adjust the volume. An example of this device is shown in Figure 10.12.

Various hard-wired systems are also available, in which a wire connects a remote microphone placed near the TV speaker to an amplifier worn by the listener.

Individuals whose hearing aids are equipped with a telecoil may purchase an induction loop system for home use. This device plugs into the TV jack and converts the audio signal to magnetic energy. This magnetic energy is delivered to the listener via a wire that functions as an induction loop that is placed around the outer perimeter of the room either in the ceiling or under the carpet. The listener then switches her hearing aid to the "T" position.

For those individuals who have difficulty understanding television programs at any volume, they may read subtitles at the bottom of the screen, if they have a closed-captioned decoder. The Television Decoder Circuitry Act of 1993 requires that all televisions with screens larger than 13 inches be equipped with these decoders. The television purchaser then has the choice of using the subtitles or not.

Group Systems for Meeting Halls, Theaters, and Places of Worship

The problems that hearing-impaired people encounter in places where large groups gather are similar to those that hearing-impaired students experience in classrooms. Poor room acoustics, dim lighting, large distances, inarticulate speakers, and audience commotion are a few of the obstacles that all listeners contend with. However, those with hearing loss are doubly handicapped in these settings. Many large-area amplification systems and services are available for meeting halls, performance theaters, and houses of worship. The Americans with Disabilities Act (ADA) of 1990 provides the legal imperative for public facilities to provide them as discussed in Chapter 1.

Many churches, temples, synagogues, and mosques equip a few seats with hardwired systems, similar to the headsets used in airline seats, so the hard-of-hearing members of the congregation can sit in these seats or pews. Any of the other technologies discussed in the "Devices for Television" section can also be adapted to houses of worship.

Large theaters and movie houses often utilize infrared systems because this technology, where the receiver must be in line of sight with the transmitter, lends itself well to the seating arrangements used. Several transmitters are built into the theater walls, and patrons borrow headsets that contain receivers and volume controls. Often the actors in live theaters wear microphones hidden in their hair that are attached to FM transmitters worn on the body. The FM signals are sent to a mixer, which in turn sends an amplified signal to speakers in the room, as well as to the infrared transmitters used by the hearing-impaired audience members.

Many large meeting rooms for conventions, government hearings, or town halls are equipped with induction loop systems. In these situations, the induction loop is installed around the perimeter of the room similar to the home loop system, so that anyone seated within the loop can access the magnetic signal. Hearing aid users with a telecoil can switch into the telecoil mode, and those without hearing aids can borrow special telecoil receivers with earphones. Figure 10.13 shows the variety of ways this system can be used. As with houses of worship and theaters, hardwired, FM, or infrared systems can also be used in these settings.

Deaf persons who communicate primarily by sign language can also participate in public events, if sign language interpreters are provided. Occasionally oral interpreters are provided for oral deaf adults, who do not sign or obtain sufficient information through audition, but who require lipreading to fully understand the spoken message. The oral interpreter faces the audience at all times and "mouths" what the speaker says, without using his voice. So if the speaker moves about or is not easy to lip-read, the oral deaf audience members can still receive the message from the oral interpreter.

Signaling Devices

Many severely or profoundly hearing-impaired individuals are unable to hear acoustic signals in their homes or workplaces, such as a ringing telephone, doorbell, or smoke alarm. Making these signals louder may not be helpful or practical, so alternative solutions are needed. These individuals can utilize special systems, which signal lights to flash in one or more rooms, or special devices to vibrate, which can be placed under a

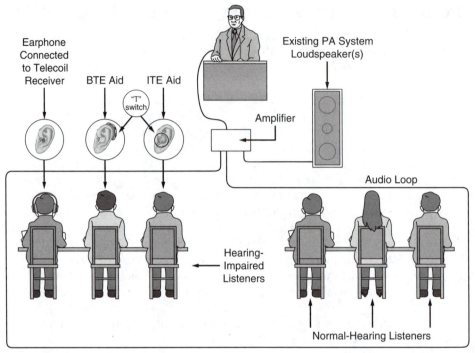

Figure 10.13 Use of an induction loop large area listening system. A coil of wire (loop) is added to existing sound system. Listeners with hearing impairment pick up sound using telecoil circuits contained in hearing aids or special receivers.

mattress or pillow. Entire systems can be installed throughout the home, so that all sounds can be signaled to the hearing-impaired family members, with coded flashes or vibrations to differentiate one sound from another. Small vibrators can be worn on the wrist, which pick up signals from transmitters placed near various sound sources, including a crying baby in another room. Special alarm clocks that vibrate are also available for deaf sleepers who cannot be aroused by loud alarms or flashing lights. Major hotels usually offer rooms equipped with signaling devices for their deaf patrons, in compliance with the Americans with Disabilities Act (ADA).

Although these electronic alerting devices are effective, some deaf individuals prefer to use specially trained hearing dogs as their signaling systems. The dog responds to people's voices and other acoustic signals, and runs back and forth between the owner and the source of the signal until the owner responds. These hearing dogs are accepted in many public places, much like Seeing Eye™ dogs for the blind.

COUNSELING

Up to this point the focus for auditory rehabilitation has been placed on hearing aids, cochlear implants, and other assistive devices. But there is another aspect of the rehabilitation process that must be considered, because it is a central component in any successful hearing aid, cochlear implant, or assistive device fitting. Dispensers and dispensing audiologists are engaged in various forms of counseling with the hearing-impaired patient and his family all along the rehabilitative process. Speech pathologists, educators, psychologists, rehabilitation counselors, and laypersons with hearing loss may also provide counseling to any given individual. These counseling roles will be discussed in four separate categories, but in reality, these distinctions often blur.

Information/Orientation

Beginning with the initial diagnosis of a hearing impairment, the audiologist must answer questions and provide information to the patient and family members about what the loss means. Where is the problem? What caused it? Can it be corrected? Will it get worse? What should I/we do about it? These are many of the questions that adult patients often ask. How will the loss affect my child's ability to speak? How can I communicate with him? Will he have to go to a special school? How will the hearing loss affect his ability to make friends, go to college, get a job? These are a few of the questions that parents often ask when a hearing loss is confirmed in their child.

The audiologist must address these concerns by providing information about the audiogram and how the hearing loss affects communication. Parents should be given information about communication and educational options and services available for their hearing-impaired child. Other professionals, such as the otolaryngologist, may provide information as to the cause of the hearing loss and prognosis for future progression. And some questions cannot be fully answered at the initial evaluation, but will continue to be addressed in subsequent sessions and as more information becomes available over time.

As an individual is fit with hearing aids, a cochlear implant or other kind of assistive device, information is provided to orient the patient and family members to the operation and maintenance of this equipment. Topics often included in this type of counseling include: battery insertion, device controls, device insertion and removal, use of the device with the telephone, cleaning and daily maintenance, and troubleshooting problems that may arise in the future. In addition, the patient and family members are counseled on what to expect from the equipment and how to monitor its success or failure. In postfitting sessions, the patient and family will report on their experiences with the equipment. This helps the dispenser to make any necessary adjustments to the fitting, while providing encouragement and counseling on appropriate expectations.

Communication Strategies

Another important area of counseling involves strategies to improve communication. Amplification devices do not restore hearing to normal, so most hearing aid users and their families find that these devices do not solve all the communication problems in all situations. Therefore, dispensers need to make them aware of simple strategies and compensations that can be used to maximize understanding by the hearing-impaired individual, and minimize the number of repetitions required by the family. Dispensers and rehabilitation therapists may also teach repair strategies for both parties to use when communication breaks down. A listing of several commonsense strategies for the

Table 10.2   Communication tips for the hard-of-hearing

1. Your hearing loss is your responsibility. Although others may assist you in communicating more easily, you are ultimately responsible for how you hear.

2. Communication involves combining all information received with thinking. General knowledge, previous experiences, and memories of past conversations can aid you in understanding what is being said.

3. Practice listening "selectively." Relearning to focus on one conversation while ignoring background noise is a skill that takes practice.

4. Make a conscious effort to pay close attention to conversation. Concentrate.

5. Watch the lips, facial expressions, and gestures of the person you are listening to. A course in speechreading may contribute to your ability to utilize these cues.

6. Learn to "stage manage." When at church, concerts, the theater, etc., find the seating location that is best for you. This will probably be nearest the speaker. Do not hesitate to move to a better location, if necessary.

7. Saying "What?" repeatedly is an annoying habit. When asking for more information, include the part of the message that you did hear. Example: "Which day were you planning to shop?"—rather than "What?"

8. When joining a group, ask someone present to clue you into the topic of conversation.

9. People cannot see a hearing loss. You need to let them know what they can do to help you. The manner in which you ask determines the way in which others respond to you.

10. You need to ask others to:
    a. Get your attention before they speak to you.
    b. Speak a little slower and in a normal tone of voice. Shouting often makes understanding more difficult.
    c. Keep their hands away from their faces when talking to you, so that you may utilize the visual cues in their message.
    d. Not talk from another room or while distractions like the television, radio, or running water are present.
    e. Rephrase rather than repeat. Having the message said differently often helps understanding.

11. Be patient with your mistakes and those of others.

hearing-impaired individual can be found in Table 10.2. Strategies for family members are listed in Table 10.3. These techniques, if applied consistently, will add to the success of the hearing aid fitting and reduce frustration and tension in the family.

Psychological Adjustment to Hearing Loss

A more nebulous area of counseling, although no less important, centers around helping the patient and family members come to grips with the hearing loss and its impact on their lives. Imagine the shock that parents must experience when they first learn that their child is deaf or hard-of-hearing. Even if their own suspicions are confirmed and

Table 10.3   Tips for talking to the hard-of-hearing

1. Speak clearly and naturally without shouting. Speaking slower often helps.

2. Look at the hard-of-hearing person, making sure that your face is easily seen while you are speaking.

3. Make sure that the amount of light is adequate, and see that the light is not shining in the eyes of the hard-of-hearing person.

4. Do not overemphasize your speech sounds or lip movements.

5. If the person does not understand what you are saying, find a different way of saying the same thing, rather than repeat the original words over and over. Rephrase rather than repeat.

6. If you are eating, chewing, or smoking while talking, your speech will be more difficult to understand.

7. Keep your hands away from your face while talking.

8. Never talk from another room.

9. Be sure to get the person's attention before you start speaking.

10. Reduce background noises when communicating. Turn off the television or radio. Move to a quieter place, if possible.

11. If you are going out to a restaurant, choose a quiet one so the noise level is not intolerable to the hard-of-hearing person. Sit away from the kitchen or entrance, if possible.

12. Remember that a hard-of-hearing person will hear and understand less when he or she is tired or ill.

13. Understanding conversation in large groups is difficult for the hard-of-hearing person. Be sure to give the person a clue to the topic of conversation in these situations.

14. Be patient with mistakes. Many speech sounds are easily confused by the hard-of-hearing person, and it is a strain for him or her to try to sort them out.

they finally have a diagnosis that explains their child's inattentiveness or language delay or behavioral problem, the news of a permanent hearing loss is extremely difficult to digest. Many parents report that when they first heard that their child was hearing-impaired, they felt faint, had trouble breathing, and just could not hear anything that was said after that.

Parents will usually go through stages of grief, very much like those described by Elizabeth Kubler-Ross in her book *On Death and Dying* (1997). After the shock wears off, they may go through a period of denial, when they seek second, third, and fourth opinions in an effort to find a different diagnosis. When they hear the same story enough times, they will usually go through a period of anger, followed by depression and grief. Eventually they will arrive at some level of acceptance or resignation, when they will be psychologically ready to get on with the business of helping their child.

The role of the professional is to listen, show compassion, and help the parents get through these stages, so that they can become advocates and partners in their child's habilitation process. Often other parents who have already gone through the process are excellent counselors, because they have greater credibility and can provide hope that there is life after a diagnosis of hearing loss. The audiologist must temper the psychological needs of the parents with the needs of the child for immediate intervention with hearing aids, therapy, and educational programs. Parents often report going through these early months of intervention in a state of numbness as they try to cope with their grief. Occasionally psychologists will be needed if the parents' grief is prolonged and gets in the way of the habilitation needs of their child.

With adults, it's usually the individual with the hearing loss who goes through difficulty adjusting to the loss. He may not be aware of the problem for some time if the loss progresses gradually. Once he does become aware, he usually goes through a period of denial, when he accuses his loved ones of mumbling. Anger, depression, and withdrawal may set in for several years before he is ready to seek help. Family members are usually frustrated at having to repeat themselves and angry that he will not get the help that he obviously needs. By the time the couple or family gets to the audiologist's office, relationships may be seriously damaged and a great deal of tension may be present. The audiologist needs to diffuse the situation by acknowledging the feelings of all parties, providing useful information, and guiding them through the steps required to improve communication.

Support Groups

Counseling in auditory rehabilitation is often provided in group sessions. For the audiologist, the group format is an effective and efficient way to orient patients and their families to hearing impairment, communication strategies, hearing aid operation, and appropriate expectations for amplification. The patients and family members have a chance to meet with others going through a similar adjustment process, which can reduce anxiety and encourage perseverance. Many schools for the hearing-impaired offer formal parent education programs or more loosely structured parent support groups.

This need for information and psychological support is frequently not fully met by professionals in auditory rehabilitation, as is evidenced by the proliferation of many patient and parent self-help groups throughout the nation (see Appendix B for a list of organizations). These self-help groups offer compassion, consolation, information, and encouragement in an accepting and sharing atmosphere. They do not take the place of professional counseling, but they offer additional resources to help individuals and families cope with problems and take responsibility for solutions to those problems.

TRADITIONAL REHABILITATIVE APPROACHES

Before body-worn amplification systems became available, hearing-impaired individuals had to make do with their residual hearing by using various acoustic horns and non-electronic devices that could only provide minimal boost of auditory signals. Those individuals who wanted to function in the hearing world had two different but related approaches to pursue, in order to maintain or develop their communicative skills: auditory training and speechreading training. Those who preferred to function in the deaf world or who could not succeed in the hearing world learned sign language and became members of the deaf community. Now that hearing aids, cochlear implants, and assistive devices provide much better reception of speech and environmental sounds, these other traditional approaches are not needed for many patients with mild and moderate hearing impairments. However, these approaches are still used for many patients with severe and profound impairments, as part of more extensive rehabilitation programs, and in conjunction with the fitting of appropriate amplification devices.

Auditory Training

There are various kinds of auditory training methods, but the goal of all is to maximize patients' hearing and understanding of their auditory environment. This can be as basic as learning to distinguish soft sounds from loud sounds, low-pitched sounds from high-pitched sounds, short sounds from long sounds—and as complex as learning to extract a speech message from a sea of background noise.

For adults with gradually progressive hearing loss who have sustained a long period of auditory deprivation or reduced auditory stimulation, the sounds received from hearing aids can be confusing and bothersome at first. They need time for the ears and brain to adjust or acclimatize to the new auditory input, but they may also need some formal auditory training to help this process along. Even adults who have already adjusted to their hearing aids may get limited benefit if their auditory systems distort the amplified sound and make speech difficult to understand at any volume. For these individuals, auditory training may be of some help.

A child who has been deafened at birth has no auditory memory for sound, and thus will need to be taught much of what comes naturally to a normal hearing child. Therefore, rehabilitative audiologists, speech pathologists, and deaf educators will be involved in developing the auditory system, so that children can utilize and make sense of the information their hearing aids or cochlear implant provide. This auditory training often goes hand in hand with speech and language therapy. Even children who are deafened sometime after birth may need formal auditory training to make the most of their amplification system.

Key factors to look at in determining if an individual needs auditory training are the severity of the loss, including speech discrimination ability and loudness tolerance levels, age of onset of the loss, length of auditory deprivation, and performance with various amplification systems. Although many individuals could benefit from auditory training, the bulk of services available today in this area are provided to children. However, Listening and Auditory Communication Enhancement, or LACE (Sweetow, 2005) is a new computerized auditory training program that adults can use at home to help them acclimatize to new amplification.

Speechreading Training

The traditional term lipreading involves watching a speaker's lips, tongue, and jaw movements in order to understand the spoken message. The newer term speechreading incorporates lipreading and adds information from other visual cues such as facial expressions, gestures, and body posture. Normal-hearing people use these visual cues to enhance understanding in difficult listening situations, such as large groups or noisy environments. However, those with hearing loss need to use visual cues to a greater extent, because of the impaired auditory system, even if that system has been optimized with hearing aids or other devices.

No one can obtain all the information in spoken language through vision alone, because there are many limitations to the speechreading process. Some limitations have to do with the nature of the spoken message. As many as 60% of speech sounds are obscure or invisible, because they are produced in the back of the mouth or with little lip, tongue, and jaw movements. Other sounds are visible, yet look identical to other sounds. For example, it is impossible to distinguish the difference between the words math, path, or bath through vision alone. In addition, speech is very rapid and fleeting, which means we often produce sounds faster than the eye can see, and there is no way to stop the speech process to have a better look.

Other limitations with the speechreading process have to do with the speaker or the environment. Some speakers are harder to read than others, because of their reduced lip, tongue, and jaw movements, their style of gesturing, or perhaps obstacles such as facial hair or braces on their teeth. And speakers do not always face the person who needs to speechread them. Environmental problems such as distance from the speaker, angle of the face, dim lighting, or glare from the sun are other confounding variables that can make speechreading a greater challenge.

Still other limitations have to do with the speechreader himself. An older patient may have visual impairment in addition to hearing impairment; he may not have the mental flexibility needed to follow rapid speech; and he may not be motivated to learn new speechreading skills. However, there are some deaf and hard-of-hearing individuals who have become excellent speechreaders, due to an inherent ability, significant need, and extraordinary motivation. These "star" speechreaders seem to defy conventional wisdom by grasping far more than 40% of spoken language, primarily through vision.

Professionals disagree on the benefits of speechreading training. Few controlled research studies have been undertaken to demonstrate improvement with training, yet many patients have reported an improvement in their communication ability and overall quality of life. Testing one's speechreading ability is possible, but the tests by their very nature alter the speechreading process and may not predict how well an individual will perform in a more natural setting. Many individuals who feel that speechreading training has helped them have shown no significant improvement on standardized tests administered before and after training. Perhaps they derive a psychological benefit from focusing on the problem and receiving attention from professionals or other group members.

Because of these and other limitations, few professionals provide formal speechreading training these days. Instead, many counsel their patients on the need to focus on visual cues to enhance understanding, as part of their overall counseling on ways to improve communication. Group classes in speechreading can still be found, although these are primarily for adults. Children are taught speechreading in some educational programs, but many other programs do not emphasize this and children seem to pick up the visual cues anyway.

SUMMARY

A Glimpse into the Profession Revisited

The rehabilitation process for Mr. Barnes, introduced in the beginning of this chapter, consisted of three main areas:

- *At the initial visit, the audiologist solicited and acknowledged the feelings of both Mr. and Mrs. Barnes concerning the hearing problem and its effects on communication and their relationship. The results of the audiological evaluation were discussed, in terms of the degree and configuration of the hearing loss, as well as how it impacts communication and lifestyle. A demonstration of what speech sounds he does not hear helped Mr. Barnes realize the extent of the problem and the need for intervention. Further counseling outlined several commonsense strategies (see Tables 10.2 and 10.3) for both parties to use, in order to maximize understand and minimize frustration.*

- *Mr. Barnes was fitted with two digital signal processing behind-the-ear instruments with noise suppression, directional microphones, direct audio input capability, and appropriate earmolds. He was counseled on their operation, care, and maintenance and both parties were counseled on appropriate expectations from amplification. Real-ear measurement using a probe microphone demonstrated good fit to target gain and output curves. Mr. Barnes was seen for several follow-up visits, where small program adjustments were made and additional information on operation and expectations was given. After a few weeks, Mr. Barnes reported that he was hearing better in most situations and that he was becoming adjusted to his "new" hearing.*

- *Because both Mr. and Mrs. Barnes reported continuing difficulty communicating in the cab of their RV and Mr. Barnes still noticed that he missed important words in group lectures, he was fitted with an additional assistive listening device, a personal FM system. Mrs. Barnes wears the microphone and transmitter and the wireless receiver is coupled directly to one of Mr. Barnes' hearing aids using a direct audio input boot. When they attend lectures, Mr. Barnes now asks the lecturer or tour guide to wear the microphone and transmitter and he finds that most people are happy to comply with his request.*

CHAPTER REVIEW

- ❑ The field of hearing rehabilitation covers any device or service that can help hearing-impaired patients and their families adjust to the handicap, optimize their communication ability, and improve their quality of life in educational, vocational, and social situations.

- ❑ For many patients, the fitting of appropriate hearing aids, orientation to the operation, maintenance of the instruments, and periodic follow-up care constitute the entire rehabilitation program.

- ❑ Other patients may need additional assistive listening devices to improve function in specific communicative situations.

- ❑ Many patients with severe or profound hearing loss who obtain little benefit with conventional hearing aids find greater help through the use of a cochlear implant.

❑ Still others will require more extensive rehabilitation in the form of auditory training and/or speechreading training.

❑ Throughout the rehabilitation process for any of these patients, the dispensers and other rehabilitation specialists will provide counseling. This counseling may take the form of information about the loss and its impact on communication and lifestyle; orientation to the operation and care of amplification devices; strategies to improve communication; or help in making the psychological adjustment to hearing loss.

❑ Any professional who engages in these activities can be considered a rehabilitation specialist. Because the numbers of hearing-impaired individuals in our society is growing, the demand for these specialists is growing proportionally every year. Those already working with hearing-impaired individuals and families—as audiologists, dispensers, speech pathologists, teachers, psychologists, rehabilitation counselors, and various kinds of aids—report high levels of job satisfaction and personal rewards. This is because they are having a positive impact and improving the lives of hearing-impaired individuals and their families.

ACTIVITIES FOR DISCUSSION

1. Can you think of any other areas of aural rehabilitation that might help Mr. Barnes and his wife?

2. Based on the levels of hearing aid technology discussed in this chapter, what other kinds of improvements or technological developments are needed?

3. If implantable hearing devices such as the cochlear implant, bone conduction implant, and middle ear implant become more commonplace, how do you think this development will impact the field of aural rehabilitation and the future careers of audiologists, dispensers, and aides?

REFERENCES

Ahlman, M. (Jan./Feb., 2006). On the go: Prepare for the age wave by understanding the "new" hearing aid compatibility and augmenting your services with cellular assistance. *Advance for Audiologists*, 8(1).

Alpiner, J. C., Chevrette, G., Glascoe, G., Metz, M., & Olsen, B. (1974). *The Denver scale of communication function*, Unpublished Study, University of Denver.

Americans with Disabilities Act of 1990, S.933.

American National Standards Institute (ANSI) S12.60. (2002). Acoustical performance criteria, design requirements, and guidelines for schools.

American National Standards Institute (ANSI) C63.19. (2001). American national standard for methods of measurement of compatibility between wireless communications devices and hearing aids.

Compton, C. L. (1989). *Assistive devices: Doorways to independence*. Washington, DC: Assistive Device Center, Gallaudet University.

Cox, R. M., & Alexander, G. C. (1995). The abbreviated profile of hearing aid benefit (APHAB). *Ear and Hearing, 16*, 176–186.

Gengel, R. W. (1971). Acceptable signal-to-noise ratios for aided speech discrimination by hearing-impaired, *Journal of Auditory Research*, 11, 219–222.

Hearing Aid Compatibility Act, 47 U.S.C. 610(b)(l)(B), 1988.

Hearing Aid Dispensers Examining Committee (HADEC). (1996), *Laws and rules and regulations relating to the practice of hearing aid dispensing*, Department of Consumer Affairs, State of California, Sacramento, CA.

High, W. S., Fairbanks, G. & Glorig, A. (1964). Scale for Self-Assessment. In J. Jeffers & M. Barley (1978), *Speechreading (Lipreading)*, 6th printing. Springfield, IL: Charles C. Thomas Publisher.

Holmes, A. E. (2002). Cochlear implants and other rehabilitative areas. In R.L. Schow, and M. A. Nerbonne,(Eds.) *Introduction to audiologic rehabilitation,*(4th ed.). Allyn & Bacon, Boston, MA.

Kirkwood, D. H. (Dec, 2006). Led by BTEs, sales rise for fourth straight year to surpass 2.3 million, in *The Hearing Journal, 59*(12).

Kirkwood, D. H. (Dec., 2005). Hearing aid sales slip back to norm, but leaders see growth potential. *The Hearing Journal, 58*(12).

Kubler-Ross, E. (1997). *On Death and Dying* (reprint ed.), Scribner.

National Institutes of Health, Medical Arts and Photography Branch, Bethesda, MD.

Newman, C. W., Weinstein, B. E., Jacobson, G. P., & Hug, G. A. (1991). Test-retest reliability of the Hearing Handicap Inventory for Adults, *Ear & Hearing, 12,* 355–357.

Olsen, W. (1988), Classroom acoustics for hearing-impaired in children. In F. H. Bess (Ed.) *Hearing impairment in children*. Parkton, MD: York Press.

Pollack, M. (1988), Electroacoustic characteristics. In M. Pollack (Ed.), *Amplification for the hearing impaired* (3rd ed.). Orlando, FL: Brune & Stratton.

Schow, R. L., and Nerbonne, M. A. (2002). *Introduction to Audiologic Rehabilitation* (4th ed.). Boston, MA: Allyn & Bacon.

Scheetz, N. A. (1993), *Orientation to deafness*, Allyn & Bacon, Needham Heights, MA.

Sinclair, J. S., et al (1980). Classroom noise in schools for the hearing impaired. Presented to Tennessee Speech and Hearing Association annual convention, Nashville.

Schow, R. L., & Nerbonne, M. A. (1982). Communication screening profile: Use with elderly clients. *Ear and Hearing, 3,* 135–147.

Schow, R. L., & Nerbonne, M. A. (1977). Assessment of Hearing Handicap by Nursing Home Residents and Staff, *Journal of the Academy of Rehabilitative Audiology, 10,* 2–12.

Staab, W., & Lybarger, S. (1994). Characteristics and use of hearing aids, in J. Katz (Ed.), *Handbook of clinical audiology* (4th ed.). Baltimore: Williams & Wilkins.

Strom, K. E. (2001). *An Industry in transformation: technology & consolidation lead the field into a new milennium, The Hearing Review,* CurAnt Communications, Inc., Los Angeles, CA.

Sweetow, R. (2005). Post hearing aid fitting, counseling and training, ASHA audiology presentation, Palm Springs.

Television Decoder Circuitry Act of 1990.

U.S. Food and Drug Administration (FDA). (1977). Hearing aid devices; conditions for sale, 21 Code of Federal Regulations, Part 801.421.

Ventry, I. M., & Weinstein, B. E. (1983). Identification of elderly people with hearing problems. *American Speech Language Hearing Association, 25,* 37.

Ventry, I. M., & Weinstein, B. E. (1982). The hearing handicap inventory for the elderly: A new tool, *Ear and Hearing, 3,* 128–134.

Wilson, B. S. (2000). Cochlear implant technology. In J. K. Niparko, et. al. (Eds.). *Cochlear implants: principles and practices*. Philadelphia: Lippincott, Williams & Wilkins.

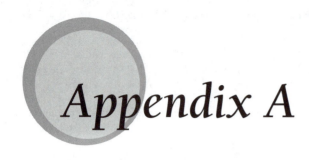

Appendix A

Web Links and Readings for Further Exploration

Chapter 1

Web Links

American Academy of Audiology
  http://audiology.org/

American Speech-Language-Hearing Association
  http://asha.org/default.htm

U.S. Bureau of Labor Statistics
  http://stats.bls.gov/oco/ocos085.htm
  http://stats.bls.gov/emp/emptab3.htm

Audiology Online
  http://www.audiologyonline.com

Healthy Hearing
  http://www.healthyhearing.com

Comm. Science and Disorders Dome
  http://www.Comdisdome.com

  www.audiology.org/professional/gov/hlfacts.
    pdf
  www.advocacyinc.org/linkdeaf.htm

www.deafandhh.com
www.gohear.com
www.gpoaccess.gov/cfr/index.html
www.hearinglossnetwork.org

Suggested Readings

Tucker, B. P. (1997). *IDEA advocacy for children who are deaf or hard of hearing.* Singular: San Diego.

Schirmer, B. R. (2001). *Psychological, social, and educational dimensions of deafness.* Boston: Allyn & Bacon.

Chapter 2

Web Links

Acoustics and Vibration Animations
  http://www.kettering.edu/~drussell/Demos.html

Decibel Calculator
  http://www.web-ee.com/Downloads/
    Calculator/db_calc.xls

Acoustical Society of America
http://asa.aip.org/

House Ear Institute
www.hei.org

Animation for Acoustics
http://www.acs.psu.edu/users/sparrow/movies/
animations9.html

Physics and Psychophysics of Music
http://www.avatar.com.au/courses/PPofM/

Chapter 3

Web Links

Animations for Processes Within the Ear
http://www.neurophys.wisc.edu/animations/

Soundwaves and the Eardrum
http://www.glenbrook.k12.il.us/gbssci/phy/
mmedia/waves/edl.html

Computer Models of the Middle Ear
http://funsan.biomed.mcgill.ca/~funnell/
Open-House96/me_model.html

Promenade 'round the Cochlea
iurc.montp.inserm.fr/cric/audition/English/
start.htm

Basilar Membrane Oscillations
http://www.blackwellpublishing.com/
matthews/ear.html

3-D Model of Brainstem
http://www.3-dmodels.com/3-dmodel_files/
371m761.htm

Audition Mechanics Laboratory
http://audilab.bmed.mcgill.ca/~funnell/
Audiolab/

Chapter 4

Web Links

http://www.geneclinics.org/profiles/
deafness-overview/details.html
www.aoa.gov/prof/statistics/statistics.asp
http://www.hopeforkids.com/
http://www.boystownhospital.org/Hearing/
index.asp

Chapter 5

Web Links

Audiology Awareness Campaign
http://www.audiologyawareness.com

Better Hearing Institute
http://www.betterhearing.org/

Self-Help for Hard of Hearing
www.hearingloss.org/html/hearing_loss_fact_
sheets.html

American Speech-Language-Hearing Association
www.asha.org/public/hearing/disorders/
causes.htm

Boystown National Research Hospital
www.babyhearing.org/HearingAmplification/
Glossary/index.asp

Suggested Readings

Harrell, R. W. (2002). Puretone evaluation. In Jack
Katz (Ed.), *Handbook of clinical audiology* (5th
ed.) Philadelphia: Lippincott, Williams &
Wilkins.

Chapter 6

Web Links

www.chclibrary.org/micromed/00039010.html
www.ehendrick.com/healthy/000170.htm
www.umm.edu/ency/article/003341.htm
www.umm.edu/medical-terms/07298.htm
web.pdx.edu/martindo/Demopages/
audiometry/audiometry.htm
www.ahealthyme.com/article/gale/100084281
www.ansi.org

Suggested Readings

Brandy, W. T. (2002). Speech audiometry. In Jack
Katz (Ed.), *Handbook of clinical audiology*
(5th ed.). Philadelphia: Lippincott, Williams
& Wilkins.

Harrell, R. W. (2002). Puretone evaluation. In Jack
Katz (Ed.), *Handbook of clinical audiology* (5th
ed.). Philadelphia: Lippincott, Williams &
Wilkins.

Nicolosi, L., Harryman, E., & Krescheck, J., 1989. *Terminology of communication disorders: Speech-language-hearing* (3rd ed.). Baltimore: Williams & Wilkins.

Chapter 7

Web Links

www.hei.org
http://www.blsc.com/hearing/index.html
http://www.babyhearing.org/

Chapter 8

Web Links

www.audiologynet.com/ped-audiology.html
www.audiology.org/professional/positions/jcih-early
www.audiology.org/professional/gov/hlfacts
www.cdc.gov/ncbddd/ehdi/default.htm
www.infanthearing.org
www.lhh.org/earlyid

Suggested Readings

Diefendorf, A. O. (2002). Detection and assessment of hearing loss in infants and children. In J. Katz (Ed.), *Handbook of clinical audiology,* (5th ed.). Baltimore: Lippincott, Williams & Wilkins.

American Speech-Language-Hearing Association Audiologic Assessment Panel 1996. (1997). *Guidelines for audiologic screening.* Rockville, MD: Author.

California Department of Health Services, (2001). *Manual for the school audiometrist.*

Johnson, C. D. (2002). Hearing and immittance screening. In J. Katz (Ed.), *Handbook of clinical audiology,* (5th ed.). Baltimore: Lippincott, Williams & Wilkins.

Joint Committee on Infant Hearing Year 2000 Position Statement. Principles and guidelines for early hearing detection and intervention programs.

Kenworthy, O. T. (1993). Early identification: Principles and practices. In J. G. Alpiner & P. A. MacCarthy, *Rehabilitative audiology: Children and adults,* Baltimore: Williams & Wilkins.

Chapter 9

Web Links

www.audiologyonline.com
www.va.gov/621quillen/clinics/asp/Products/PRIMER
www.comdisdome.com
www.healthypeople.gov/document/

Suggested Readings

Martin, F. N. (2002). Pseudohypacusis. In J. Katz (Ed.), *Handbook of clinical audiology,* (5th ed.). Baltimore: Lippincott, Williams & Wilkins.

Rintelmann, W. F., & Schwan, S. A. (1999). Pseudohypacusis. In F. E. Musiek & W. F. Rintelmann (Eds.), *Contemporary perspectives in hearing assessment* (pp. 415–435). Boston: Allyn & Bacon.

Chapter 10

Web Links

www.nidcd.nih.gov/health/hearing/hearingaid.asp
www.asha.org/public/hearing/treatment/hearing_aids.htm
http://www.earinfo.com/
www.fcc.gov/cgb/consumerfacts/hac.html
http://www.audiologynet.com/hearing-aids.html
http://ctl.augie.edu/perry/ar/ar.htm

Suggested Readings

Alpiner, J. G., & McCarthy, P. A. (2000). *Rehabilitative audiology: Children and adults* (3rd ed.). Philadelphia: Lippincott Willimas & Wilkins.

Dillon, H. (2001). *Hearing aids.* New York: Thieme Medical Publishers.

Flexer, C. (1999). *Facilitating Hearing and Listening in Young Children.* San Diego Singular.

Himber, C. (2002). *How to survive hearing loss.* Washington, DC: Gallaudet University Press.

Schow, R. L., & Nerbonne, M. A. (2002). *Introduction to audiologic rehabilitation* (4th ed.). Boston: Allyn & Bacon.

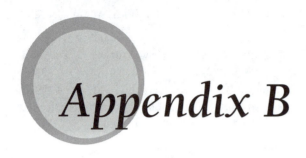

Appendix B

Professional Organizations and Advocacy Groups

American Academy of Audiology (AAA)

AAA was founded in 1988 by a group of 32 audiologists who concluded that a separate organization from ASHA would more effectively represent the specific interests of audiologists and the advancement of the profession. AAA has rapidly become a major organization representing the interests of the audiology profession with a membership of over 12,000.

> http://www.audiology.org
> 11730 Plaza America Drive, Suite 300
> Reston, VA 20190
> (800)222-2336, (703)790-8466
> (703)790-8631 (fax)

American Speech-Language-Hearing Association (ASHA)

ASHA is the oldest organization for audiologists and speech-language pathologists and also governs the national certification and accreditation for educational programs. The American Speech Correction Association adopted the new profession of Audiology in 1947 and changed its name to The American Speech and Hearing Association (ASHA). This organization was later renamed The American Speech-Language-Hearing Association in 1978 although it retained its traditional acronym of ASHA.

> http://www.asha.org
> 10801 Rockville Pike
> Rockville, MD 20852-3279

(301)897-5700

Professionals/Students: (800)498-2071

Public: (800)638-8255

American Auditory Society

http://www.amauditorysoc.org

352 Sundial Ridge Circle

Dammeron Valley, UT 84783

(435)574-0062

(435)574-0063 (fax)

Academy of Dispensing Audiology

http://www.audiologist.org

3008 Millwood Avenue

Columbia, SC 29205

(803)252-5646

(800)445-8629

(803)765-0860 (fax)

Academy of Rehabilitative Audiology

http://www.audrehab.org

ARA National Office

PO Box 26532

Minneapolis, MN 55426

(952)920-0484

(952)920-6098 (fax)

Educational Audiology Association

http://www.edaud.org

13153 N Dale Mabry Hwy, Suite 105

Tampa, FL 33618

(800)460-7322

National Association of Future Doctors of Audiology

http://www.nafda.org

National Student Speech-Language-Hearing Association

http://www.nsslha@asha.org

10801 Rockville Pike

Rockville, MD 20852

(800)498-2071

(301)571-0481 (fax)

A. G. Bell Association for the Deaf

The Alexander Graham Bell Association for the Deaf and Hard of Hearing (AG Bell) is the world's oldest and largest membership organization promoting the use of spoken language by children and adults with hearing loss. Members include parents of children with hearing loss, adults who are deaf or hard of hearing, educators, audiologists, speech-language pathologists, physicians, and other professionals in fields related to hearing loss and deafness. Through advocacy, publications, financial aid and scholarships, and numerous programs and services, AG Bell promotes its mission: Advocating Independence through Listening and Talking.

http://www.agbell.org

3714 Volta Pl, NW

Washington, DC 20007

(202)337-5220 (phone)

(202)337-5221 (TDD)

(202)337-8314 (fax)

Parents Section, A. G. Bell Association for the Deaf

Founded in 1958, the Parents Section is a division whose members promote advocating independence through listening and talking. It is concerned with continuing education about the necessity of early diagnosis and auditory, language, and speech training for children who are deaf or hard-of-hearing. The association also works to preserve parents' and children's rights by advocating auditory-oral and auditory-verbal education, and serves as clearinghouse to dispense information and exchange ideas.

American Society for Deaf Children

This national organization founded in 1967 currently has 120 affiliates. It provides information and support for parents and families with children who are deaf or hard-of-hearing. A quarterly magazine and biennial conventions are also part of its services.

> http://www.deafchildren.org
> PO Box 3355
> Gettysburg, PA 17325
> (800)942-2732 (voice/TDD)
> (717)334-7922 (TDD)
> (717)334-8808 (fax)
> Email: asdc1@aol.com

Association of Late-Deafened Adults (ALDA)

ALDA was founded in 1987 in Chicago, Illinois, for people who became deaf as adults. Within a few years, the organization had chapters in over 15 regions across the United States and today, ALDA's membership is international in scope. ALDA holds annual conventions (ALDAcon) and publishes a monthly newsletter, the ALDA News. ALDA works collaboratively with other organizations around the world serving the needs of late-deafened people.

> http://www.alda.org
> ALDA Inc.
> 1131 Lake St, #204
> Oak Park, IL 60301
> (877)907-1738 (voice/fax) (Cont. US only)
> (708)358-0135 (TDD)

Auditory-Verbal International, Inc.

This international network was founded in 1987 with an aim to provide the choice of listening and speaking as a way of life for children and adults who are deaf or hard-of-hearing. Services provided as part of the annual dues are a newsletter, networking, literature, phone support, information, and referrals. There are also networking opportunities and links for parents of deaf children as well referrals to certified auditory-verbal therapists.

> http://www.auditory-verbal.org
> 2121 Eisenhower Ave, Suite 402
> Alexandria, VA 22314
> (703)739-1049 (phone, day/eve)
> (703)739-0874 (TDD)
> (703)739-0395 (fax)
> Email: audiverb@aol.com

CODA (Children of Deaf Adults International)

CODA is an international association founded in 1983. It provides mutual support for hearing children of deaf parents and promotes family awareness and individual growth through self-help groups, educational programs, advocacy, and resource development. A newsletter, referral information, and assistance in starting a new groups is also provided.

> http://www.coda-international.org
> PO Box 30715
> Santa Barbara, CA 93130
> (805)682-0997 (voice/TDD 9 am–9 pm PST)

Cochlear Implant Association

This international association currently has 30 affiliated groups in the United States and Canada. It was founded in 1981 to offer support through fellowship for cochlear implant recipients and their families. The quarterly magazine provides pre- and postoperation counseling, and information on new technology.

> http://www.cici.org
> 5335 Wisconsin Ave NW, Suite 440
> Washington, DC 20015-2052
> (202)895-2781 (Dr. Peg Williams, voice/TTY)
> (202)895-2782 (fax)
> Email: pwms.cici@worldnet.att.net

Cochlear Implant Club International

Cochlear Implant Club International (CICI) is a nonprofit organization for cochlear implant recipients, their families, professionals, and other individuals interested in cochlear implants. CICI provides support and information to anyone who has a cochlear implant, has a child with an implant, or is interested in information about implants. CICI also advocates for rights and services for people with hearing loss.

> http://www.cici.org
> 5335 Wisconsin Ave NW, Suite 440
> Washington, DC 20015-2052
> (202)895-2781 (voice/TTY)
> (202)895-2782 (fax)

Hearing Loss Association of America (formerly SHHH)

In November of 2005, Self-Help for Hard-of-Hearing (SHHH) changed its name to the Hearing Loss Association of America. With 250 chapters and groups, this organization is the largest support network in the country. It was founded in 1979 with an aim to open the world of communication to people with hearing loss by providing a bimonthly journal of information, education, support, and advocacy.

> https://www.shhh.org
> 7910 Woodmont Ave, Suite 1200
> Bethesda, MD 20814
> (301)657-2248 (phone)
> (301)657-2249 (TDD)
> (301)913-9413 (fax)
> Email: bthomas@shhh.org

National Association of The Deaf

Founded in 1880, the National Association of the Deaf is the nation's largest constituency organization safeguarding the accessibility and civil rights for 28 million deaf and hard-of-hearing Americans in education, employment, health care, and telecommunications. Its primary areas of focus include grassroots, advocacy, empowerment, captioned media, deafness-related information, publications, legal assistance, policy development, research, public awareness, and youth leadership programs.

> http://www.nad.org
> 814 Thayer Ave, Suite 250
> Silver Spring, MD 20910-4500
> (301)587-1788 (voice)
> (301)587-1789 (TTY)
> (301)587-1791 (fax)
> Email: nadinfo@nad.org

National Fraternal Society of The Deaf

This national society has 72 divisions and was founded in 1901. It is a self-help organization for deaf and hard-of-hearing persons, their families, and concerned professionals. It also provides low-cost life insurance, scholarships for students, a quarterly newsletter, information and referrals, fellowship, and advocacy.

> http://www.nfsd.com
> 1118 S Sixth St
> Springfield, IL 62703
> (217)789-7429 (phone)
> (217)789-7438 (TDD)

(217)789-7489 (fax)

Email: thefrat@nfsd.com

SHHH (Self Help for Hard of Hearing People, Inc.

See Hearing Loss Association of America

Subject Index

A

ABR (auditory brainstem
        response), 164, 186–191,
        188*f*, 190*f*, 198, 200, 201
Absolute latency, 189
Absolute sensitivity, 99
Absolute threshold, 43
Absorption, 35–36
Acoustic admittance, 171, 174*t*
Acoustic immittance measures,
        164–179, 166*f*, 167*f*
Acoustic neuroma, 90–91
Acoustic reflex testing, 168–169,
        176–178
Acoustic trauma, 88
Acoustics, 34
    classroom, 253–256
Action potential, 56
Active exudate, 77
Acute otitis media, 78
Adaptation, 59
Adaptive testing, 43
Admittance, 37, 165
    acoustic, 171, 174*t*
AEP (auditory evoked potential),
        184–185
Afferent nerve fibers, 58
Age-related hearing loss, 16–18,
        18*f*, 62–63, 89–90
Air conduction hearing aids, 238*f*
Air conduction testing, 102, 141*f*
    masking during, 144–145, 145*f*
Alport Syndrome, 82
Alzheimer's disease, 224
American Sign Language, 14, 253
Amplifier, 237
Amplitude, 38
Ampulla, 64

Anechoic, defined, 36
Animated toys, 212*f*
Anterior, defined, 50
Antihelix, 51
Antinode, 42
Antitragus, 51
Anvil. *See* Incus
AOM (acute otitis media), 78
AP (action potential), 56
Apert Syndrome, 80
ARHL (age-related hearing loss),
        16–18, 18*f*, 62–63, 89–90
Articulation index, 106–107, 107*f*
ASL (American Sign Language),
        14, 253
Assistive listening devices, 24–25,
        256. *See also* Hearing aids
Atresia, 72–73
Attenuation, interaural, 144–146
AuD doctorate degree, 6, 10, 11
Audibility, threshold of, 98–99
Audibility curve, minimal,
        99, 100*f*
Audibility index, 106–107, 107*f*
Audible angle, minimum, 62
Audiogram, 100–101, 101*f*
    count-the-dot, 107*f*
    thresholds depicted in, 140*f*
Audiologic habilitation/
        rehabilitation. *See*
        Rehabilitation therapy
Audiological evaluation, 2
    case history in, 120, 122–224
Audiologist, 3–4, 10
Audiology, 2–4
    defined, 3
    degrees in, 5–6
    history, 4–6
    licenses for, 12

professional interactions
        in, 8–10
professional societies, 12
specialties in, 7–8
subspecialties in, 6–7
terminology for, 13–14
web resources for, 270–273
work settings in, 8*f*
Audiology assistant, 6–7, 11
Audiology practice
    academic requirements for, 10–11
    clinical requirements for, 11
    national certification for, 11–12
Audiometer, 4, 127–134
    automatic, 127, 129
    calibrating equipment for, 133*f*
    clinical, 127, 128*f*
    components, 129*f*
    manual, 127, 129
    portable, 124, 128*f*, 129*f*
Audiometric symbols, 102–105
Audiometric zero, 99–100
Audiometrist, 6, 10
Audiometry, 7
    conditioned play, 201
    conventional, modifications
        to, 217
    evoked potential, 184–191
    pure tone, 102*f*, 104*f*, 134–140
    speech, 154–158
    visual reinforcement, 201,
        211–214, 212*f*, 214*f*
Auditory brainstem response, 164,
        186–191, 188*f*, 190*f*, 198,
        200, 201
Auditory cortex, primary, 60*f*
Auditory dyssynchrony, 91–92
Auditory evoked potential, 184–185
Auditory nerve, 90–93

Name Index

A

A. G. Bell Association for the Deaf, 275
   Parents Section, 275–276
Abemayer, E., 75
Academy of Dispensing Audiologists (ADA), 6, 7, 275
Academy of Rehabilitative Audiology, 275
Adams, P.F., 16, 17, 18, 19
Ades, H.W., 57
Administration on Aging, 16, 17, 89
Adour, K., 85
Aguilar, C., 22, 23
Ahlman, M., 256, 257
Albright, K., 198
Alexander, G.C., 156
Alpiner, J.C., 248
Amado, A.N., 224
American Academy of Audiology (AAA), 3, 6, 7, 165, 198, 274
American Academy of Family Physicians, 77, 78
American Academy of Ophthalmology and Otolaryngology (AAO/ACO), 108
American Academy of Otolaryngology, 108
American Academy of Otoloryngology-Head and Neck Surgery, 198
American Academy of Pediatrics, 78, 198
American Audiology Society, 275

American Board of Audiology (ABA), 11–12
American College of Medical Genetics, 81
American Council of Otolaryngology, 108
American National Standards Institute (ANSI), 40, 41, 99, 100, 129, 133, 135, 143, 167, 169, 203, 256
American Society for Deaf Children, 276
American Speech-Language-Hearing Association (ASHA), 3, 5, 7, 10, 11–12, 99, 101, 101f, 102, 102f, 104f, 105, 105t, 124, 136, 138, 139, 154–155, 164, 165, 172, 187f, 190, 195, 198, 200–202, 203, 204, 206–207, 256, 274
Americans with Disabilities Act (ADA), 26–27, 224, 259, 260
Anderson, H., 144
Anderson, K.L., 106
Arnos, K., 80, 81
Association of Late-Deafened Adults (ALDA), 276
Auditory-verbal International, Inc., 276

B

Backus, J., 41
Bacon, S.P., 62
Bader, C., 180
Baldwin, M., 19
Baloh, R, 88
Baran, J., 92

Barlow, N.N., 22
Barry, S.J., 148
Batsuuri, J., 86
Beattie, R.C., 157
Beauchaine, K., 170
Behrens, T.R., 19
Békésy, 61, 62, 179–180
Benson, R., 155
Benson, V, 15, 16
Bentler, R., 15, 22, 23, 220
Beranek, L.L., 40
Berg, A., 198
Bergman, M., 4
Berlin, C., 91
Bess, F.H., 22, 203, 206
Betrand, D., 180
Beyer, C., 7
Bilger, R.C., 62
Bjorkman, G., 144
Blair, J.C., 15, 106, 203, 206
Bluestone, C., 76, 78, 202
Bonfils, P., 182
Bowling, L.S., 155
Brackett, D., 105
Bradley, M., 198
Brandy, W.T., 155, 156
Bray, C.W., 61
Bridges, J., 23
Briggs, R., 59
Brody, D.J., 203
Brookhouser, P., 83, 84
Brown, C., 92
Brown, O., 75
Brownell, W., 180
Buchman, C., 92
Burggraaff, B., 220
Burk, M.H., 138
Burney, P., 178
Burns, D., 83